Contemporary Endocrinology

Series Editor
Leonid Poretsky, Division of Endocrinology
Lenox Hill Hospital
New York, NY, USA

Contemporary Endocrinology offers an array of titles covering clinical as well as bench research topics of interest to practicing endocrinologists and researchers. Topics include obesity management, androgen excess disorders, stem cells in endocrinology, evidence-based endocrinology, diabetes, genomics and endocrinology, as well as others. Series Editor Leonid Poretsky, MD, is Chief of the Division of Endocrinology and Associate Chairman for Research at Lenox Hill Hospital, and Professor of Medicine at Hofstra North Shore-LIJ School of Medicine.

Lewis S. Blevins Jr. • Manish K. Aghi
Editors

Acromegaly

A Guide to Diagnosis and Treatment

Springer

Editors
Lewis S. Blevins Jr.
Department of Neurological Surgery
University of San Francisco
San Francisco, CA, USA

Manish K. Aghi
Department of Neurological Surgery
University of San Francisco
San Francisco, CA, USA

ISSN 2523-3785 ISSN 2523-3793 (electronic)
Contemporary Endocrinology
ISBN 978-3-031-16257-2 ISBN 978-3-031-16258-9 (eBook)
https://doi.org/10.1007/978-3-031-16258-9

This Springer imprint is published by the registered company Springer Nature Switzerland AG
The registered company address is: Gewerbestrasse 11, 6330 Cham, Switzerland

Preface

People with acromegaly are probably not much different today than they were when the earliest ancestors similar to modern-day *Homo sapiens* lived. Perhaps that is not really accurate. I suspect that modern dietary and societal factors and activities of daily living have led to a higher prevalence of diabetes mellitus and hypertension than were likely present in our affected early ancestors. In general, however, it can probably be assumed that those early persons with acromegaly, much like those in our time with the disorder, looked, well, acromegalic. The most dramatic changes are in our understanding of every facet of the disorder including its causes, molecular genetics, manifestations, diagnosis, treatments, and much more. In the 33 years or so since I first saw a patient with acromegaly we have seen a great number of changes. One of the most remarkable sets of changes that come to mind are those where our molecular understanding of the disease has led to drug development and multiple avenues for medical management of patients with residual and recurrent disease. When I saw the first patient mentioned, we only had one drug available that worked in 10% of patients. Today, there are three main classes of pharmacologic agents to treat acromegaly, encompassing at least eight different medications, and newer agents are on the way. It used to be next to impossible to control IGF-1 levels in patients with active disease. Today, uncontrolled acromegaly is the exception rather than the rule. Also, our recognition of the long-term morbidity and mortality seen in patients with residual and recurrent disease, coupled with advances in laboratory medicine, led to refinement of criteria employed to determine those patients who need additional treatment after surgery and radiotherapy. We better understand the biochemical goals of medical management of patients with acromegaly. A treatise of the historical aspects of the disorder is beyond the scope of this book. It is always useful, however, to have an appreciation of where we were and how far we have come to truly appreciate the contents and recommendations in this book. If you learn a few things in review of this body of work please share it with colleagues so that, together, we can facilitate knowledge and improve the lot of patients afflicted with this condition.

San Francisco, CA, USA
July 19, 2022

Lewis S. Blevins Jr.

Preface

Acromegaly, well described in antiquity, was recognized as a distinct clinical syndrome by Marie in 1886. The pituitary source of the disorder was confirmed in 1909 by Cushing, who postulated the excessive secretion of growth-promoting hormone by a hyperfunctioning pituitary gland. Soon thereafter, clinicians began to appreciate that the external manifestations that had first led to interest and fascination with the condition were also associated with devasting internal manifestations of excessive growth hormone in nearly every organ system. Despite its relative rarity, with only 3–14 of every 100,000 people diagnosed with acromegaly, research into the disease has had far-reaching implications on the medical care of a vast number of patients by improving our understanding of topics such as normal growth in children and the safe use of growth hormone to treat hypopituitarism. In this book, we review our understanding of every aspect of acromegaly, including its molecular etiology, manifestations, diagnosis, and therapies. We have presented this information in a manner that emphasizes the opinions, practice patterns, and decision makings of our team of experts. We encourage you to share this book with colleagues to enhance the medical community's continued development of new insights into acromegaly.

San Francisco, CA, USA
July 20, 2022

Manish K. Aghi

Contents

Chapter 1
The Molecular Biology and Pathology of Acromegaly

Luis R. Carrete and Manish K. Aghi

Introduction

Acromegaly is a disorder characterized by anatomical disfigurement and metabolic dysregulation caused by a state of chronic sustained growth hormone (GH) hypersecretion. GH is a peptide hormone produced in somatotroph cells of the anterior pituitary in response to stimulation from growth hormone-releasing hormone (GHRH) of the hypothalamus [1]. GH induces the production of insulin-like growth factor 1 (IGF1), a mediator of cellular processes that promote tissue growth and differentiation [2]. In acromegaly, chronic overexposure to GH and IGF1 results in excessive skeletal growth and enlargement of soft tissues, classically described as frontal bossing, prognathism, macroglossia, and acral growth [3, 4]. Subtle clinical manifestations of acromegaly are also common, including menstrual disturbances, erectile dysfunction, hyperhidrosis, headaches, and visual disturbances from pituitary tumor mass effect [3]. Furthermore, the systemic effects of GH hypersecretion increases the likelihood of mortality and causes multiple medical comorbidities, including diabetes, hypertension, cardiovascular disease, and visceromegaly [5].

The clinical manifestations of acromegaly can be insidious and may result in delayed recognition of disease with diagnosis often occurring 5–10 years after disease onset [3]. The estimated prevalence of acromegaly is ten cases per one million persons [6, 7] and has an average age at diagnosis between 40 and 50 years of age [3]. Over 95% of cases of GH hypersecretion stem from somatotrophic pituitary adenomas, while other causes include excessive GHRH production from hypothalamic tumors or ectopic sources (i.e., neuroendocrine tumors) [5, 8]. While

L. R. Carrete
University of California San Francisco, San Francisco, CA, USA
e-mail: luis.carrete@ucsf.edu

M. K. Aghi (✉)
Department of Neurological Surgery, University of California, San Francisco, CA, USA
e-mail: manish.aghi@ucsf.edu

L. S. Blevins Jr., M. K. Aghi (eds.), *Acromegaly*, Contemporary Endocrinology,
https://doi.org/10.1007/978-3-031-16258-9_1

somatotroph adenomas occur sporadically in over 90% of cases, familial syndromes, such as McCune-Albright syndrome, multiple endocrine neoplasia type 1 (MEN1), Carney complex, and familial isolated pituitary adenoma (FIPA), can also lead to the development of acromegaly from adenoma formation [5, 9, 10].

Treatment of acromegaly from somatotrophic pituitary adenomas involves a multi-faceted approach, often combining surgery, medical management, and in some cases radiotherapy. Surgical resection of somatotroph adenomas through transsphenoidal approach is recommended as a first-line therapeutic modality in most patients, with high reported rates of long-term biochemical remission based on postoperative GH and IGH1 levels at the time of follow-up [11–13]. Persistent disease is managed through the use of dopamine agonists, GH antagonists, somatotropin analogs, and, in some cases, radiotherapy [11].

Postoperative pathologic staining and hormonal levels are suggested features of somatotroph adenomas that may be of prognostic value. Cellular morphology, staining for multiple hormones, and somatotroph receptor expression are all factors that influence response to surgical and medical management [10, 14]. Furthermore, tumoral factors such as tumor size and cavernous sinus invasion are predictors of postoperative biochemical remission [15]. Understanding the biochemical processes involved in determining tumor response to treatment is important in order to refine therapeutic approaches and improve patient outcomes.

This chapter will discuss the molecular biology underlying the development of GH hypersecretion in acromegaly as well as the significance of histopathologic findings in somatotroph adenomas in helping to predict postoperative outcomes and guiding pharmacologic management.

Physiological Features of GH and IGF1

GH Physiology

GH is a peptide hormone secreted by somatotrophs in the anterior pituitary. During development, specific transcription factors orchestrate differentiation of adenohypophysial cells arising from Rathke's pouch into subtypes with specialized hormonal production, including corticotrophs, gonadotrophs, thyrotrophs, lactotrophs, and somatotrophs [16]. Somatotrophs are part of the Pit-1 (POI1F1) transcription factor lineage, along with lactotrophs and thyrotrophs [17]. In the case of somatotroph development, Pit-1 acts by binding to nuclear GH promoters, leading to somatotroph proliferation and development as well as GH transcription. After translation, secretion of the GH peptide is mediated hypothalamic hormones GHRH and somatostatin, which bind to somatotroph surface receptors and induce or inhibit GH secretion, respectively [10].

GH is secreted in a pulsatile fashion and can be highly variable in healthy individuals. Usually GH serum levels are less than 0.2 ng/mL at baseline; however, these levels are often higher due to stimulation from a variety of factors, including exercise, stress, fasting, and sleep [18]. Particularly at night or after vigorous exercise, levels of GH can rise to as high as 30 ng/mL, overlapping with the elevated range observed in patients with acromegaly.

Once in circulation, GH binds to growth hormone receptors (GHRs), a class I pleiotropic cytokine receptor, expressed primarily on liver, cartilage, fat, and muscle. GH binds to the GHR, which dimerizes and induces autophosphorylation of intracellular Janus kinase 2 (JAK2), activating signal transduction pathways that influence key cellular responses, such as glucose metabolism, cellular proliferation, cytoskeletal changes, and synthesis of IGF [19]. Importantly, GH-mediated JAK2 activation is necessary for inducing the STAT signaling pathway, in which phosphorylated STAT proteins are translocated to the nucleus to induce transcription of IGF1 and other GH target proteins. On the other hand, intracellular signaling induced by GH is suppressed by several proteins, notably tyrosine phosphatases and suppressors of cytokine signaling (SOCS) [20].

IGF1 Physiology

IGF1 is a polypeptide hormone that is the product of the *IGF1* gene on chromosome 12 in humans [2]. Circulating IGF1 is generated primarily in the liver and is also produced in high quantities in extrahepatic tissues, such as bone, muscle, kidney, and the pituitary gland itself. IGF1 has both endocrine and paracrine functions. Hepatically derived IGF1 under the influence of GH makes up approximately 80% of IGF1 in circulation [5]. IGF1 is transported by IGF1 binding protein 3 (IGFBP) and acid-liable subunit (ALS) in circulation, permitting IGF1 endocrine function. IGF1 produced by extrahepatic tissues has lower affinity for IGFBPs, and thus IGF1 has autocrine and paracrine activity in these tissues [2, 21, 22]. IGF1 receptors are ubiquitously expressed, allowing endocrine IGF1 activity to have widespread effects on tissue growth and metabolism. Of note, paracrine and autocrine secretion of IGF1 often serves to regulate growth of GH-target tissues.

In acromegaly, cellular processes driven by high levels of GH and IGF1 overwhelm regulatory cellular mechanisms that attenuate GH signaling. These include pathways orchestrated by SOCS, tyrosine phosphatases, and negative feedback in the form of somatostatin interacting with somatostatin receptors in the pituitary [1, 5, 23]. Disinhibited GH and IGF1 activity results in tissue overgrowth and metabolic dysregulations leading to significant comorbid conditions.

Pathogenesis of Somatotroph Adenomas

Pituitary adenomas are the second most common intracranial tumor [24]. Somatotroph adenomas compose 15–20% of pituitary adenomas. Commonly presenting as macroadenomas (>10 mm in diameter), these functional tumors oversecrete GH and are the cause of 95% of acromegaly cases [25]. Somatotroph adenomas develop as a result of unrestrained somatotroph expansion arising from inherent cell-cycle dysregulation and alterations in regulatory pathways that modulate somatotroph growth, GH synthesis, and GH secretion [5]. These adenomas are benign and, while they can be locally invasive, do not have the tendency to metastasize [26]. Pathogenesis of somatotroph adenomas is associated with genetic changes in the form of mutations, epigenetic alterations, and chromosomal instability. These observed genetic alterations provide insight into potential causal pathways that lead to somatotroph adenoma tumorigenesis [27].

Altered cAMP Signaling in Somatotroph Adenomas

The vast majority of somatotroph adenomas arise sporadically, with fewer than 5% of somatotroph adenomas having an association with familial syndromes [28]. Although the pathogenesis of somatotroph adenomas has not been fully elucidated, studying the germline mutations that result in the familial syndromes of familial isolated pituitary adenoma (FIPA) and Carney complex has served to elucidate potential pathways responsible for the formation of somatotroph adenomas [25]. Increased cAMP signaling in these germline mutations is hypothesized to play a pro-proliferative effect that generates a somatotroph adenoma. Carney complex, a syndrome associated with somatotroph adenomas, cardiac myxomas, and hyperpigmentation, is a result of an inactivating mutation in the *PRKAR1A* (protein kinase cAMP-dependent type 1 regulatory subunit alpha) tumor suppressor gene. This mutation generates elevated cAMP levels that drives activation of cAMP-dependent kinase and protein kinase A (PKA), leading to increased cell proliferation [29]. Similarly, inactivating mutations in the form of a duplication of G-coupled protein receptor 101 (GPR101) or aryl hydrocarbon receptor interacting protein (*AIP*) gene lead to increased cAMP production and accelerated cell proliferation [30, 31]. Either of these mutations is present in FIPA, an autosomal dominant disorder that results in the formation of pituitary adenomas, the majority of which are somatotroph adenomas [31].

Impaired regulation of cAMP signaling pathways is observed in sporadic somatotroph adenomas as well. Somatic mutations in the oncogene *GNAS* and transcription factor *CREB* are implicated in elevated cAMP production in sporadic somatotroph adenomas. Present in approximately 40% of somatotroph adenomas, an activating mutation of *GNAS* (the encoding gene for the stimulatory G-protein alpha subunit (Gs-α)) results in elevated cAMP levels, increased PKA activation, and increased synthesis and secretion of GH [5, 25, 32]. Whole genome sequencing of 12 human somatotroph adenomas yielded *GNAS* mutation (p.Arg201Cys) and shared chromosome losses as the only recurrent somatic events, thus reinforcing the notion that *GNAS* may play a critical role in somatotroph tumorigenesis [33]. *CREB* mutations, on the other hand, are responsible for constitutive activation of adenyl cyclase and induce elevated cAMP expression in somatotroph adenomas independent of *GNAS* mutations [34]. While *GNAS* and *CREB* mutations are undoubtedly involved in the pathophysiology of somatotroph adenomas, it is still unclear whether these mutations are inciting factors leading to tumorigenesis or a secondary events functioning to maintain tumor growth [25].

Epigenetic Gene Silencing in Somatotroph Adenomas

Epigenetic changes affecting the functionality of cell-cycle regulators are also implicated in the sporadic development of somatotroph adenomas. Silencing of p16 (also known as *CDKN2A)* and p27 through DNA hypermethylation results in diminished activation of retinoblastoma protein (Rb), leading to unchecked cell proliferation in pituitary adenomas [35, 36]. Similarly, growth arrest and DNA damage-inducible gene (*GADD45γ*) and maternal expressed 3 (*MEG3*) genes are epigenetically silenced in pituitary adenomas. Both genes play a role in negative regulation of cell growth, and hypermethylation allows for tumorigenesis [35, 37–39]. *MEG3* encodes a long noncoding RNA (lncRNA) and plays a role in inhibiting tumor proliferation in normal tissues. Although *MEG3* expression is diminished in both functioning and nonfunctioning pituitary adenomas (NFPAs), loss of expression of this gene is more strongly associated with tumorigenesis in NFPAs [40–42].

On the other hand, bromodomain-containing protein 4 (*BRD4*) is an epigenetic regulator, whose aberrant expression can lead to activation of oncogenes such as *c-Myc* and B-cell lymphoma 2(*Bcl2*) [43]. BRD4 regulates the initiation and elongation steps of transcription, and to promote cell-cycle progression. BRD4 is overexpressed in somatotroph adenomas and NFPAs, and in vivo and in vitro studies show that inhibition of BRD4 results in decreased GH production and reduced proliferation of GH-overexpressing cell lines, implicating BRD4 as a promoter of somatotroph adenoma formation [44, 45].

Gene Overexpression in Somatotroph Adenomas

In addition to impaired function of tumor suppression genes, there have also been genes whose overexpression is implicated in somatotroph tumorigenesis. Somatotroph and lactotroph adenomas are seen in transgenic mice with overexpression of the high-motility AT-hook protein, HMGA2. HMGA2 leads to cell-cycle disruption by enhancing E2F1 activity, diminishing activity of the cell-cycle inhibitor pRB, and driving pituitary cells into S phase, resulting in uncontrolled cell proliferation [46–48]. Similarly, pituitary tumor-transforming protein (PTTG) is overexpressed in almost all pituitary adenomas, and is especially plentiful in somatotroph adenomas [49]. PTTG functions to promote faithful sister chromatid separation during mitosis and plays a role in DNA damage repair and apoptosis through interactions with p53 [50, 51]. Overexpression induces aneuploidy, mitosis abnormalities, and DNA damage [52].

Significant strides have been made in the understanding of pituitary adenoma pathogenesis. However, efforts at developing novel therapeutic agents for the management of somatotroph adenomas have yet to yield a definitive target to stop the aberrant cellular proliferation that is proposed to be the cause of tumorigenesis in somatotroph adenomas.

The Impact of Histopathological Features in Somatotroph Adenoma Management

Classification of Pituitary Adenomas

Histopathological classification of surgically resected pituitary lesions is an important step in determining adenoma behavior, prognosis, and best potential choice of treatment. A structured sequence of steps is undertaken to classify pituitary lesions with hormone hypersecretion: distinguishing hyperplasia from neoplasia, identifying cell population responsible for hormone production, and using cellular features to devise an optimal treatment strategy.

One important initial step in the characterization of somatotroph adenomas is to ensure that the resected pituitary lesion is a somatotroph adenoma, rather than hyperplasia. Somatotroph hyperplasia is a rare cause of acromegaly that is usually a result of ectopic GHRH secretion from pancreatic or bronchial carcinoid tumors, or, less commonly, due to hypothalamic tumors causing ectopic GHRH hypersecretion (i.e., gangliocytoma, hamartoma, glioma, etc.) [53–55]. The resultant overstimulation of somatotrophs leads to hyperplasia and GH hypersecretion [4]. Hyperplasia can be differentiated from pituitary adenoma prior to surgery through plasma GHRH assays demonstrating excessive GHRH secretion, identification of ectopic source of tumor production, or pituitary characteristics on MRI [4]. However, differences between pituitary adenomas and hyperplasia can be subtle and overlooked, resulting in surgical resection of hyperplastic pituitary tissue [16, 56–58]. Pathological inspection of hyperplastic pituitary tissue reveals an increase in acinar size with preserved architecture of surrounding reticulin network. Conversely, pituitary adenomas exhibit widespread breakdown of the reticulin fibrin network [16].

Once the pituitary lesion is determined to be a pituitary adenoma, subclassification based on histological staining of hormone production and lineage-specific transcription factors is performed. The majority of somatotroph adenomas are monohormonal, staining for GH and Pit1; however, up to a quarter of GH-producing adenomas also exhibit positive staining for prolactin (PRL) (Fig. 1.1). Causes for this dual-staining include adenomas expressing a dimorphous population of lactotrophs and somatotrophs; development from a common progenitor of lactotrophs and somatotrophs, known as mammosomatotrophs; and, in extremely rare cases (~0.2% of dual GH/PRL-producing tumors), arising from acidophilic stem cell adenoma, a primitive and aggressive neoplasm [59, 60]. Pathological classifications, as monohormonal or dual-staining and as densely or sparsely granulated, are

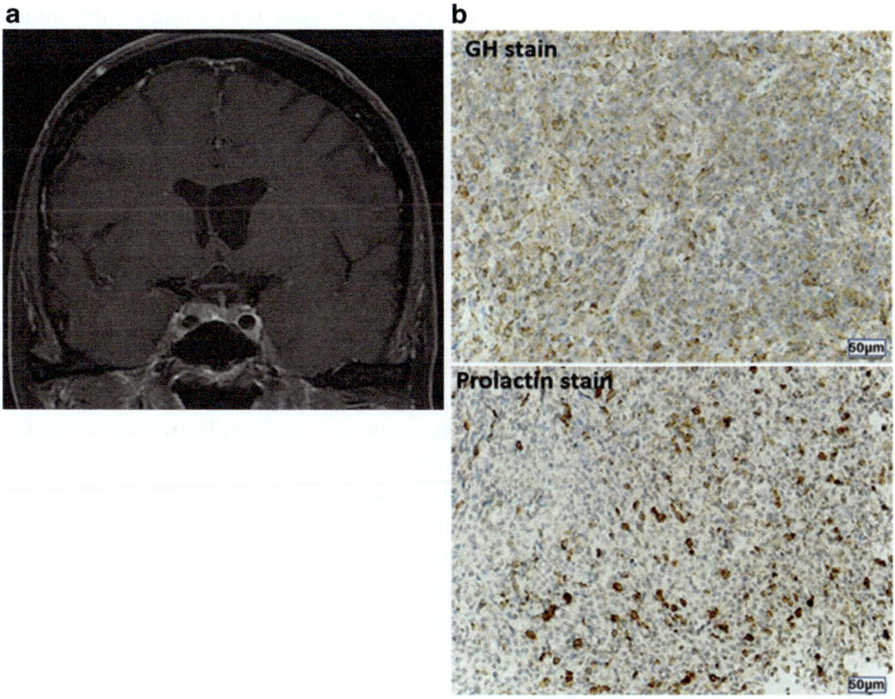

Fig. 1.1 Example of mammosomatotroph adenoma. (**a**) 72-year-old female presents with right eye vision loss. MRI with 11 × 6 × 12 mm right sellar lesion invading cavernous sinus. Prolactin = 107.4 mg/L, IGF-1 = 130 ng/mL. After 6 months of cabergoline, prolactin = 9.5 mg/L but no regression of lesion and persistence of the right vision loss. (**b**) Tumor surgically completely resected and co-stained for GH (top) and prolactin (bottom)

important subcategorizations that must be made, given that these findings play an important role in predicting response to medical treatment and other prognostic tumor behaviors.

Somatotroph Adenoma Behavior Based on Pathological Features

Somatostatin Receptor Subtypes in Somatotroph Adenomas

Somatostatin influences somatotroph signaling mechanisms by binding to somatostatin receptors (SSTRs) and modulating adenylyl cyclase activity [61]. There are five known SSTR subtypes. Most somatotroph adenomas express SSTR1 through SSTR5, with predominant expression of SSTR2 and SSTR5 [62–64]. The inhibitory effects of somatostatin analogs (SAs) on GH secretion and tumor cell proliferation can occur together or be dissociated events, depending on the tumor expression of SSTR subtypes involved in each mechanism [65, 66]. First-generation somatostatin analogs (SAs) octreotide and lanreotide bind preferentially to SSTR2 and, to a lesser extent, to SSTR5 [67–69]. The inhibitory effects of octreotide and lanreotide on somatotroph adenoma GH secretion and proliferation are highly correlated with the degree of SSTR2 expression [62, 70]. Somatotroph adenomas with a low ratio of SSTR2/SSTR5 expression are more likely to exhibit resistance to octreotide and lanreotide theapy [62, 71, 72]. Efforts in managing treatment-resistant somatotroph adenomas have led to the development of specific somatostatin subtype analogs (SAs), mainly for SSTR5, of a SSTR2-SSTR5 bispecific compound, and of a "universal" analog with high affinity to SSTR1, 2, 3, and 5, showing preliminary, albeit promising results [72–76]. One important example of said "universal" SAs is pasireotide, which exhibits highest affinity to SSTR5, followed by SSTR2, SSTR3, and SSTR1 [76, 77]. Response to pasireotide treatment is also linked to expression of SSTR subtype. There is evidence to suggest that somatotroph adenomas with high degree of immunohistochemical staining for SSTR5 are more likely to respond to pasireotide after failed treatment with first-generation SAs [78–80]. Meanwhile, very low expression of SST5 is a highly predictive of tumor nonresponse to pasireotide [80]. In sum, immunohistochemical staining for SSTRs is important as it can serve to guide personalized medical management of somatotroph adenomas.

Densely Granulated Vs Sparsely Granulated Somatotroph Adenomas

The classification of somatotroph adenomas as densely granulated (DG) or sparsely granulated (SG) is an important distinction, as this feature is known to be predictive of tumor behavior. DG somatotroph adenomas contain cells with numerous secretory granules, a property that is reflected on pathology by considerable cytoplasmic granularity. Cells are large with central nuclei and prominent nucleoli. These cells resemble somatotrophs on an ultrastructural level and display prominent immunohistochemical staining for GH and α-subunit of glycoprotein hormones [81]. SG somatotroph adenomas, on the other hand, exhibit a scarce number of secretory granules and weak staining for GH. These cells are characterized by dense aggregates of cytokeratin filaments known as fibrous bodies [82, 83].

SG somatotroph adenomas display more aggressive clinical behavior than DG adenomas. SG adenomas are more likely to be large and locally invasive and occur predominantly in younger patients [84]. Furthermore, DG somatotroph adenomas have a more pronounced response to medical management than SG somatotroph adenomas [85]. One proposed reason for this is that DG adenomas express SSTR2 to a significantly higher degree than SG adenomas (89% vs 13%), resulting in a more responsive phenotype to octreotide and lanreotide [68]. Meanwhile, pasireotide treatment in somatotroph adenomas resistant to first-generation SAs is suggested to be more effective in SG adenomas [80].

Dual-Staining Somatotroph Adenomas

Hormonal-staining profile is another feature of somatotroph adenomas that is prognostic value. Dual-staining pituitary adenomas (DSPAs) are composed of either a mixed population of somatotrophs and lactotrophs or mammosomatotrophs. DSPAs have been reported to have a distinct biochemical profile than monohormonal pituitary adenomas. One retrospective study by Rick et al. of 91 surgically resected somatotroph adenomas showed that DSPAs had significantly higher average preoperative IGF1 levels, acromegalic symptoms at presentation, and lower rates of postoperative biochemical remission relative to monohormonal (GH-staining) somatotroph adenomas. For patients, requiring adjunctive postoperative medical therapy, DSPAs were more likely to require polypharmacy and higher mean doses of lanreotide, pegvisomant, and cabergoline. Also, DSPAs required a longer time for postoperative disease remission, and monohormonal staining for GH was found to be independently associated with surgical remission of acromegaly [14].

A subsequent retrospective study by Lv et al. investigated differences in clinical behavior between monohormonal and DSPAs that were further subdivided into groups of mammosomatotrophs (MSAs) and mixed somatotroph-lactotroph adenomas (MSLAs). MSLAs were found to be larger on average and had lower gross total resection (GTR) rates and higher postoperative GH levels. MSAs, on the other hand, were significantly smaller on average, had lower rates of cavernous sinus invasion, and had the greatest rates of tumor resection among all three groups. It is likely that due to these properties, MSAs have higher rates of short-term and long-term biological remission with tumor size being identified as an independent predictor of biological remission. Response to postoperative pharmacological management was not reported in this study [86].

These studies suggest that rates of biological remission and response to medication are lower in DSPAs (esp. MSLAs). MSAs and MSLAs exhibit similar expression of SSTR2 and SSTR5 to somatotroph adenomas with monohormonal staining; however, the extent of literature published in this topic is limited [69, 87]. Further investigation into response of MSAs and MSLAs to postoperative medical intervention is warranted. Moreover, there is no definitive evidence to suggest that DSPAs lead to significantly higher rates of recurrence relative to monohormonal somatotroph adenomas. Ultimately, the biological behavior of DSPAs requires further characterization to definitively guide clinical decision-making.

Conclusions

In summary, excess production of GH and IGF1 in acromegaly is the result of somatotroph adenoma in most cases. The pathophysiology of somatotroph adenomas is not completely understood but is known to be correlated to excess production of cAMP and disrupted cell-cycle regulation. Surgical resection is the preferred first step of treatment in patients who are surgical candidates, followed by pharmacological treatment and radiotherapy (usually in the form of SRS) in select patients. Response to treatment predicted through postoperative histopathological characterization is an important clinical consideration when managing patients with somatotroph adenoma-induced acromegaly. While features such as DG and SG tumor morphologies as well as SSTR2 expression are predictors of medical treatment success, a similar association has yet to be definitively made in the case of MSAs and MSLAs. Further studies aimed at utilizing pathological features of somatotroph adenomas to guide personalized patient care are warranted.

References

1. Lu M, Flanagan JU, Langley RJ, Hay MP, Perry JK. Targeting growth hormone function: strategies and therapeutic applications. Signal Transduct Target Ther. 2019;4:3. https://doi.org/10.1038/s41392-019-0036-y.
2. Delafontaine P, Song YH, Li Y. Expression, regulation, and function of IGF-1, IGF-1R, and IGF-1 binding proteins in blood vessels. ATVB. 2004;24(3):435–44. https://doi.org/10.1161/01.ATV.0000105902.89459.09.
3. Vilar L, Vilar CF, Lyra R, Lyra R, Naves LA. Acromegaly: clinical features at diagnosis. Pituitary. 2017;20(1):22–32. https://doi.org/10.1007/s11102-016-0772-8.
4. Chanson P, Salenave S, Kamenicky P. Acromegaly. Handb Clin Neurol. 2014;124:197–219. https://doi.org/10.1016/B978-0-444-59602-4.00014-9.
5. Melmed S. Acromegaly pathogenesis and treatment. J Clin Invest. 2009;119(11):3189–202. https://doi.org/10.1172/JCI39375.
6. Melmed S. Pituitary-tumor endocrinopathies. N Engl J Med. 2020;382(10):937–50. https://doi.org/10.1056/NEJMra1810772.
7. Burton T, Le Nestour E, Neary M, Ludlam WH. Incidence and prevalence of acromegaly in a large US health plan database. Pituitary. 2016;19(3):262–7. https://doi.org/10.1007/s11102-015-0701-2.
8. Chin SO. Epidemiology of functioning pituitary adenomas. Endocrinol Metab. 2020;35(2):237–42. https://doi.org/10.3803/EnM.2020.35.2.237.
9. Eugster E. Gigantism. In: Feingold KR, Anawalt B, Boyce A, et al., editors. Endotext. MDText.com, Inc.; 2000. http://www.ncbi.nlm.nih.gov/books/NBK279155/. Accessed 3 Apr 2022.
10. Melmed S. Medical progress: acromegaly. N Engl J Med. 2006;355(24):2558–73. https://doi.org/10.1056/NEJMra062453.
11. Katznelson L, Laws ER, Melmed S, et al. Acromegaly: an endocrine society clinical practice guideline. J Clin Endocrinol Metab. 2014;99(11):3933–51. https://doi.org/10.1210/jc.2014-2700.
12. Abu Dabrh AM, Mohammed K, Asi N, et al. Surgical interventions and medical treatments in treatment-naïve patients with acromegaly: systematic review and meta-analysis. J Clin Endocrinol Metab. 2014;99(11):4003–14. https://doi.org/10.1210/jc.2014-2900.
13. Freda PU, Bruce JN, Reyes-Vidal C, et al. Prognostic value of nadir GH levels for long-term biochemical remission or recurrence in surgically treated acromegaly. Pituitary. 2021;24(2):170–83. https://doi.org/10.1007/s11102-020-01094-4.
14. Rick J, Jahangiri A, Flanigan PM, et al. Growth hormone and prolactin-staining tumors causing acromegaly: a retrospective review of clinical presentations and surgical outcomes. J Neurosurg. 2019;131(1):147–53. https://doi.org/10.3171/2018.4.JNS18230.
15. Yao S, Chen WL, Tavakol S, et al. Predictors of postoperative biochemical remission in acromegaly. J Neurooncol. 2021;151(2):313–24. https://doi.org/10.1007/s11060-020-03669-4.

16. Al-Brahim NYY, Asa SL. My approach to pathology of the pituitary gland. J Clin Pathol. 2006;59(12):1245–53. https://doi.org/10.1136/jcp.2005.031187.
17. Scully KM, Rosenfeld MG. Pituitary development: regulatory codes in mammalian organogenesis. Science. 2002;295(5563):2231–5. https://doi.org/10.1126/science.1062736.
18. Iranmanesh A, Grisso B, Veldhuis JD. Low basal and persistent pulsatile growth hormone secretion are revealed in normal and hyposomatotropic men studied with a new ultrasensitive chemiluminescence assay. J Clin Endocrinol Metab. 1994;78(3):526–35. https://doi.org/10.1210/jcem.78.3.8126122.
19. Argetsinger LS, Campbell GS, Yang X, et al. Identification of JAK2 as a growth hormone receptor-associated tyrosine kinase. Cell. 1993;74(2):237–44. https://doi.org/10.1016/0092-8674(93)90415-m.
20. Greenhalgh CJ, Rico-Bautista E, Lorentzon M, et al. SOCS2 negatively regulates growth hormone action in vitro and in vivo. J Clin Invest. 2005;115(2):397–406. https://doi.org/10.1172/JCI22710.
21. Delafontaine P. Insulin-like growth factor I and its binding proteins in the cardiovascular system. Cardiovasc Res. 1995;30(6):825–34. https://doi.org/10.1016/S0008-6363(95)00163-8.
22. Jones JI, Clemmons DR. Insulin-like growth factors and their binding proteins: biological actions. Endocr Rev. 1995;16(1):3–34. https://doi.org/10.1210/edrv-16-1-3.
23. Lanning NJ, Carter-Su C. Recent advances in growth hormone signaling. Rev Endocr Metab Disord. 2006;7(4):225–35. https://doi.org/10.1007/s11154-007-9025-5.
24. Ostrom QT, Patil N, Cioffi G, Waite K, Kruchko C, Barnholtz-Sloan JS. Corrigendum to: CBTRUS statistical report: primary brain and other central nervous system tumors diagnosed in the United States in 2013–2017. Neuro Oncol. 2022;24(7):1214. https://doi.org/10.1093/neuonc/noaa269.
25. Faltermeier CM, Magill ST, Blevins LS, Aghi MK. Molecular biology of pituitary adenomas. Neurosurg Clin N Am. 2019;30(4):391–400. https://doi.org/10.1016/j.nec.2019.05.001.
26. Colao A, Grasso LFS, Giustina A, et al. Acromegaly. Nat Rev Dis Primers. 2019;5(1):20. https://doi.org/10.1038/s41572-019-0071-6.
27. Melmed S. Mechanisms for pituitary tumorigenesis: the plastic pituitary. J Clin Invest. 2003;112(11):1603–18. https://doi.org/10.1172/JCI20401.
28. Melmed S. Pituitary medicine from discovery to patient-focused outcomes. J Clin Endocrinol Metab. 2016;101(3):769–77. https://doi.org/10.1210/jc.2015-3653.
29. Correa R, Salpea P, Stratakis CA. Carney complex: an update. Eur J Endocrinol. 2015;173(4):M85–97. https://doi.org/10.1530/EJE-15-0209.
30. Tuominen I, Heliövaara E, Raitila A, et al. AIP inactivation leads to pituitary tumorigenesis through defective Gαi-cAMP signaling. Oncogene. 2015;34(9):1174–84. https://doi.org/10.1038/onc.2014.50.
31. Caimari F, Korbonits M. Novel genetic causes of pituitary adenomas. Clin Cancer Res. 2016;22(20):5030–42. https://doi.org/10.1158/1078-0432.CCR-16-0452.
32. Vallar L, Spada A, Giannattasio G. Altered Gs and adenylate cyclase activity in human GH-secreting pituitary adenomas. Nature. 1987;330(6148):566–8. https://doi.org/10.1038/330566a0.
33. Välimäki N, Demir H, Pitkänen E, et al. Whole-genome sequencing of growth hormone (GH)-secreting pituitary adenomas. J Clin Endocrinol Metab. 2015;100(10):3918–27. https://doi.org/10.1210/jc.2015-3129.
34. Bertherat J, Chanson P, Montminy M. The cyclic adenosine 3',5'-monophosphate-responsive factor CREB is constitutively activated in human somatotroph adenomas. Mol Endocrinol. 1995;9(7):777–83. https://doi.org/10.1210/mend.9.7.7476961.
35. Farrell WE. Pituitary tumours: findings from whole genome analyses. Endocr Relat Cancer. 2006;13(3):707–16. https://doi.org/10.1677/erc.1.01131.
36. Farrell WE. Epigenetic mechanisms of tumorigenesis. Horm Metab Res. 2005;37(6):361–8. https://doi.org/10.1055/s-2005-870153.

37. Binse I, Ueberberg B, Sandalcioglu IE, et al. Expression analysis of GADD45γ, MEG3, and p8 in pituitary adenomas. Horm Metab Res. 2014;46(9):644–50. https://doi.org/10.1055/s-0034-1383566.
38. Zhang X, Sun H, Danila DC, et al. Loss of expression of GADD45 gamma, a growth inhibitory gene, in human pituitary adenomas: implications for tumorigenesis. J Clin Endocrinol Metab. 2002;87(3):1262–7. https://doi.org/10.1210/jcem.87.3.8315.
39. Bahar A, Bicknell JE, Simpson DJ, Clayton RN, Farrell WE. Loss of expression of the growth inhibitory gene GADD45gamma, in human pituitary adenomas, is associated with CpG island methylation. Oncogene. 2004;23(4):936–44. https://doi.org/10.1038/sj.onc.1207193.
40. Gejman R, Batista DL, Zhong Y, et al. Selective loss of MEG3 expression and intergenic differentially methylated region hypermethylation in the MEG3/DLK1 locus in human clinically nonfunctioning pituitary adenomas. J Clin Endocrinol Metab. 2008;93(10):4119–25. https://doi.org/10.1210/jc.2007-2633.
41. Cheunsuchon P, Zhou Y, Zhang X, et al. Silencing of the imprinted DLK1-MEG3 locus in human clinically nonfunctioning pituitary adenomas. Am J Pathol. 2011;179(4):2120–30. https://doi.org/10.1016/j.ajpath.2011.07.002.
42. Mezzomo LC, Gonzales PH, Pesce FG, et al. Expression of cell growth negative regulators MEG3 and GADD45γ is lost in most sporadic human pituitary adenomas. Pituitary. 2012;15(3):420–7. https://doi.org/10.1007/s11102-011-0340-1.
43. Wadhwa E, Nicolaides T. Bromodomain inhibitor review: bromodomain and extra-terminal family protein inhibitors as a potential new therapy in central nervous system tumors. Cureus. 2016;8(5):e620. https://doi.org/10.7759/cureus.620.
44. Yang Z, Yik JHN, Chen R, et al. Recruitment of P-TEFb for stimulation of transcriptional elongation by the bromodomain protein Brd4. Mol Cell. 2005;19(4):535–45. https://doi.org/10.1016/j.molcel.2005.06.029.
45. Shi C, Ye Z, Han J, et al. BRD4 as a therapeutic target for nonfunctioning and growth hormone pituitary adenoma. Neuro Oncol. 2020;22(8):1114–25. https://doi.org/10.1093/neuonc/noaa084.
46. Fedele M, Battista S, Kenyon L, et al. Overexpression of the HMGA2 gene in transgenic mice leads to the onset of pituitary adenomas. Oncogene. 2002;21(20):3190–8. https://doi.org/10.1038/sj.onc.1205428.
47. Fedele M, Visone R, De Martino I, et al. HMGA2 induces pituitary tumorigenesis by enhancing E2F1 activity. Cancer Cell. 2006;9(6):459–71. https://doi.org/10.1016/j.ccr.2006.04.024.
48. Fedele M, Pierantoni GM, Visone R, Fusco A. E2F1 activation is responsible for pituitary adenomas induced by HMGA2 gene overexpression. Cell Div. 2006;1:17. https://doi.org/10.1186/1747-1028-1-17.
49. Hunter JAC, Skelly RH, Aylwin SJB, et al. The relationship between pituitary tumour transforming gene (PTTG) expression and in vitro hormone and vascular endothelial growth factor (VEGF) secretion from human pituitary adenomas. Eur J Endocrinol. 2003;148(2):203–11. https://doi.org/10.1530/eje.0.1480203.
50. Pei L, Melmed S. Isolation and characterization of a pituitary tumor-transforming gene (PTTG). Mol Endocrinol. 1997;11(4):433–41. https://doi.org/10.1210/mend.11.4.9911.
51. Zou H, McGarry TJ, Bernal T, Kirschner MW. Identification of a vertebrate sister-chromatid separation inhibitor involved in transformation and tumorigenesis. Science. 1999;285(5426):418–22. https://doi.org/10.1126/science.285.5426.418.
52. Vlotides G, Eigler T, Melmed S. Pituitary tumor-transforming gene: physiology and implications for tumorigenesis. Endocr Rev. 2007;28(2):165–86. https://doi.org/10.1210/er.2006-0042.
53. Gola M, Doga M, Bonadonna S, Mazziotti G, Vescovi PP, Giustina A. Neuroendocrine tumors secreting growth hormone-releasing hormone: pathophysiological and clinical aspects. Pituitary. 2006;9(3):221–9. https://doi.org/10.1007/s11102-006-0267-0.
54. Melmed S, Ezrin C, Kovacs K, Goodman RS, Frohman LA. Acromegaly due to secretion of growth hormone by an ectopic pancreatic islet-cell tumor. N Engl J Med. 1985;312(1):9–17. https://doi.org/10.1056/NEJM198501033120103.

55. Biermasz NR, Smit JWA, Pereira AM, Frölich M, Romijn JA, Roelfsema F. Acromegaly caused by growth hormone-releasing hormone-producing tumors: long-term observational studies in three patients. Pituitary. 2007;10(3):237–49. https://doi.org/10.1007/s11102-007-0045-7.
56. Srirangam Nadhamuni V, Iacovazzo D, Evanson J, et al. GHRH secretion from a pancreatic neuroendocrine tumor causing gigantism in a patient with MEN1. Endocrinol Diabetes Metab Case Rep. 2021;2021:EDM200208. https://doi.org/10.1530/EDM-20-0208.
57. Ezzat S, Asa SL, Stefaneanu L, et al. Somatotroph hyperplasia without pituitary adenoma associated with a long standing growth hormone-releasing hormone-producing bronchial carcinoid. J Clin Endocrinol Metab. 1994;78(3):555–60. https://doi.org/10.1210/jcem.78.3.8126126.
58. Othman NH, Ezzat S, Kovacs K, et al. Growth hormone-releasing hormone (GHRH) and GHRH receptor (GHRH-R) isoform expression in ectopic acromegaly: GHRH and GHRH-R in lung endocrine tumour. Clin Endocrinol. 2001;55(1):135–40. https://doi.org/10.1046/j.1365-2265.2001.01268.x.
59. Day RN, Koike S, Sakai M, Muramatsu M, Maurer RA. Both Pit-1 and the estrogen receptor are required for estrogen responsiveness of the rat prolactin gene. Mol Endocrinol. 1990;4(12):1964–71. https://doi.org/10.1210/mend-4-12-1964.
60. Annapurni A, Rathi M. Acidophil stem cell pituitary adenoma: a case report and literature review. Hormones (Athens). 2019;18(4):507–12. https://doi.org/10.1007/s42000-019-00154-0.
61. O'Toole TJ, Sharma S. Physiology, somatostatin. In: StatPearls. StatPearls Publishing; 2022. http://www.ncbi.nlm.nih.gov/books/NBK538327/. Accessed 20 Apr 2022.
62. Taboada GF, Luque RM, Neto LV, et al. Quantitative analysis of somatostatin receptor subtypes (1-5) gene expression levels in somatotropinomas and correlation to in vivo hormonal and tumor volume responses to treatment with octreotide LAR. Eur J Endocrinol. 2008;158(3):295–303. https://doi.org/10.1530/EJE-07-0562.
63. Fougner SL, Casar-Borota O, Heck A, Berg JP, Bollerslev J. Adenoma granulation pattern correlates with clinical variables and effect of somatostatin analogue treatment in a large series of patients with acromegaly. Clin Endocrinol (Oxf). 2012;76(1):96–102. https://doi.org/10.1111/j.1365-2265.2011.04163.x.
64. Panetta R, Patel YC. Expression of mRNA for all five human somatostatin receptors (hSSTR1-5) in pituitary tumors. Life Sci. 1995;56(5):333–42. https://doi.org/10.1016/0024-3205(94)00956-2.
65. Weckbecker G, Lewis I, Albert R, Schmid HA, Hoyer D, Bruns C. Opportunities in somatostatin research: biological, chemical and therapeutic aspects. Nat Rev Drug Discov. 2003;2(12):999–1017. https://doi.org/10.1038/nrd1255.
66. Danila DC, Haidar JNS, Zhang X, Katznelson L, Culler MD, Klibanski A. Somatostatin receptor-specific analogs: effects on cell proliferation and growth hormone secretion in human somatotroph tumors. J Clin Endocrinol Metab. 2001;86(7):2976–81. https://doi.org/10.1210/jcem.86.7.7620.
67. Lamberts SW, van der Lely AJ, de Herder WW, Hofland LJ. Octreotide. N Engl J Med. 1996;334(4):246–54. https://doi.org/10.1056/NEJM199601253340408.
68. Kato M, Inoshita N, Sugiyama T, et al. Differential expression of genes related to drug responsiveness between sparsely and densely granulated somatotroph adenomas. Endocr J. 2012;59(3):221–8. https://doi.org/10.1507/endocrj.ej11-0177.
69. Greenman Y, Melmed S. Expression of three somatostatin receptor subtypes in pituitary adenomas: evidence for preferential SSTR5 expression in the mammosomatotroph lineage. J Clin Endocrinol Metab. 1994;79(3):724–9. https://doi.org/10.1210/jcem.79.3.7521350.
70. Fougner SL, Borota OC, Berg JP, Hald JK, Ramm-Pettersen J, Bollerslev J. The clinical response to somatostatin analogues in acromegaly correlates to the somatostatin receptor subtype 2a protein expression of the adenoma. Clin Endocrinol. 2008;68(3):458–65. https://doi.org/10.1111/j.1365-2265.2007.03065.x.
71. Jaquet P, Saveanu A, Gunz G, et al. Human somatostatin receptor subtypes in acromegaly: distinct patterns of messenger ribonucleic acid expression and hormone suppression identify different tumoral phenotypes. J Clin Endocrinol Metab. 2000;85(2):781–92. https://doi.org/10.1210/jcem.85.2.6338.

72. Saveanu A, Gunz G, Dufour H, et al. Bim-23244, a somatostatin receptor subtype 2- and 5-selective analog with enhanced efficacy in suppressing growth hormone (GH) from octreotide-resistant human GH-secreting adenomas. J Clin Endocrinol Metab. 2001;86(1):140–5. https://doi.org/10.1210/jcem.86.1.7099.
73. Reubi JC, Eisenwiener KP, Rink H, Waser B, Mäcke HR. A new peptidic somatostatin agonist with high affinity to all five somatostatin receptors. Eur J Pharmacol. 2002;456(1-3):45–9. https://doi.org/10.1016/s0014-2999(02)02651-1.
74. Lewis I, Bauer W, Albert R, et al. A novel somatostatin mimic with broad somatotropin release inhibitory factor receptor binding and superior therapeutic potential. J Med Chem. 2003;46(12):2334–44. https://doi.org/10.1021/jm021093t.
75. van der Hoek J, de Herder WW, Feelders RA, et al. A single-dose comparison of the acute effects between the new somatostatin analog SOM230 and octreotide in acromegalic patients. J Clin Endocrinol Metab. 2004;89(2):638–45. https://doi.org/10.1210/jc.2003-031052.
76. Schmid HA. Pasireotide (SOM230): development, mechanism of action and potential applications. Mol Cell Endocrinol. 2008;286(1-2):69–74. https://doi.org/10.1016/j.mce.2007.09.006.
77. Schmid HA, Schoeffter P. Functional activity of the multiligand analog SOM230 at human recombinant somatostatin receptor subtypes supports its usefulness in neuroendocrine tumors. Neuroendocrinology. 2004;80(Suppl 1):47–50. https://doi.org/10.1159/000080741.
78. Gatto F, Arvigo M, Ferone D. Somatostatin receptor expression and patients' response to targeted medical treatment in pituitary tumors: evidences and controversies. J Endocrinol Invest. 2020;43(11):1543–53. https://doi.org/10.1007/s40618-020-01335-0.
79. Chiloiro S, Giampietro A, Mirra F, et al. Pegvisomant and pasireotide LAR as second line therapy in acromegaly: clinical effectiveness and predictors of response. Eur J Endocrinol. 2021;184(2):217–29. https://doi.org/10.1530/EJE-20-0767.
80. Iacovazzo D, Carlsen E, Lugli F, et al. Factors predicting pasireotide responsiveness in somatotroph pituitary adenomas resistant to first-generation somatostatin analogues: an immunohistochemical study. Eur J Endocrinol. 2016;174(2):241–50. https://doi.org/10.1530/EJE-15-0832.
81. Horvath E, Kovacs K. Pathology of acromegaly. Neuroendocrinology. 2006;83(3-4):161–5. https://doi.org/10.1159/000095524.
82. Lopes MBS. Growth hormone-secreting adenomas: pathology and cell biology. Neurosurg Focus. 2010;29(4):E2. https://doi.org/10.3171/2010.7.FOCUS10169.
83. Obari A, Sano T, Ohyama K, et al. Clinicopathological features of growth hormone-producing pituitary adenomas: difference among various types defined by cytokeratin distribution pattern including a transitional form. Endocr Pathol. 2008;19(2):82–91. https://doi.org/10.1007/s12022-008-9029-z.
84. Ku CR, Lim H, Lee YJ, et al. Novel somatic variants involved in biochemical activity of pure growth hormone-secreting pituitary adenoma without GNAS variant. Sci Rep. 2021;11(1):16530. https://doi.org/10.1038/s41598-021-95829-3.
85. Gadelha MR, Kasuki L, Korbonits M. Novel pathway for somatostatin analogs in patients with acromegaly. Trends Endocrinol Metab. 2013;24(5):238–46. https://doi.org/10.1016/j.tem.2012.11.007.
86. Lv L, Jiang Y, Yin S, et al. Mammosomatotroph and mixed somatotroph-lactotroph adenoma in acromegaly: a retrospective study with long-term follow-up. Endocrine. 2019;66(2):310–8. https://doi.org/10.1007/s12020-019-02029-1.
87. Thodou E, Kontogeorgos G, Theodossiou D, Pateraki M. Mapping of somatostatin receptor types in GH or/and PRL producing pituitary adenomas. J Clin Pathol. 2006;59(3):274–9. https://doi.org/10.1136/jcp.2005.026914.

Chapter 2
Growth Hormone-Releasing Hormone-Secreting Neuroendocrine Tumors

Thomas M. Fandel and Lewis S. Blevins Jr.

Introduction

The neuroendocrine system in mammals plays an integral role in supporting multiple biological and physiological activities. Growth hormone (GH) is a pleiotropic hormone produced in somatotroph cells of the anterior pituitary that regulates body growth and metabolic activity [1]. Expression and release of GH is governed by the counter-regulatory effects of hypothalamic growth hormone-releasing hormone (GHRH) and somatostatin (SST), respectively [2]. In addition, several other hormonal factors impact the GH axis [3].

Acromegaly is a rare condition characterized by GH excess [4]. The incidence of acromegaly across several geographic areas ranges between 0.2 and 1.1 cases/100,000 people per year, and the total prevalence ranges between 2.8 and 13.7 cases/100,000 people [5]. While benign pituitary adenomas producing GH are the most common cause for acromegaly, ectopic GH hypersecretion and excess production of growth hormone-releasing hormone (GHRH) by extrapituitary tumors are rare causes, accounting for less than 1% of cases [6].

Neuroendocrine neoplasias are a heterogeneous group of tumors derived from neuroendocrine cells that may potentially develop anywhere in the human body but are most commonly found in the intestine, pancreas, and lung [7, 8]. These tumors are classified according to their origin, extension, and histological differentiation, with their grading being based on the mitotic count and KI-67 index [9]. Neuroendocrine

T. M. Fandel
Division of Endocrinology and Metabolism, Department of Medicine, University of California, San Francisco, CA, USA

L. S. Blevins Jr. (✉)
Department of Neurological Surgery, University of California, San Francisco, CA, USA
e-mail: lewis.blevins@ucsf.edu

L. S. Blevins Jr., M. K. Aghi (eds.), *Acromegaly*, Contemporary Endocrinology,
https://doi.org/10.1007/978-3-031-16258-9_2

neoplasias are categorized as well-differentiated (grade 1 and 2) neuroendocrine tumors (NETs) and poorly differentiated (grade 3) neuroendocrine carcinomas (NECs). Ectopic GHRH secretion may be due to neuroendocrine tumors (NETs) [10]. In addition to sporadic cases, familial syndromes, such as multiple endocrine neoplasia type 1 (MEN1), have been linked to GHRH-secreting NETs [11–14].

The association of acromegaly with bronchial carcinoids is recognized by Altman and Schütz in 1959 [15]. Achieving cure of acromegaly following removal of a bronchial carcinoid tumor with no evidence of tumoral GH excess, Sönksen et al. propose in 1976 the ectopic secretion of a growth hormone-releasing substance [15]. Similarly, in 1982 Thorner describes normalization of GH levels following removal of a pancreatic islet cell tumor in a patient with acromegaly, with subsequent identification of a GH-releasing factor in the tumor [16]. The structure of human GH-releasing factor (also termed GHRH) has been characterized from pancreatic islet cell tumor extracts, which are shown to stimulate GH release both in vitro and in vivo [17, 18].

Causes of Ectopic GHRH Production

While ectopic GHRH production by hypothalamic gangliocytomas is rare, the ectopic production of GHRH is well recognized [19, 20]. Ectopic acromegaly is mainly due to NETs of pancreatic or bronchial origin [21]. Indeed, published case reports suggest that over 50% of NETs leading to ectopic acromegaly are located in the lung, which are almost exclusively carcinoids. One third of tumors are found in the pancreas. Few GHRH-secreting tumors are described in the gastrointestinal tract and in adrenal pheochromocytomas, with singular reports in other locations, such as the thymus, medullary pituitary, mediastinum, endometrium, breast, and ovary [10, 22, 23]. In contrast, results from a single registry in France reveal a higher proportion of GHRH-secreting pancreas tumors (57% of cases), of which 80% are found to have an MEN-1 gene mutation [22]. A bronchial carcinoid is found in 33% of cases. Of note, about 25% of NETs express GHRH in vitro, including carcinoid tumors of the lung and gastrointestinal tract, pancreatic tumors, pheochromocytomas and paragangliomas, small cell lung carcinomas, medullary thyroid carcinomas, endometrial tumors, and breast tumors. However, only a small proportion of those hormonally active tumors lead to acromegaly, which is thought to be due to disordered tissue processing of GHRH by tumors or impaired bioactivity of GHRH [24].

Clinical Presentation of Ectopic GHRH Production

Patients with *ectopic* acromegaly are typically diagnosed at the beginning of their fifth decade of life, with a female gender predilection (M:F ratio of 1:2) [10, 25]. In contrast, patients with *pituitary* acromegaly from a Danish registry show no gender disparity, although results of a meta-analysis point to changes in gender distribution over publication time with a female predominance in earlier studies [26]. The time to diagnosis of ectopic acromegaly is approximately 8 years, which is in line with the reported diagnostic delay of 5–10 years for patients with pituitary acromegaly [22, 26].

GH stimulates synthesis and secretion of insulin-like growth factor (IGF-1), which promotes cell proliferation and inhibits apoptosis, resulting in soft tissue enlargement, skeletal, and organ growth [4]. The clinical spectrum of ectopic acromegaly is wide with features ranging from subtle to severe. The most common characteristics at presentation are acral enlargement and coarse facial features. However, the classic manifestations of acromegaly are indistinguishable from those caused by GH-secreting pituitary adenomas [4]. Instead, neuroendocrine tumors may cause symptoms associated with local tumor mass, such as obstructive jaundice, cough, or unilateral wheezing. Hypothalamic gangliocytomas may cause compression of the optic chiasm [27]. Pancreatic carcinoids tend to occur in the pancreatic tail, which may explain the late development of symptoms for such tumors. Also, symptoms at presentation may be linked to hormonal hypersecretion by the NET. Co-secretion of GHRH and other hormones is described for calcitonin [28], ACTH [29, 30], serotonin [31, 32], prolactin [33], insulin [31], and catecholamines [34]. In addition, co-secretion of GHRH and prolactin is described in a patient with diffuse large B-cell lymphoma [35].

Diagnostic Workup of Ectopic GHRH Syndrome

The presentation of clinical acromegaly requires biochemical evaluation and careful assessment for the primary process, which will dictate the appropriate therapeutic approach. The rarity of NETs across various sites, lack of awareness by health-care workers, and difficulties with obtaining a diagnosis, present particular problems, often resulting in diagnostic delay [22, 36].

The initial screening for acromegaly entails documentation of elevated IGF-1 levels in combination with failure to suppress GH during an oral glucose tolerance test [37]. However, the potential for pituitary versus extrapituitary acromegaly poses a diagnostic challenge, as the aforementioned tests are not useful in making this distinction [24]. Likewise, dynamic pituitary tests are not helpful [38]. Instead, the GHRH assay has been proposed as a precise and straightforward method to measure the biological activity of GHRH in blood [39]. Healthy adults have low levels of GHRH in the systemic circulation, with a mean fasting plasma level of 10.3 ng/L and no significant sex difference in the level [40]. In patients with peripheral GHRH secretion, levels are elevated, reaching values hundreds or thousands-fold normal values [22]. In one series of patients with peripheral GHRH production using the same laboratory for all test results, the median GHRH at diagnosis is elevated with a value of 548 ng/L [25]. Of note, patients with a hypothalamic gangliocytoma may have normal plasma GHRH levels due to secretion of excess ectopic GHRH into the hypophyseal portal system, which suggests that the peptide hormone does not appreciably enter the systemic circulation under these conditions [41].

Imaging modalities are used for localization and further characterization of any suspected tumor. An MRI is helpful to assess for pituitary pathology. In ectopic acromegaly, the extrapituitary GHRH secretion leads to stimulation of the pituitary with subsequent production and release of GH. Thus, the pituitary should appear symmetrically enlarged and hyperplastic without any indication for a distinct pituitary tumor [6]. Localized gadolinium enhancement may be indicative for the presence of a tumor with less vascularity. In a series of 99 patients with ectopic GHRH secretion, MRI of the pituitary reveals a spectrum of presentation showing imaging features consistent with hyperplasia, adenoma, empty sella, and normal microcystic lesions [22]. Pituitary hyperplasia may be difficult to distinguish from pituitary adenoma, leading to unnecessary transsphenoidal surgeries [42]. Hypothalamic gangliocytomas are often incidental findings on MRI, in one case series showing a sellar mass with cavernous sinus invasion and a thin attachment to the hypothalamus [19, 20].

CT is the imaging modality of choice in the evaluation of patients with suspected NETs, providing information regarding localization and staging of ectopic NETs. Pulmonary carcinoid tumors typically arise within the central airways as endobronchial masses [43]. The detection rate of solitary pulmonary nodules on helical CT is high [44]. In addition to signs of airway obstruction, characteristic features of carcinoid tumors include an ovoid/round shape with regular margins, although peripheral tumors may appear as lobulated nodules with hyper-attenuation on contrast-enhanced CT and calcifications [44, 45]. Pancreatic NETs appear often as well-circumscribed, solid lesions with hyperattenuation due to rich vascularity. They are often larger in size and may demonstrate cyst formation [46]. In addition to multiple NETs larger than 0.5 cm, pancreatic microadenomatosis is a typical finding in familial syndromes [47]. The incidence of gastrointestinal NETs appears to be rising, due in part to heightened awareness of the disease, improved diagnostic techniques, and an increased rate of incidental diagnoses due to investigation for other conditions [48]. The various imaging features of carcinoids occurring along the gastrointestinal tract are summarized in [49]. Hepatic lesions with hypervascularity, large size, and intralesional hemorrhage or necrosis may be suggestive of metastasis from pancreatic NETs [50]. CT features suggestive of a pheochromocytoma include a spherical shape, a "ring-sign," and a sharply demarcated intralesional necrosis [51]. MRI is preferred over CT for imaging hepatic metastases [52].

While CT and MRI provide structural imaging, nuclear imaging modalities afford new potential detecting and characterizing NETs. The overexpression of specific peptide hormone receptors on the tumor surface, such as the somatostatin receptor (SSTR), is a characteristic feature of NETs [53]. The five receptors of the SSTR family belong to the G-protein coupled receptor superfamily. NETs including GHRH-secreting NETs typically express a high number of SSTRs on the cell surface, in particular the subtypes 2, 3, and 5 [54, 55]. The receptor setup in ectopic GHRH-producing tumors is lesser known. There is indication that GHRH-producing carcinoids of the lung express SSTR1, SSTR2, and SSTR5 in vitro [56]; however, others report the presence of only SSTR2 in GHRH-producing bronchial carcinoid and pancreatic NET [13, 57]. By combining positron emission tomography (PET)/computer tomography (CT) with radiotracers geared toward the SSTR, it allows for molecular imaging. Since approval of ^{111}In-diethylenetriamine pentaacetate-conjugated octreotide in 1994, several radiolabeled somatostatin analogs (SSA) have been proposed [58]. Newer SSA labeled with ^{68}Ga- or ^{64}Cu-tetraxetan (DOTA) have shown superior image quality, with ^{68}Ga-DOTA-conjugated peptides currently being the gold standard for localization and staging of SSTR-expressing NETs [59]. This imaging modality has been employed in the evaluation of GHRH-producing NETs [12, 60–62]. NETs with variable-to-low SSTRs, such as pheochromocytoma and abdominal paraganglioma, may be detected by ^{18}F-DOPA [63]. In more aggressive tumors, including high-grade NETs and undifferentiated forms, ^{18}F-FDG is superior. Several new pharmaceuticals are currently evaluated for their potential role to detect NETs by exploiting different targets on the tumor cells [59, 64].

Immunohistochemical evaluation of the surgical specimen is used to aide in the determination of the tumor origin. Neuroendocrine markers used to characterize NETs include chromogranin A [65], synaptophysin [66], neuron-specific enolase [67], cytokeratins AE1/AE3 [68], somatostatin [69], and S-100 [70]. GHRH expression of the tumor can be determined by positive tumor specimen GHRH immunostaining [71]. If inconclusive, additionally positive bioassay (ability of cultured rat pituitary cells to produce GH in response to tumor extract), A-V gradient of GHRH across the tumor, detection of GHRH mRNA, and GHRH extraction from tumor may be used [22]. Of note, hypothalamic gangliocytoma are very difficult to diagnose based on biochemical and radiologic findings, being often misinterpreted as pituitary adenomas, with the eventual diagnosis made during histological examination [72].

Differential Diagnosis for NETs According to Site

A proper differential diagnosis for NETs is imperative prior to treatment, because several benign and malignant conditions can mimic the presence of such a tumor. Diagnostic challenges often require an interdisciplinary approach.

Hypothalamic gangliocytomas, resembling normal hypothalamic magnocellular neurons, are a rare occurrence [19, 20]. Other tumor types developing in the hypothalamic region, including those derived from hypothalamic neurons, glia, and stromal cells, as well as infiltrating primary pituitary tumors, and metastases need to be considered [73]. Immunohistochemistry of the resected tumor may be needed to distinguish between these entities.

Lung NETs account for approximately 25% of primary lung neoplasms [74]. The distinction between well-differentiated carcinoids, small cell lung carcinoma, and large cell neuroendocrine carcinoma is challenging, requiring the utilization of novel immunohistochemistry markers [75]. The differential diagnosis for pulmonary carcinoid tumors includes salivary gland-type tumors [76], paragangliomas

[77], metastases from breast cancer [78], and metastatic carcinoids from other locations, such as the gastrointestinal tract.

In the gastrointestinal tract, NETs represent 2% of all malignant tumors, and approximately 40% of NETs are hormone secreting [79]. Flushing and diarrhea may be the prominent clinical features at presentation, with an extensive list of differential diagnoses [80, 81]. The imaging differential diagnosis for small intestinal carcinoids includes metastatic disease, primary small intestinal adenocarcinomas, lymphoma, and gastrointestinal stromal tumors [82].

Neoplasms of the neuroendocrine pancreas comprise about 2% of pancreatic tumors [83]. Pancreatic hypervascular lesions, which can mimic the appearance of NETs, include serous cystadenomas, an accessory spleen, as well as metastases, in particular those from a renal cell carcinoma, thyroid cancer, and melanoma [84]. However, MRI imaging characteristics and the absence of ^{68}Ga-DOTA-conjugated peptide uptake may distinguish a serous cystadenoma and an accessory spleen from NETs, while the pancreatic tumor enhancement pattern on contrast-enhanced CT may discriminate metastases from NETs [85]. Hypervascular peripancreatic lesions may include gastrointestinal stroma tumors and paraganglioma [86]. Irregular tumor margins and hypovascular appearance of poorly differentiated neuroendocrine carcinomas can mimic pancreatic ductal adenocarcinoma.

Of patients with an adrenal incidentaloma, 4% are diagnosed with a pheochromocytoma [87]. Adenomas, primary carcinomas, metastases, and myelolipomas are part of the differential diagnosis [88]. However, distinguishing features at presentation, such as patient age, size and laterality of the lesion, lipid content, as well as presence of intratumoral necrosis and hemorrhage, may guide the diagnostic process [89].

Treatment Options for NETs

Patients with NETs, including functional NETs with GHRH overproduction, require a multidisciplinary team approach in their care, often including surgery, nuclear medicine, radiotherapy, and medical therapy [90]. Goals are aimed at treating the primary tumor and normalizing GH levels.

The treatment of choice for patients with NETs is surgical resection with curative intent, whenever possible [52, 91]. By removing the offending tumor, normalization of GH and IGF-1 levels can be achieved [14, 57, 92, 93]. Debulking surgery in combination with other interventions may be considered as a second-line therapy in patients with an unresectable NET and extensive metastases.

SST is a key regulator of endocrine function by inhibiting the secretion of various hormones, including GH [94]. The overexpression of SSTR on the cell membrane of NETs provides the basis for the treatment with SST and its synthetic analogues. While the natural compound has a very short half-life [95], the development of long-acting SSAs, such as octreotide [96], lanreotide [97], and pasireotide [98], has greatly advanced the clinical management of patients with NETs. A dual action of SSAs in patients with NETs is reported, showing antisecretory and antitumoral effects, although the latter one is less robust [99, 100]. Combination therapies of SSA with antiangiogenic drugs, kinase inhibitors, and interferon are studied [101]. In GHRH-producing NETs, SSA therapy reduces GHRH secretion and suppresses both basal and GHRH-stimulated GH release but does not affect GH biosynthesis [10, 102]. SSA therapy has no significant effect on the primary tumor mass [10, 25]. The variable expression of SSTRs on NETs and the receptor-specific affinity to SSAs pose therapeutic challenges, rendering this therapy mainly palliative [100].

SSTR-targeted therapy using radioisotope-coupled molecules represents a new advance in the treatment of NETs. By combining an SSA with a therapeutic isotope, peptide-receptor radionuclide therapy for patients with unresectable or metastasized NETs is feasible [8]. Lutetium 177 (^{177}Lu) is a beta- and gamma-emitting radionuclide, characterized by a low particle range of 2mm and a half-life of 160 h [103]. In the phase 3 Neuroendocrine Tumors Therapy (NETTER-1) trial, ^{177}Lu-DOTATATE is superior to long-acting repeatable octreotide in patients with advanced, progressive, SSTR-positive midgut NETs [104]. Likewise, ^{177}Lu-DOTATATE proves favorable to other treatment options in patients with advanced or metastasized G1-G2 gastroenteropancreatic NETs and bronchial NETs [105]. Treatment for SSTR-negative G1-G2 pancreatic NETs is less clear, but a trial with SSA may be considered [106]. It is uncertain whether the results from the NETTER-1 trial are generalizable to all SSTR-positive NETs, and randomized clinical trials regarding advanced or metastasized bronchial carcinoids and pheochromocytoma/paraganglioma are lacking. Nevertheless, small clinical trials regarding pulmonary NETs are encouraging, and the current guidelines support the use of peptide receptor radionuclide therapy for SSTR-positive pulmonary NETs [91]. Although preliminary data suggest potential clinical efficacy of ^{177}Lu-DOTATATE for metastatic pheochromocytoma/paraganglioma, currently no clear treatment recommendation is given [107, 108]. Instead, radionuclide therapy with iodine-metaiodobenzylguanidine (I-MIBG) may be considered, given that catecholaminergic cells express the norepinephrine transporter for uptake of amines into cell vesicles [109]. If a metastatic pheochromocytoma/paraganglioma demonstrates robust uptake during a ^{123}I-MIBG scintigraphy, therapy with ^{131}I-MIBG may be considered [110].

Systemic treatment using cytotoxic chemotherapy may be considered for advanced and metastatic NETs. Phase 3 clinical trials in patients with pancreatic NETs demonstrate that sunitinib and everolimus improve progression-free survival by approximately 6 months [111, 112]. For pulmonary NETs, no clear guidance is given for the use of a particular chemotherapy agent, with several agents being considered [91, 113]. However, chemotherapy directed at GHRH-producing carcinoid tumors is generally unsuccessful controlling the activated GH axis [24]. For metastasized pheochromocytoma and paraganglioma, no clinical trials exist. Small studies suggest the use of cyclophosphamide/vincristine/dacarbazine or temozolomide-based treatments [114, 115].

Radiation therapy, ethanol ablation, radiofrequency ablation, and embolization of NETs may be considered for local control and symptom control [52, 91, 108, 116, 117]; however, available data is only based on case reports and small series.

Prognosis

Functional NETs producing GHRH are typically well-differentiated with slow progression and a low rate of metastases, providing an excellent prognosis [10]. In one series, surgical removal of the primary tumor results in a 2-year disease-free survival of 87% [118]. In a French series, survival rate is 85% after a median of 5 years [25]. In contrast, the 5-year survival rate of the total population with NETs is 72% [119]. It appears that the presence of SSTR2 is an independent prognostic marker associated with progression-free survival in patients treated with SSA [55, 120]. GHRH may be used for monitoring of disease progression [10].

References

1. Ranke MB, Wit JM. Growth hormone—past, present and future. Nat Rev Endocrinol. 2018;14:285–300.
2. Colao A, Grasso LFS, Giustina A, Melmed S, Chanson P, Pereira AM, Pivonello R. Acromegaly. Nat Rev Dis Primers. 2019;5:20.
3. Devesa J. The complex world of regulation of pituitary growth hormone secretion: the role of Ghrelin, Klotho, and Nesfatins in it. Front Endocrinol (Lausanne). 2021;12:636403.
4. Melmed S. Medical progress: acromegaly. N Engl J Med. 2006;355:2558–73.
5. Lavrentaki A, Paluzzi A, Wass JA, Karavitaki N. Epidemiology of acromegaly: review of population studies. Pituitary. 2017;20:4–9.
6. Akirov A, Asa SL, Amer L, Shimon I, Ezzat S. The clinicopathological spectrum of acromegaly. J Clin Med. 2019;8:1962.
7. Oronsky B, Ma PC, Morgensztern D, Carter CA. Nothing but NET: a review of neuroendocrine tumors and carcinomas. Neoplasia. 2017;19:991–1002.
8. Refardt J, Hofland J, Kwadwo A, Nicolas GP, Rottenburger C, Fani M, Wild D, Christ E. Theranostics in neuroendocrine tumors: an overview of current approaches and future challenges. Rev Endocr Metab Disord. 2021;22:581–94.
9. Rindi G, Mete O, Uccella S, Basturk O, La Rosa S, Brosens LAA, Ezzat S, de Herder WW, Klimstra DS, Papotti M, Asa SL. Overview of the 2022 WHO classification of neuroendocrine neoplasms. Endocr Pathol. 2022;33:115–54.
10. Borson-Chazot F, Garby L, Raverot G, Claustrat F, Raverot V, Sassolas G. GTE group. Acromegaly induced by ectopic secretion of GHRH: a review 30 years after GHRH discovery. Ann Endocrinol (Paris). 2012;73:497–502.
11. Saleem TF, Santhanam P, Hamoudeh E, Hassan T, Faiz S. Acromegaly caused by growth hormone releasing hormone (GHRH) secreting tumor in multiple endocrine neoplasia (MEN-1). W V Med J. 2012;108:26–30.
12. Sala E, Ferrante E, Verrua E, Malchiodi E, Mantovani G, Filopanti M, Ferrero S, Pietrabissa A, Vanoli A, La Rosa S, Zatelli MC, Beck-Peccoz P, Verga U. Growth hormone-releasing hormone-producing pancreatic neuroendocrine tumor in a multiple endocrine neoplasia type 1 family with an uncommon phenotype. Eur J Gastroenterol Hepatol. 2013;25:858–62.
13. Srirangam Nadhamuni V, Iacovazzo D, Evanson J, Sahdev A, Trouillas J, McAndrew L, Kurzawinski R, T, Bryant D, Hussain K, Bhattacharya S, Korbonits M. GHRH secretion from a pancreatic neuroendocrine tumor causing gigantism in a patient with MEN1. Endocrinol Diabetes Metab Case Rep. 2021;2021:20–0208.
14. Koivikko M, Ebeling T, Mäkinen M, Leppäluoto J, Raappana A, Ahtiainen P, Salmela P. Acromegaly caused by a GHRH-producing pancreatic neuroendocrine tumor: a rare manifestation of MEN1 syndrome. Endocrinol Diabetes Metab Case Rep. 2022;2022:21-0079.

15. Sönksen PH, Ayres AB, Braimbridge M, Corrin B, Davies DR, Jeremiah GM, Oaten SW, Lowy C, West TE. Acromegaly caused by pulmonary carcinoid tumours. Clin Endocrinol (Oxf). 1976;5:503–13.
16. Thorner MO, Perryman RL, Cronin MJ, Rogol AD, Draznin M, Johanson A, Vale W, Horvath E, Kovacs K, Somatotroph hyperplasia. Successful treatment of acromegaly by removal of a pancreatic islet tumor secreting a growth hormone-releasing factor. J Clin Invest. 1982;70:965–77.
17. Frohman LA, Szabo M, Berelowitz M, Stachura ME. Partial purification and characterization of a peptide with growth hormone-releasing activity from extrapituitary tumors in patients with acromegaly. J Clin Invest. 1980;65:43–54.
18. Rivier J, Spiess J, Thorner M, Vale W. Characterization of a growth hormone-releasing factor from a human pancreatic islet tumour. Nature. 1982;300:276–8.
19. Asa SL, Ezzat S. An update on pituitary neuroendocrine tumors leading to acromegaly and gigantism. J Clin Med. 2021;10:2254.
20. Asa SL, Ezzat S. Hypothalamic hormone-producing tumors. Handb Clin Neurol. 2021;181:67–74.
21. Biermasz NR, Smit JW, Pereira AM, Frölich M, Romijn JA, Roelfsema F. Acromegaly caused by growth hormone-releasing hormone-producing tumors: long-term observational studies in three patients. Pituitary. 2007;10:237–49.
22. Ghazi AA, Amirbaigloo A, Dezfooli AA, Saadat N, Ghazi S, Pourafkari M, Tirgari F, Dhall D, Bannykh S, Melmed S, Cooper O. Ectopic acromegaly due to growth hormone releasing hormone. Endocrine. 2013;43:293–302.
23. Ozkaya M, Sayiner ZA, Kiran G, Gul K, Erkutlu I, Elboga U. Ectopic acromegaly due to a growth hormone-secreting neuroendocrine-differentiated tumor developed from ovarian mature cystic teratoma. Wien Klin Wochenschr. 2015;127:491–3.
24. Gola M, Doga M, Bonadonna S, Mazziotti G, Vescovi PP, Giustina A. Neuroendocrine tumors secreting growth hormone-releasing hormone: pathophysiological and clinical aspects. Pituitary. 2006;9:221–9.
25. Garby L, Caron P, Claustrat F, Chanson P, Tabarin A, Rohmer V, Arnault G, Bonnet F, Chabre O, Christin-Maitre S, du-Boullay H, Murat A, Nakib I, Sadoul JL, Sassolas G, Claustrat B, Raverot G, Borson-Chazot F, GTE Group. Clinical characteristics and outcome of acromegaly induced by ectopic secretion of growth hormone-releasing hormone (GHRH): a French nationwide series of 21 cases. J Clin Endocrinol Metab. 2012;97:2093–104.
26. Dal J, Skov BG, Andersen M, Feldt-Rasmussen U, Feltoft CL, Karmisholt J, Nielsen EH, Dekkers OM, Jørgensen JOL. Sex differences in acromegaly at diagnosis: a nationwide cohort study and meta-analysis of the literature. Clin Endocrinol (Oxf). 2021;94:625–35.
27. Donadille B, Villa C, Gaillard S, Christin-Maitre S. Gangliocytoma: outcome of a rare silent pituitary tumour. BMJ Case Rep. 2017;2017:bcr2016218859.
28. Zornitzki T, Rubinfeld H, Lysyy L, Schiller T, Raverot V, Shimon I, Knobler H. pNET co-secreting GHRH and calcitonin: ex vivo hormonal studies in human pituitary cells. Endocrinol Diabetes Metab Case Rep. 2016;2016:150134.
29. Southgate HJ, Archbold GP, el-Sayed ME, Wright J, Marks V. Ectopic release of GHRH and ACTH from an adenoid cystic carcinoma resulting in acromegaly and complicated by pituitary infarction. Postgrad Med J. 1988;64:145–8.
30. Jansson JO, Svensson J, Bengtsson BA, Frohman LA, Ahlman H, Wängberg B, Nilsson O, Nilsson M. Acromegaly and Cushing's syndrome due to ectopic production of GHRH and ACTH by a thymic carcinoid tumour: in vitro responses to GHRH and GHRP-6. Clin Endocrinol (Oxf). 1998;48:243–50.
31. Furrer J, Hättenschwiler A, Komminoth P, Pfammatter T, Wiesli P. Carcinoid syndrome, acromegaly, and hypoglycemia due to an insulin-secreting neuroendocrine tumor of the liver. J Clin Endocrinol Metab. 2001;86:2227–30.
32. Babiker T, Kyrodimou E, Berney DM, Gurnell M, Drake WM, Brooke A. Acromegaly and Cushing's syndrome caused by a neuroendocrine tumor arising within a sacrococcygeal teratoma. Clin Case Rep. 2017;5:1768–71.

33. Riedl S, Frisch H. Diagnosis of growth hormone excess and hyperprolactinemia. In: Ranke MB, Mullis P-E, editors. Diagnostics of endocrine function in children and adolescents. 4th ed. Basel: Karger; 2011. p. 183–93.
34. Roth KA, Wilson DM, Eberwine J, Dorin RI, Kovacs K, Bensch KG, Hoffman AR. Acromegaly and pheochromocytoma: a multiple endocrine syndrome caused by a plurihormonal adrenal medullary tumor. J Clin Endocrinol Metab. 1986;63:1421–6.
35. Ravindra VM, Raheja A, Corn H, Driscoll M, Welt C, Simmons DL, Couldwell WT. Primary pituitary diffuse large B-cell lymphoma with somatotroph hyperplasia and acromegaly: case report. J Neurosurg. 2017;126:1725–30.
36. Feinberg Y, Law C, Singh S, Wright FC. Patient experiences of having a neuroendocrine tumour: a qualitative study. Eur J Oncol Nurs. 2013;17:541–5.
37. Katznelson L, Laws ER Jr, Melmed S, Molitch ME, Murad MH, Utz A, Wass JA, Endocrine Society. Acromegaly: an endocrine society clinical practice guideline. J Clin Endocrinol Metab. 2014;99:3933–51.
38. Barkan AL, Shenker Y, Grekin RJ, Vale WW, Lloyd RV, Beals TF. Acromegaly due to ectopic growth hormone (GH)-releasing hormone (GHRH) production: dynamic studies of GH and ectopic GHRH secretion. J Clin Endocrinol Metab. 1986;63:1057–64.
39. Frank-Heinrich JA, Xia Y, Chadha-Mohanty P, Wagner FW, Grotjan HE. Bioassay for growth hormone releasing hormone (GHRH) using a recombinant receptor and cAMP-responsive reporter system. Mol Cell Endocrinol. 1999;150(1–2):65–72.
40. Saito H, Hosoi E, Yamasaki R, Kameyama K, Irahara M, Ohno Y, Saito S. Immunoreactive growth hormone-releasing hormone (IR-GHRH) in the feto-placental circulation and differential effects of L-dopa, L-arginine and somatostatin-14 on the plasma levels of IR-GHRH in normal adults. Horm Metab Res. 1997;29:184–9.
41. Doga M, Bonadonna S, Burattin A, Giustina A. Ectopic secretion of growth hormone-releasing hormone (GHRH) in neuroendocrine tumors: relevant clinical aspects. Ann Oncol. 2001;12(Suppl 2):S89–94.
42. De Sousa SM, Earls P, McCormack AI. Pituitary hyperplasia: case series and literature review of an under-recognised and heterogeneous condition. Endocrinol Diabetes Metab Case Rep. 2015;2015:150017.
43. Modlin IM, Lye KD, Kidd M. A 5-decade analysis of 13,715 carcinoid tumors. Cancer. 2003;97:934–59.
44. Stefani A, Franceschetto A, Nesci J, Aramini B, Proli C, Kaleci S, Casolo A, Massi L, Casali C, Morandi U. Integrated FDG-PET/CT imaging is useful in the approach to carcinoid tumors of the lung. J Cardiothorac Surg. 2013;8:223.
45. Meisinger QC, Klein JS, Butnor KJ, Gentchos G, Leavitt BJ. CT features of peripheral pulmonary carcinoid tumors. AJR Am J Roentgenol. 2011;197:1073–80.
46. Lee NJ, Hruban RH, Fishman EK. Pancreatic neuroendocrine tumor: review of heterogeneous spectrum of CT appearance. Abdom Radiol (NY). 2018;43:3025–34.
47. Klöppel G. Classification and pathology of gastroenteropancreatic neuroendocrine neoplasms. Endocr Relat Cancer. 2011;18(Suppl 1):S1–16.
48. Xu Z, Wang L, Dai S, Chen M, Li F, Sun J, Luo F. Epidemiologic trends of and factors associated with overall survival for patients with gastroenteropancreatic neuroendocrine tumors in the United States. JAMA Netw Open. 2021;4:e2124750.
49. Ganeshan D, Bhosale P, Yang T, Kundra V. Imaging features of carcinoid tumors of the gastrointestinal tract. AJR Am J Roentgenol. 2013;201:773–86.
50. Debray MP, Geoffroy O, Laissy JP, Lebtahi R, Silbermann-Hoffman O, Henry-Feugeas MC, Cadiot G, Mignon M, Schouman-Claeys E. Imaging appearances of metastases from neuroendocrine tumours of the pancreas. Br J Radiol. 2001;74:1065–70.
51. Ctvrtlik F, Tudos Z, Szasz P, Sedlackova Z, Hartmann I, Schovanek J, Frysak Z, Macova I, Zelinka T, Hora M, Kocova E, Pacovsky J, Krsek M, Lehotska V, Mojtova E, Molnar J, Vanek V, Pacak K, Baxa J. Characteristic CT features of pheochromocytomas—probability model calculation tool based on a multicentric study. Biomed Pap Med Fac Univ Palacky Olomouc Czech Repub. 2019;163:212–9.

52. Howe JR, Merchant NB, Conrad C, Keutgen XM, Hallet J, Drebin JA, Minter RM, Lairmore TC, Tseng JF, Zeh HJ, Libutti SK, Singh G, Lee JE, Hope TA, Kim MK, Menda Y, Halfdanarson TR, Chan JA, Pommier RF. The North American Neuroendocrine Tumor Society consensus paper on the surgical management of pancreatic neuroendocrine tumors. Pancreas. 2020;49:1–33.
53. Moody TW, Ramos-Alvarez I, Jensen RT. Neuropeptide G protein-coupled receptors as oncotargets. Front Endocrinol (Lausanne). 2018;9:345.
54. Krenning EP, Kwekkeboom DJ, Bakker WH, Breeman WA, Kooij PP, Oei HY, van Hagen M, Postema PT, de Jong M, Reubi JC, et al. Somatostatin receptor scintigraphy with [111In-DTPA-D-Phe1]- and [123I-Tyr3]-octreotide: the Rotterdam experience with more than 1000 patients. Eur J Nucl Med. 1993;20:716–31.
55. Qian ZR, Li T, Ter-Minassian M, Yang J, Chan JA, Brais LK, Masugi Y, Thiaglingam A, Brooks N, Nishihara R, Bonnemarie M, Masuda A, Inamura K, Kim SA, Mima K, Sukawa Y, Dou R, Lin X, Christiani DC, Schmidlin F, Fuchs CS, Mahmood U, Ogino S, Kulke MH. Association between somatostatin receptor expression and clinical outcomes in neuroendocrine tumors. Pancreas. 2016;45:1386–93.
56. Zatelli MC, Maffei P, Piccin D, Martini C, Rea F, Rubello D, Margutti A, Culler MD, Sicolo N, degli Uberti EC. Somatostatin analogs in vitro effects in a growth hormone-releasing hormone-secreting bronchial carcinoid. J Clin Endocrinol Metab. 2005;90:2104–9.
57. Kyriakakis N, Trouillas J, Dang MN, Lynch J, Belchetz P, Korbonits M, Murray RD. Diagnostic challenges and management of a patient with acromegaly due to ectopic growth hormone-releasing hormone secretion from a bronchial carcinoid tumour. Endocrinol Diabetes Metab Case Rep. 2017;2017:16-0104.
58. Park S, Parihar AS, Bodei L, Hope TA, Mallak N, Millo C, Prasad K, Wilson D, Zukotynski K, Mittra E. Somatostatin receptor imaging and theranostics: current practice and future prospects. J Nucl Med. 2021;62:1323–9.
59. Fortunati E, Argalia G, Zanoni L, Fanti S, Ambrosini V. New PET radiotracers for the imaging of neuroendocrine neoplasms. Curr Treat Options Oncol. 2022;23(5):703–20. https://doi.org/10.1007/s11864-022-00967-z.
60. Krug S, Boch M, Rexin P, Pfestroff A, Gress T, Michl P, Rinke A. Acromegaly in a patient with a pulmonary neuroendocrine tumor: case report and review of current literature. BMC Res Notes. 2016;9:326.
61. Lamback EB, Henriques DG, Vazquez-Borrego MC, de Azeredo Lima CH, Kasuki L, Luque RM, Chimelli L, Gadelha MR. Growth hormone-releasing hormone-secreting pulmonary neuroendocrine tumor associated with pituitary hyperplasia and somatotropinoma. Arch Endocrinol Metab. 2021;65:648–63.
62. Daya R, Seedat F, Purbhoo K, Bulbulia S, Bayat Z. Acromegaly with empty sella syndrome. Endocrinol Diabetes Metab Case Rep. 2021;2021:21-0049.
63. Bozkurt MF, Virgolini I, Balogova S, Beheshti M, Rubello D, Decristoforo C, Ambrosini V, Kjaer A, Delgado-Bolton R, Kunikowska J, Oyen WJG, Chiti A, Giammarile F, Sundin A, Fanti S. Guideline for PET/CT imaging of neuroendocrine neoplasms with ^{68}Ga-DOTA-conjugated somatostatin receptor targeting peptides and ^{18}F-DOPA. Eur J Nucl Med Mol Imaging. 2017;44:1588–601.
64. Fani M, Mansi R, Nicolas GP, Wild D. Radiolabeled somatostatin analogs—a continuously evolving class of radiopharmaceuticals. Cancers (Basel). 2022;14:1172.
65. Deftos LJ. Chromogranin A: its role in endocrine function and as an endocrine and neuroendocrine tumor marker. Endocr Rev. 1991;12:181–7.
66. Wiedenmann B, Franke WW, Kuhn C, Moll R, Gould VE. Synaptophysin: a marker protein for neuroendocrine cells and neoplasms. Proc Natl Acad Sci U S A. 1986;83:3500–4.
67. Tapia FJ, Polak JM, Barbosa AJ, Bloom SR, Marangos PJ, Dermody C, Pearse AG. Neuron-specific enolase is produced by neuroendocrine tumours. Lancet. 1981;1(8224):808–11.
68. Gal AA, Koss MN, Hochholzer L, DeRose PB, Cohen C. Pigmented pulmonary carcinoid tumor. An immunohistochemical and ultrastructural study. Arch Pathol Lab Med. 1993;117:832–6.

69. Rehfeld JF. Radioimmunoassay in diagnosis, localization and treatment of endocrine tumours in gut and pancreas. Scand J Gastroenterol Suppl. 1979;53:33–8.
70. Ishiguro Y, Kato K, Ito T, Nagaya M. Determination of three enolase isozymes and S-100 protein in various tumors in children. Cancer Res. 1983;43:6080–4.
71. Asa SL, Kovacs K, Thorner MO, Leong DA, Rivier J, Vale W. Immunohistological localization of growth hormone-releasing hormone in human tumors. J Clin Endocrinol Metab. 1985;60:423–7.
72. Cossu G, Daniel RT, Messerer M. Gangliocytomas of the sellar region: a challenging diagnosis. Clin Neurol Neurosurg. 2016;149:122–35.
73. Asa SL, Mete O. Hypothalamic endocrine tumors: an update. J Clin Med. 2019;8:1741.
74. Hendifar AE, Marchevsky AM, Tuli R. Neuroendocrine tumors of the lung: current challenges and advances in the diagnosis and management of well-differentiated disease. J Thorac Oncol. 2017;12:425–36.
75. Rekhtman N. Lung neuroendocrine neoplasms: recent progress and persistent challenges. Mod Pathol. 2022;35(Suppl 1):36–50.
76. Wang M, Gilani S, Xu H, Cai G. Salivary gland-type tumors of the lung. Arch Pathol Lab Med. 2021;145:1379–86.
77. Aubertine CL, Flieder DB. Primary paraganglioma of the lung. Ann Diagn Pathol. 2004;8:237–41.
78. Darvishian F, Ginsberg MS, Klimstra DS, Brogi E. Carcinoid tumorlets simulate pulmonary metastases in women with breast cancer. Hum Pathol. 2006;37:839–44.
79. Ahmed M. Gastrointestinal neuroendocrine tumors in 2020. World J Gastrointest Oncol. 2020;12:791–807.
80. Hannah-Shmouni F, Stratakis CA, Koch CA. Flushing in (neuro)endocrinology. Rev Endocr Metab Disord. 2016;17:373–80.
81. Eads JR, Reidy-Lagunes D, Soares HP, Chan JA, Anthony LB, Halfdanarson TR, Naraev BG, Wolin EM, Halperin DM, Li D, Pommier RF, Zacks JS, Morse MA, Metz DC, From the Carcinoid Syndrome Control Collaborative. Differential diagnosis of diarrhea in patients with neuroendocrine tumors. Pancreas. 2020;49:1123–30.
82. Levy AD, Sobin LH. From the archives of the AFIP: gastrointestinal carcinoids: imaging features with clinicopathologic comparison. Radiographics. 2007;27:237–57.
83. Guilmette JM, Nosé V. Neoplasms of the neuroendocrine pancreas: an update in the classification, definition, and molecular genetic advances. Adv Anat Pathol. 2019;26:13–30.
84. Khanna L, Prasad SR, Sunnapwar A, Kondapaneni S, Dasyam A, Tammisetti VS, Salman U, Nazarullah A, Katabathina VS. Pancreatic neuroendocrine neoplasms: 2020 update on pathologic and imaging findings and classification. Radiographics. 2020;40:1240–62.
85. Bicci E, Cozzi D, Ferrari R, Grazzini G, Pradella S, Miele V. Pancreatic neuroendocrine tumours: spectrum of imaging findings. Gland Surg. 2020;9(6):2215–24.
86. Raman SP, Hruban RH, Cameron JL, Wolfgang CL, Fishman EK. Pancreatic imaging mimics: part 2, pancreatic neuroendocrine tumors and their mimics. AJR Am J Roentgenol. 2012;199:309–18.
87. Strosberg JR. Update on the management of unusual neuroendocrine tumors: pheochromocytoma and paraganglioma, medullary thyroid cancer and adrenocortical carcinoma. Semin Oncol. 2013;40:120–33.
88. Ctvrtlík F, Herman M, Student V, Tichá V, Minarík J. Differential diagnosis of incidentally detected adrenal masses revealed on routine abdominal CT. Eur J Radiol. 2009;69:243–52.
89. Leung K, Stamm M, Raja A, Low G. Pheochromocytoma: the range of appearances on ultrasound, CT, MRI, and functional imaging. AJR Am J Roentgenol. 2013;200:370–8.
90. Giustina A, Barkhoudarian G, Beckers A, Ben-Shlomo A, Biermasz N, Biller B, Boguszewski C, Bolanowski M, Bollerslev J, Bonert V, Bronstein MD, Buchfelder M, Casanueva F, Chanson P, Clemmons D, Fleseriu M, Formenti AM, Freda P, Gadelha M, Geer E, Gurnell M, Heaney AP, Ho KKY, Ioachimescu AG, Lamberts S, Laws E, Losa M, Maffei P, Mamelak A, Mercado M, Molitch M, Mortini P, Pereira AM, Petersenn S, Post K, Puig-Domingo M,

Salvatori R, Samson SL, Shimon I, Strasburger C, Swearingen B, Trainer P, Vance ML, Wass J, Wierman ME, Yuen KCJ, Zatelli MC, Melmed S. Multidisciplinary management of acromegaly: a consensus. Rev Endocr Metab Disord. 2020;21:667–78.

91. Singh S, Bergsland EK, Card CM, Hope TA, Kunz PL, Laidley DT, Lawrence B, Leyden S, Metz DC, Michael M, Modahl LE, Myrehaug S, Padda SK, Pommier RF, Ramirez RA, Soulen M, Strosberg J, Sung A, Thawer A, Wei B, Xu B, Segelov E. Commonwealth Neuroendocrine Tumour Research Collaboration and the North American Neuroendocrine Tumor Society guidelines for the diagnosis and management of patients with lung neuroendocrine tumors: an International Collaborative Endorsement and Update of the 2015 European Neuroendocrine Tumor Society expert consensus guidelines. J Thorac Oncol. 2020;15:1577–98.
92. Kałużny M, Polowczyk B, Bladowska J, Kubicka E, Bidlingmaier M, Bolanowski M. Acromegaly due to ectopic growth hormone-releasing hormone secretion by lung carcinoid. Pol Arch Intern Med. 2020;130:685–7.
93. Mumby C, Davis JR, Trouillas J, Higham CE. Phaeochromocytoma and acromegaly: a unifying diagnosis. Endocrinol Diabetes Metab Case Rep. 2014;2014:140036.
94. Masuda A, Shibasaki T, Kim YS, Imaki T, Hotta M, Demura H, Ling N, Shizume K. The somatostatin analog octreotide inhibits the secretion of growth hormone (GH)-releasing hormone, thyrotropin, and GH in man. J Clin Endocrinol Metab. 1989;69:906–9.
95. O'Toole TJ, Sharma S. Physiology, somatostatin. 2021 Jul 26. In: StatPearls. Treasure Island (FL): StatPearls Publishing; 2022.
96. Lamberts SW, van der Lely AJ, de Herder WW, Hofland LJ. Octreotide. N Engl J Med. 1996;334:246–54.
97. Caplin ME, Pavel M, Ćwikła JB, Phan AT, Raderer M, Sedláčková E, Cadiot G, Wolin EM, Capdevila J, Wall L, Rindi G, Langley A, Martinez S, Blumberg J, Ruszniewski P, CLARINET Investigators. Lanreotide in metastatic enteropancreatic neuroendocrine tumors. N Engl J Med. 2014;371:224–33.
98. Ferolla P, Brizzi MP, Meyer T, Mansoor W, Mazieres J, Do Cao C, Léna H, Berruti A, Damiano V, Buikhuisen W, Grønbæk H, Lombard-Bohas C, Grohé C, Minotti V, Tiseo M, De Castro J, Reed N, Gislimberti G, Singh N, Stankovic M, Öberg K, Baudin E. Efficacy and safety of long-acting pasireotide or everolimus alone or in combination in patients with advanced carcinoids of the lung and thymus (LUNA): an open-label, multicentre, randomised, phase 2 trial. Lancet Oncol. 2017;18:1652–64.
99. Cives M, Strosberg JR. Gastroenteropancreatic neuroendocrine tumors. CA Cancer J Clin. 2018;68:471–87.
100. Grozinsky-Glasberg S, Shimon I, Korbonits M, Grossman AB. Somatostatin analogues in the control of neuroendocrine tumours: efficacy and mechanisms. Endocr Relat Cancer. 2008;15:701–20.
101. Kaderli RM, Spanjol M, Kollár A, Bütikofer L, Gloy V, Dumont RA, Seiler CA, Christ ER, Radojewski P, Briel M, Walter MA. Therapeutic options for neuroendocrine tumors: a systematic review and network meta-analysis. JAMA Oncol. 2019;5:480–9.
102. Giustina A, Veldhuis JD. Pathophysiology of the neuroregulation of growth hormone secretion in experimental animals and the human. Endocr Rev. 1998;19:717–97.
103. van der Zwan WA, Bodei L, Mueller-Brand J, de Herder WW, Kvols LK, Kwekkeboom DJ. GEPNETs update: radionuclide therapy in neuroendocrine tumors. Eur J Endocrinol. 2015;172:R1–8.
104. Strosberg J, El-Haddad G, Wolin E, Hendifar A, Yao J, Chasen B, Mittra E, Kunz PL, Kulke MH, Jacene H, Bushnell D, O'Dorisio TM, Baum RP, Kulkarni HR, Caplin M, Lebtahi R, Hobday T, Delpassand E, Van Cutsem E, Benson A, Srirajaskanthan R, Pavel M, Mora J, Berlin J, Grande E, Reed N, Seregni E, Öberg K, Lopera Sierra M, Santoro P, Thevenet T, Erion JL, Ruszniewski P, Kwekkeboom D, Krenning E, NETTER-1 Trial Investigators. Phase 3 trial of ^{177}Lu-Dotatate for midgut neuroendocrine tumors. N Engl J Med. 2017;376:125–35.
105. Brabander T, van der Zwan WA, Teunissen JJM, Kam BLR, Feelders RA, de Herder WW, van Eijck CHJ, Franssen GJH, Krenning EP, Kwekkeboom DJ. Long-term efficacy, survival, and

safety of [^{177}Lu-DOTA^{0},Tyr^{3}]octreotate in patients with gastroenteropancreatic and bronchial neuroendocrine tumors. Clin Cancer Res. 2017;23:4617–24.

106. Halfdanarson TR, Strosberg JR, Tang L, Bellizzi AM, Bergsland EK, O'Dorisio TM, Halperin DM, Fishbein L, Eads J, Hope TA, Singh S, Salem R, Metz DC, Naraev BG, Reidy-Lagunes DL, Howe JR, Pommier RF, Menda Y, Chan JA. The North American Neuroendocrine Tumor Society consensus guidelines for surveillance and medical management of pancreatic neuroendocrine tumors. Pancreas. 2020;49(7):863–81.
107. Zandee WT, Feelders RA, Smit Duijzentkunst DA, Hofland J, Metselaar RM, Oldenburg RA, van Linge A, Kam BLR, Teunissen JJM, Korpershoek E, Hendriks JM, Abusaris H, Slagter C, Franssen GJH, Brabander T, De Herder WW. Treatment of inoperable or metastatic paragangliomas and pheochromocytomas with peptide receptor radionuclide therapy using 177Lu-DOTATATE. Eur J Endocrinol. 2019;181(1):45–53.
108. Fishbein L, Del Rivero J, Else T, Howe JR, Asa SL, Cohen DL, Dahia PLM, Fraker DL, Goodman KA, Hope TA, Kunz PL, Perez K, Perrier ND, Pryma DA, Ryder M, Sasson AR, Soulen MC, Jimenez C. The North American Neuroendocrine Tumor Society consensus guidelines for surveillance and management of metastatic and/or unresectable pheochromocytoma and paraganglioma. Pancreas. 2021;50:469–93.
109. Bayer M, Kuçi Z, Schömig E, Gründemann D, Dittmann H, Handgretinger R, Bruchelt G. Uptake of mIBG and catecholamines in noradrenaline- and organic cation transporter-expressing cells: potential use of corticosterone for a preferred uptake in neuroblastoma- and pheochromocytoma cells. Nucl Med Biol. 2009;36:287–94.
110. Jha A, Taïeb D, Carrasquillo JA, Pryma DA, Patel M, Millo C, de Herder WW, Del Rivero J, Crona J, Shulkin BL, Virgolini I, Chen AP, Mittal BR, Basu S, Dillon JS, Hope TA, Mari Aparici C, Iagaru AH, Hicks RJ, Avram AM, Strosberg JR, Civelek AC, Lin FI, Pandit-Taskar N, Pacak K. High-specific-activity-^{131}I-MIBG versus ^{177}Lu-DOTATATE targeted radionuclide therapy for metastatic pheochromocytoma and paraganglioma. Clin Cancer Res. 2021;27:2989–95.
111. Yao JC, Shah MH, Ito T, Bohas CL, Wolin EM, Van Cutsem E, Hobday TJ, Okusaka T, Capdevila J, de Vries EG, Tomassetti P, Pavel ME, Hoosen S, Haas T, Lincy J, Lebwohl D, Öberg K, RAD001 in Advanced Neuroendocrine Tumors, Third Trial (RADIANT-3) Study Group. Everolimus for advanced pancreatic neuroendocrine tumors. N Engl J Med. 2011;364:514–23.
112. Raymond E, Dahan L, Raoul JL, Bang YJ, Borbath I, Lombard-Bohas C, Valle J, Metrakos P, Smith D, Vinik A, Chen JS, Hörsch D, Hammel P, Wiedenmann B, Van Cutsem E, Patyna S, Lu DR, Blanckmeister C, Chao R, Ruszniewski P. Sunitinib malate for the treatment of pancreatic neuroendocrine tumors. N Engl J Med. 2011;364:501–13.
113. Chan DL, Singh S. Current chemotherapy use in neuroendocrine tumors. Endocrinol Metab Clin North Am. 2018;47:603–14.
114. Niemeijer ND, Alblas G, van Hulsteijn LT, Dekkers OM, Corssmit EP. Chemotherapy with cyclophosphamide, vincristine and dacarbazine for malignant paraganglioma and pheochromocytoma: systematic review and meta-analysis. Clin Endocrinol (Oxf). 2014;81:642–51.
115. Koumarianou A, Kaltsas G, Kulke MH, Oberg K, Strosberg JR, Spada F, Galdy S, Barberis M, Fumagalli C, Berruti A, Fazio N. Temozolomide in advanced neuroendocrine neoplasms: pharmacological and clinical aspects. Neuroendocrinology. 2015;101:274–88.
116. Rowland NC, Aghi MK. Radiation treatment strategies for acromegaly. Neurosurg Focus. 2010;29:E12.
117. Rolston JD, Blevins LS Jr. Gamma knife radiosurgery for acromegaly. Int J Endocrinol. 2012;2012:821579.
118. Losa M, Schopohl J, von Werder K. Ectopic secretion of growth hormone-releasing hormone in man. J Endocrinol Invest. 1993;16:69–81.
119. Kim SJ, Kim JW, Oh DY, Han SW, Lee SH, Kim DW, Im SA, Kim TY, Heo DS, Bang YJ. Clinical course of neuroendocrine tumors with different origins (the pancreas, gastrointestinal tract, and lung). Am J Clin Oncol. 2012;35:549–56.

120. Brunner P, Jörg AC, Glatz K, Bubendorf L, Radojewski P, Umlauft M, Marincek N, Spanjol PM, Krause T, Dumont RA, Maecke HR, Müller-Brand J, Briel M, Schmitt A, Perren A, Walter MA. The prognostic and predictive value of $sstr_2$-immunohistochemistry and $sstr_2$-targeted imaging in neuroendocrine tumors. Eur J Nucl Med Mol Imaging. 2017;44:468–75.

Chapter 3
Diagnosis of Acromegaly

Nicholas A. Tritos

Introduction

Acromegaly is a consequence of long-term exposure to growth hormone (GH) excess, which is almost always secreted autonomously from a somatotroph pituitary adenoma [1–3]. Acromegaly is associated with substantial morbidity and mortality, if inadequately treated [4]. On the other hand, patients who achieve adequate control of GH excess experience mortality rates that are indistinguishable from those in the general population [4–6].

It is therefore critical that acromegaly be diagnosed and treated promptly in order to optimize patient outcomes [7]. Of note, a longer interval between estimated disease onset and diagnosis of acromegaly has been associated with higher morbidity and mortality [8].

The present chapter aims at reviewing all diagnostic aspects of acromegaly, including clinical evaluation, laboratory testing, and imaging. To compile the literature cited in this manuscript, electronic literature searches were conducted using the keywords: acromegaly, diagnosis, pituitary adenoma. Studies were included in the bibliography at the author's judgment and discretion.

N. A. Tritos (✉)
Neuroendocrine Unit and Neuroendocrine and Pituitary Tumor Clinical Center, Massachusetts General Hospital, Boston, MA, USA

Harvard Medical School, Boston, MA, USA
e-mail: ntritos@mgh.harvard.edu

L. S. Blevins Jr., M. K. Aghi (eds.), *Acromegaly*, Contemporary Endocrinology,
https://doi.org/10.1007/978-3-031-16258-9_3

Physiology and Pathophysiology

Growth hormone is a 191-amino acid polypeptide that is secreted in a pulsatile manner, predominantly during slow-wave sleep, with additional secretory events occurring during exercise or in the fasting state [9, 10]. In addition to the major 22 kDa species, there are several GH isoforms present in the systemic circulation, arising from alternative splicing or various posttranslational modifications [11]. Different immunoassays may variably detect distinct GH isoforms, which may partly account for the considerable inter-assay variability of GH levels measured across various immunoassay platforms [11–13]. In healthy individuals, GH secretion is stimulated by growth hormone-releasing hormone (GHRH) of hypothalamic origin and ghrelin, secreted mainly from the stomach [9]. On the other hand, somatostatin, also of hypothalamic origin, decreases GH secretion [9]. Glucose administration suppresses GH secretion and blunts GH levels in healthy individuals but not in patients with acromegaly [14, 15].

Growth hormone acts via its cognate receptor to exert its diverse effects, either directly or via the stimulation of insulin-like growth factor I (IGF-I) secretion [9]. Although may tissues synthesize IGF-I, the majority of circulating IGF-I is of hepatic origin. The serum IGF-I level does not fluctuate during the day and serves as an accurate measure of GH action in vivo [9, 16]. In patients with acromegaly, GH is secreted autonomously by a pituitary adenoma (or rarely by an ectopic tumor), leading to elevated IGF-I levels [17].

Clinical Evaluation

Acromegaly is quite uncommon in the general population, which often results in substantial diagnostic delays, since the diagnosis is often not considered during the initial patient encounter [18, 19]. A high index of suspicion is required in order to consider the diagnosis of acromegaly early in the course of the disease [20]. Although acral enlargement and headache are common presenting manifestations, there is substantial variation in presenting symptoms, which can be subtle and relatively nonspecific [21, 22]. Patients with acromegaly often present to their primary care physician but may also present to anyone of a variety of non-endocrine subspecialists, who may not consider the diagnosis of acromegaly. Patients with a cluster of suggestive symptoms and signs, including acral enlargement, frequent headache, hypertension, diabetes mellitus, sleep apnea, oligomenorrhea, arthropathy, carpal tunnel syndrome, and hyperhidrosis, among others, should be considered for endocrine testing in order to evaluate the presence of GH excess [1, 23]. Increased linear growth before epiphyseal closure should also suggest the diagnosis and the need for endocrine testing. It may be recognized that several presenting symptoms of acromegaly are common in the general population. Indeed, widespread endocrine evaluation of patients with solitary symptoms, such as sleep apnea occurring in isolation, does not appear to be justified, since the diagnostic yield for acromegaly is likely to be low in unselected populations [24].

The absence of typical facial features should not serve as a means of excluding the diagnosis, since abnormalities in facial features can be quite subtle in patients with acromegaly of recent onset. It is often helpful to compare the patient's appearance to that in older photographs, which may reveal mild changes in facial features associated with acromegaly. Face classification software appears promising as a diagnostic tool that may assist physicians in detecting acromegaly early in its course [25]. It has been suggested that the utilization of artificial intelligence, including machine learning algorithms used for face classification analysis, may have high diagnostic accuracy in patients with acromegaly [26]. Maintaining respect for patient confidentiality is important when using such technologies.

A thorough history and physical examination may additionally uncover clues to the presence of a pituitary adenoma, such as visual field defects, or other manifestations of chronic GH excess, such as prognathism, wide dental spacing, or multiple skin tags. Patients with incidentally discovered sellar masses may have underlying acromegaly and should be considered for evaluation of possible GH excess [27].

Laboratory Testing

Growth Hormone Endocrine testing represents the cornerstone in making the diagnosis of acromegaly (Table 3.1). Growth hormone secretion retains some pulsatility in acromegaly. However, it is the basal GH levels, rather than GH pulse mass, that correlate with serum IGF-I levels in this population [28]. Random GH levels below 0.4 mcg/L suggest that acromegaly is unlikely. However, there is a substantial overlap in random GH levels between patients with acromegaly and healthy individuals, such that randomly obtained GH levels are of limited diagnostic utility [1, 2, 28].

Oral Glucose Tolerance Test *G*lucose-suppressed GH levels are of diagnostic value in patients with suspected acromegaly. The oral glucose tolerance test (OGTT) is performed by administering 75 g of glucose orally after an 8-h fast and obtaining serum specimens every 30 min for 2 h, which are submitted for GH and glucose assays. The availability of increasingly sensitive GH immunoassays has led to the identification of patients with acromegaly who suppress GH to very low levels during the test, leading to a gradual decrease in proposed diagnostic cut points for nadir GH levels during the OGTT; over the past several decades, these have declined from 2 mcg/L to 1 mcg/L and then to 0.4 mcg/L [29, 30]. Of note, nadir GH levels below 0.4 mcg/L have been reported in some patients with acromegaly who exhibit minimally elevated GH secretory output [15]. Healthy individuals generally suppress GH levels to even lower values (around 0.1 mcg/L), using sensitive immunoassays [31]. Among healthy subjects, nadir GH values are higher in lean patients and women on combination oral contraceptives [31].

Table 3.1 Endocrine tests that have been proposed for use in making the diagnosis of acromegaly

Test	Diagnostic cut point	Comments
Random serum GH levels	Random GH <0.4 mcg/L suggest that acromegaly is unlikely	Limited diagnostic value in light of substantial overlap in random GH levels between patients with acromegaly and healthy individuals
Nadir GH during OGTT	Nadir GH <0.4 mcg/L in healthy individuals; nadir GH >0.4 mcg/L in the majority of patients with acromegaly[a]	Some overlap in nadir GH levels exists between patients with acromegaly and healthy individuals, using either 0.4 mcg/L or 1.0 mcg/L as the diagnostic cut point; also consider conditions that may influence GH response during this test[b]
Serum IGF-I	Age and assay-dependent	IGF-I represents the best available test in the diagnosis of acromegaly; consider conditions that may influence test results[b]
Serum IGFBP-3	Assay-dependent	Cannot be recommended for clinical use in light of insufficient diagnostic accuracy
Serum acid labile subunit	Assay-dependent	Cannot be recommended for clinical use in light of insufficient diagnostic accuracy
TRH stimulation test	Peak GH increases <50% over baseline in healthy individuals; peak GH increases >50% over baseline in patients with acromegaly	TRH is currently unavailable in the United States
Serum GHRH level	Assay-dependent	Very high levels (several times above the upper end of the normal range) in patients with ectopic GHRH-secreting tumors

GH growth hormone, *GHRH* growth hormone-releasing hormone, *IGF-I* insulin-like growth factor I, *IGFBP-3* insulin-like growth factor binding protein 3, *OGTT* oral glucose tolerance test, *TRH* thyrotropin-releasing hormone

[a]A GH cut point of 1.0 mcg/L has been proposed in the latest Endocrine Society guidelines, recognizing that many commercially available immunoassays have limited analytical accuracy at low GH levels. Healthy individuals suppress GH levels to <0.1 mcg/L using sensitive immunoassays

[b]Starvation, anorexia, liver or kidney disease, hypothyroidism, poorly controlled diabetes mellitus, and combination oral contraceptive use may lead to lack of GH suppression during OGTT and abnormally low serum IGF-I levels

As some commercially available GH assays may lack sufficient analytical accuracy at low GH levels, it has been recommended to use 1 mcg/L as the diagnostic cut point for nadir GH levels during OGTT in routine clinical care [1]. It should be recognized, however, that some patients with acromegaly may suppress GH to lower levels (below 1 mcg/L) during the test. Different GH immunoassays vary with regard to detection of various GH isoforms and some may use nonuniform reference standard preparations, partly accounting for observed variations in diagnostic performance across GH assay platforms [12–14, 17, 32, 33]. Patients with anorexia, starvation, severe liver or kidney disease, and poorly controlled diabetes mellitus and women on combination oral contraceptives may all fail to suppress GH levels during OGTT in the absence of acromegaly (Table 3.1) [23, 32].

Insulin-Like Growth Factor I The serum IGF-I level serves as an integrated measure of GH action and is of substantial diagnostic value in patients with suspected acromegaly, representing the best, currently available, diagnostic test [1, 34]. It should be noted that IGF-I assays are technically challenging and require separation of IGF-I from its binding proteins before assay [17, 33]. Serum IGF-I levels vary considerably by age, increasing during adolescence and then gradually declining throughout adult life, thus requiring meticulous attention in establishing age-appropriate reference ranges [17, 33].

Considerable variation in serum IGF-I levels has been reported using different immunoassays, leading to variable diagnostic performance across IGF-I immunoassay platforms [35]. More recently, liquid chromatography-tandem mass spectrometry (LC/MS-MS) has been introduced to measure serum IGF-I levels [36]. However, IGF-I data obtained using LC/MS-MS may vary considerably from those obtained using immunoassays. It is therefore advisable to use the same assay consistently when measuring IGF-I levels longitudinally in patients, if possible [37].

Patients with anorexia, starvation, poorly controlled diabetes mellitus, severe hypothyroidism, and severe liver or kidney disease and women on combination oral contraceptives may have abnormally low IGF-I levels in the absence of acromegaly (Table 3.1) [23, 33]. On the other hand, healthy adolescents, pregnant women, or some patients receiving pharmacological doses of glucocorticoids may have abnormally elevated IGF-I levels [23, 33]. Discordant data between IGF-I and nadir GH levels during OGTT are not uncommon, both during initial patient assessment and on postoperative testing of patients with acromegaly, and their significance is uncertain [16, 29, 30, 38, 39]. Therefore, laboratory data should always be placed in proper clinical context in order to avoid errors in test interpretation. Of note, discordance between IGF-I and nadir GH levels during OGTT is very common in patients on somatostatin receptor ligand therapy [40]. As a corollary, it is advisable not to perform OGTT to assess disease control in patients being treated with somatostatin receptor ligands.

Insulin-Like Growth Factor Binding Protein 3 and Acid Labile Subunit Insulin-like growth factor binding protein 3 (IGFBP-3) and the acid labile subunit (ALS) form a ternary complex with IGF-I in the systemic circulation. Both the expression and systemic levels of serum IGFBP-3 and ALS are GH-dependent [41, 42]. As a corollary, both serum IGFBP-3 and ALS levels have been studied as potential biomarkers of GH action and assessed for their diagnostic utility in patients with acromegaly [41, 42]. However, the diagnostic accuracy of these tests is not sufficient to justify their clinical use at present [1, 2].

Thyrotropin-Releasing Hormone Stimulation Test The thyrotropin-releasing hormone (TRH) stimulation test can be useful in the diagnosis of acromegaly. In these patients, GH levels increase by over 50% above baseline within 30 min after the intravenous administration of TRH (500 mcg); in contrast, healthy subjects show no or little increase in GH levels after TRH administration [43]. However, TRH is not commercially available in the United States at present.

Growth Hormone-Releasing Hormone Serum levels of growth hormone-releasing hormone (GHRH) can be of diagnostic utility among the rare patients with suspected ectopic tumors that cause acromegaly by secreting GHRH [44–46]. In these patients, serum GHRH levels are generally elevated several times above the upper end of the normal range. However, serum GHRH levels are of no diagnostic utility in the vast majority of patients with acromegaly who have an evident pituitary tumor on sellar imaging.

Additional Tests A thorough evaluation of pituitary function is recommended in all patients with acromegaly. Either prolactin or, less frequently, thyrotropin (TSH) can be co-secreted by some somatotroph adenomas [47, 48]. Anterior hypopituitarism is not uncommon among patients with acromegaly, since about 70% of somatotroph tumors are macroadenomas at presentation [1, 2]. As a corollary, serum levels of prolactin, TSH, and free thyroxine should be measured in all patients with acromegaly, and morning serum cortisol (or cosyntropin stimulation testing), serum gonadotropins, and morning testosterone (in men) or estradiol (in women) should be obtained in all patients with macroadenomas and those with microadenomas who have symptoms of respective pituitary hormone deficiencies. In addition, a thorough neuro-ophthalmic evaluation is recommended for all patients with visual symptoms as well as those whose tumors abut or compress the optic chiasm, nerves, or tracts. Genetic testing should be considered for younger patients, those with gigantism, or those with a positive family history of acrogigantism or evidence of a syndromic condition (such as multiple endocrine neoplasia 1 or Carney complex). A detailed discussion of genetic testing is beyond the scope of this chapter.

Imaging Studies

In over 95% of patients with acromegaly, the underlying cause is a sellar mass, usually a benign somatotroph adenoma or, rarely, carcinoma or a GHRH-secreting gangliocytoma [1, 2, 23, 49]. Therefore, pituitary imaging is essential for tumor localization and preoperative evaluation. However, imaging studies should be deferred until the diagnosis of acromegaly is established based on clinical evaluation and endocrine testing. This is important in order to avoid potential misdiagnosis of patients with nonfunctioning pituitary lesions. Indeed, incidental sellar masses are present in approximately 10% of the general population [50].

In patients with acromegaly, magnetic resonance imaging (MRI) of the sella is advisable as the imaging study of choice and should be performed using a dedicated, high-resolution, pituitary protocol. Pituitary MRI will readily detect a sellar mass in the large majority of patients with acromegaly, since 70% of somatotroph tumors are macroadenomas at diagnosis (Fig. 3.1) [1, 2, 51]. As an alternative, a high-resolution examination of the sella by computed tomography (CT) can be obtained in patients who have contraindications to MRI, including some patients with older pacemakers or those with metal shrapnel.

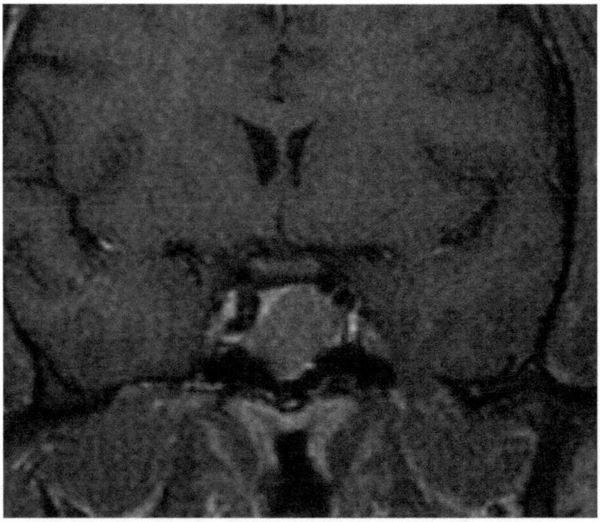

Fig. 3.1 Coronal, postcontrast, T1-weighted magnetic resonance image of a 36-year-old male patient with acromegaly, showing a pituitary macroadenoma, likely extending into the left cavernous sinus

In a small minority of patients with acromegaly, there is no evidence of a pituitary tumor on MRI. Most of these patients likely have a somatotroph adenoma that is below the resolution of modern imaging techniques. However, a small proportion of them have an ectopic neuroendocrine tumor in the chest or abdomen, which is secreting GHRH or, even more rarely, GH [44–46, 52]. Ectopic GH secretion from non-Hodgkin's lymphoma has also been reported [53]. Cross-sectional imaging, including CT examinations of the chest and abdomen as well as positron emission tomography (PET)-CT examinations using gallium 68-labelled dodecane tetraacetic acid tyrosine-3-octreotate (DOTATATE), will usually demonstrate ectopic neuroendocrine tumors in these patients [45].

Approach to the Patient

Delays in considering the diagnosis of acromegaly likely account for the substantial interval between disease onset and diagnosis, which has been estimated to be approximately 5.5 years (mean value) but may exhibit wide variation [8]. This long interval can be explained by the slow, insidious onset and the nonspecific nature of several symptoms, some of which can be attributed to aging by patients or lead to unrelated investigations by non-endocrine subspecialists who may have relatively little familiarity with acromegaly.

Once the diagnosis of acromegaly is considered, serum IGF-I levels should be measured using a well-validated assay (Fig. 3.2). In the presence of typical disease manifestations and unequivocally elevated serum IGF-I levels, the diagnosis of acromegaly can be made with confidence and pituitary imaging obtained (preferably by MRI). Careful attention is needed to the presence of factors or conditions that

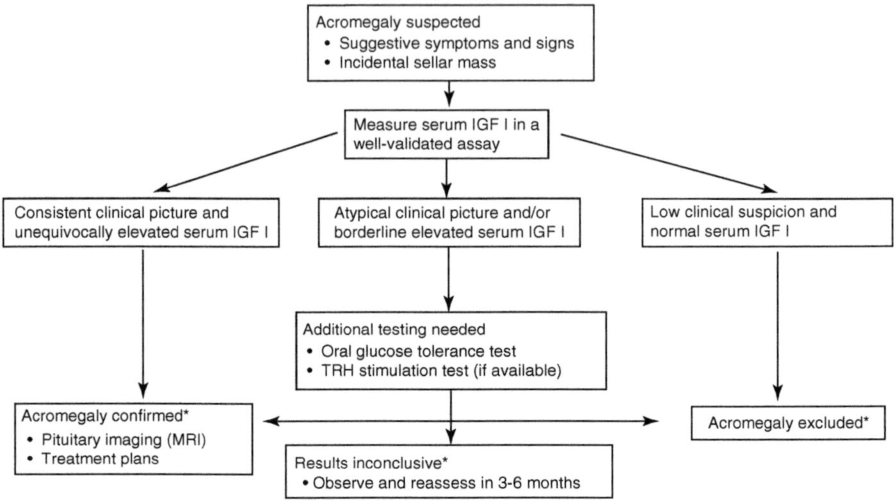

Fig. 3.2 A diagnostic algorithm for the evaluation of patients with suspected acromegaly *IGF-I* insulin-like growth factor I, *MRI* magnetic resonance imaging, *TRH* thyrotropin-releasing hormone. *Always consider conditions that can influence IGF-I and GH data in the absence of acromegaly

can influence the results of IGF-I levels and GH levels during OGTT, such as liver or kidney disease or combination oral contraceptive use, when interpreting test data. If the clinical presentation is atypical or serum IGF-I levels are borderline high (below 1.5 times above the upper end of the normal range), then additional investigations are warranted, including a 2-h OGTT or a TRH stimulation test (in countries where TRH is available). If test results are still inconclusive, the patient can be observed and reassessed in several months.

Once the diagnosis is established and a pituitary mass is identified on MRI, treatment can begin without delay, including transsphenoidal surgery or, in some cases, primary medical therapy [7]. If no sellar mass is demonstrated on high-resolution pituitary imaging, then a search for an ectopic tumor is advisable by means of measuring serum GHRH levels and obtaining cross-sectional imaging (CT of the chest and abdomen and, if needed, whole body PET-CT using Ga 68 DOTATATE) [44–46, 52]. Ectopic tumors may be treated with surgery and somatostatin receptor ligand therapy.

If no evidence of an ectopic lesion is found despite appropriate testing, then it is likely that a very small pituitary adenoma is present, which is below the resolution of MRI (smaller than 2–3 mm in diameter). In such cases, postcontrast, volumetric interpolated breath-hold examination (VIBE), thin slice, MRI images may demonstrate a tumor and facilitate surgical resection [54].

The diagnosis of acromegaly is very difficult to make during pregnancy owing to physiological changes associated with normal gestation [1, 55]. The placenta secretes a GH variant, which is not distinguishable from pituitary GH by many commercially available immunoassays [1, 55]. Of note, GH levels may not be suppressible on OGTT during pregnancy. Placental GH stimulates maternal IGF-I secretion, which may lead to elevated serum IGF-I levels in late pregnancy, despite the development of estrogen-induced GH resistance during gestation [1, 55]. In the absence of evidence of mass effect, such as vision loss or unremitting headache, it is generally best to defer evaluation of possible acromegaly in women during gestation and perform appropriate endocrine testing in the postpartum state.

Summary and Future Directions

A systematic approach to the evaluation of patients with suspected acromegaly is essential in order to optimize clinical outcomes. Measuring serum IGF-I levels and performing OGTT in selected cases will generally help establish or exclude the diagnosis. Once a biochemical diagnosis of acromegaly is made, high-resolution pituitary imaging is advisable for tumor localization before initiating treatment.

Raising awareness of the disease in the medical community is important in order to facilitate the early detection of acromegaly. Use of face classification software may also assist clinicians in making a timely diagnosis. Harmonization of GH and IGF-I assays across test platforms and identification of novel biomarkers of GH action may lead to further refinements in our ability to accurately diagnose this serious condition.

References

1. Katznelson L, Laws ER Jr, Melmed S, et al. Acromegaly: an endocrine society clinical practice guideline. J Clin Endocrinol Metab. 2014;99:3933–51.
2. Colao A, Grasso LFS, Giustina A, Melmed S, Chanson P, Pereira AM, Pivonello R. Acromegaly. Nat Rev Dis Primers. 2019;5:20.
3. Capatina C, Wass JA. 60 years of neuroendocrinology: acromegaly. J Endocrinol. 2015;226:T141–60.
4. Holdaway IM, Bolland MJ, Gamble GD. A meta-analysis of the effect of lowering serum levels of GH and IGF-I on mortality in acromegaly. Eur J Endocrinol. 2008;159:89–95.
5. Swearingen B, Barker FG 2nd, Katznelson L, et al. Long-term mortality after transsphenoidal surgery and adjunctive therapy for acromegaly. J Clin Endocrinol Metab. 1998;83:3419–26.
6. Tritos NA, Mattsson AF, Vila G, et al. All-cause mortality in patients with acromegaly treated with pegvisomant: an ACROSTUDY analysis. Eur J Endocrinol. 2020;182:285–92.
7. Melmed S, Bronstein MD, Chanson P, et al. A consensus statement on acromegaly therapeutic outcomes. Nat Rev Endocrinol. 2018;14:552–61.
8. Esposito D, Ragnarsson O, Johannsson G, Olsson DS. Prolonged diagnostic delay in acromegaly is associated with increased morbidity and mortality. Eur J Endocrinol. 2020;182(6):523–53.
9. Melmed S. Pathogenesis and diagnosis of growth hormone deficiency in adults. N Engl J Med. 2019;380:2551–62.
10. Ho PJ, Friberg RD, Barkan AL. Regulation of pulsatile growth hormone secretion by fasting in normal subjects and patients with acromegaly. J Clin Endocrinol Metab. 1992;75:812–9.
11. Bidlingmaier M, Strasburger CJ. Growth hormone. Handb Exp Pharmacol. 2010;(195):187–200.

12. Bidlingmaier M, Freda PU. Measurement of human growth hormone by immunoassays: current status, unsolved problems and clinical consequences. Growth Hormon IGF Res. 2010;20:19–25.
13. Bidlingmaier M, Strasburger CJ. Growth hormone assays: current methodologies and their limitations. Pituitary. 2007;10:115–9.
14. Arafat AM, Mohlig M, Weickert MO, et al. Growth hormone response during oral glucose tolerance test: the impact of assay method on the estimation of reference values in patients with acromegaly and in healthy controls, and the role of gender, age, and body mass index. J Clin Endocrinol Metab. 2008;93:1254–62.
15. Ribeiro-Oliveira A Jr, Faje AT, Barkan AL. Limited utility of oral glucose tolerance test in biochemically active acromegaly. Eur J Endocrinol. 2011;164:17–22.
16. Subbarayan SK, Fleseriu M, Gordon MB, et al. Serum IGF-1 in the diagnosis of acromegaly and the profile of patients with elevated IGF-1 but normal glucose-suppressed growth hormone. Endocr Pract. 2012;18:817–25.
17. Clemmons DR. Clinical laboratory indices in the treatment of acromegaly. Clin Chim Acta. 2011;412:403–9.
18. Holdaway IM, Rajasoorya C. Epidemiology of acromegaly. Pituitary. 1999;2:29–41.
19. Lavrentaki A, Paluzzi A, Wass JA, Karavitaki N. Epidemiology of acromegaly: review of population studies. Pituitary. 2017;20:4–9.
20. Tritos NA. Setting the bar high for the care of patients with acromegaly. J Clin Endocrinol Metab. 2020;105:e1895–6.
21. Nachtigall L, Delgado A, Swearingen B, Lee H, Zerikly R, Klibanski A. Changing patterns in diagnosis and therapy of acromegaly over two decades. J Clin Endocrinol Metab. 2008;93:2035–41.
22. Vilar L, Vilar CF, Lyra R, Lyra R, Naves LA. Acromegaly: clinical features at diagnosis. Pituitary. 2017;20:22–32.
23. Katznelson L, Atkinson JL, Cook DM, Ezzat SZ, Hamrahian AH, Miller KK, American Association of Clinical Endocrinologists. American Association of Clinical Endocrinologists medical guidelines for clinical practice for the diagnosis and treatment of acromegaly--2011 update. Endocr Pract. 2011;17(Suppl 4):1–44.
24. Heinrich DA, Reinholz C, Bauer M, et al. IGF-1-based screening reveals a low prevalence of acromegaly in patients with obstructive sleep apnea. Endocrine. 2018;60:317–22.
25. Schneider HJ, Kosilek RP, Gunther M, et al. A novel approach to the detection of acromegaly: accuracy of diagnosis by automatic face classification. J Clin Endocrinol Metab. 2011;96:2074–80.
26. Kong X, Gong S, Su L, Howard N, Kong Y. Automatic detection of acromegaly from facial photographs using machine learning methods. EBioMedicine. 2018;27:94–102.
27. Seltzer J, Wedemeyer MA, Bonney PA, Carmichael JD, Weiss M, Zada G. Outcomes following transsphenoidal surgical management of incidental pituitary adenomas: a series of 52 patients over a 17-year period. J Neurosurg. 2018:1–9.
28. Faje AT, Barkan AL. Basal, but not pulsatile, growth hormone secretion determines the ambient circulating levels of insulin-like growth factor-I. J Clin Endocrinol Metab. 2010;95:2486–91.
29. Freda PU. Pitfalls in the biochemical assessment of acromegaly. Pituitary. 2003;6:135–40.
30. Freda PU, Reyes CM, Nuruzzaman AT, Sundeen RE, Bruce JN. Basal and glucose-suppressed GH levels less than 1 microg/L in newly diagnosed acromegaly. Pituitary. 2003;6:175–80.
31. Schilbach K, Gar C, Lechner A, et al. Determinants of the growth hormone nadir during oral glucose tolerance test in adults. Eur J Endocrinol. 2019;181:55–67.
32. de Oliveira R, Longo Schweizer J, Ribeiro-Oliveira A Jr, Bidlingmaier M. Growth hormone: isoforms, clinical aspects and assays interference. Clin Diabetes Endocrinol. 2018;4:18.
33. Clemmons DR. Consensus statement on the standardization and evaluation of growth hormone and insulin-like growth factor assays. Clin Chem. 2011;57:555–9.
34. Johannsson G, Bidlingmaier M, Biller BMK, et al. Growth Hormone Research Society perspective on biomarkers of GH action in children and adults. Endocr Connect. 2018;7:R126–R34.

35. Pokrajac A, Wark G, Ellis AR, Wear J, Wieringa GE, Trainer PJ. Variation in GH and IGF-I assays limits the applicability of international consensus criteria to local practice. Clin Endocrinol. 2007;67:65–70.
36. Bystrom C, Sheng S, Zhang K, Caulfield M, Clarke NJ, Reitz R. Clinical utility of insulin-like growth factor 1 and 2; determination by high resolution mass spectrometry. PLoS One. 2012;7:e43457.
37. Bonert V, Carmichael J, Wu Z, et al. Discordance between mass spectrometry and immunometric IGF-1 assay in pituitary disease: a prospective study. Pituitary. 2018;21:65–75.
38. Brzana JA, Yedinak CG, Delashaw JB, Gultelkin HS, Cook D, Fleseriu M. Discordant growth hormone and IGF-1 levels post pituitary surgery in patients with acromegaly naive to medical therapy and radiation: what to follow, GH or IGF-1 values? Pituitary. 2012;15:562–70.
39. Dimaraki EV, Jaffe CA, DeMott-Friberg R, Chandler WF, Barkan AL. Acromegaly with apparently normal GH secretion: implications for diagnosis and follow-up. J Clin Endocrinol Metab. 2002;87:3537–42.
40. Carmichael JD, Bonert VS, Mirocha JM, Melmed S. The utility of oral glucose tolerance testing for diagnosis and assessment of treatment outcomes in 166 patients with acromegaly. J Clin Endocrinol Metab. 2009;94:523–7.
41. Morrison KM, Wu Z, Bidlingmaier M, Strasburger CJ. Findings and theoretical considerations on the usefulness of the acid-labile subunit in the monitoring of acromegaly. Growth Hormon IGF Res. 2001;11(Suppl A):S61–3.
42. Grinspoon S, Clemmons D, Swearingen B, Klibanski A. Serum insulin-like growth factor-binding protein-3 levels in the diagnosis of acromegaly. J Clin Endocrinol Metab. 1995;80:927–32.
43. Irie M, Tsushima T. Increase of serum growth hormone concentration following thyrotropin-releasing hormone injection in patients with acromegaly or gigantism. J Clin Endocrinol Metab. 1972;35:97–100.
44. Barkan AL, Shenker Y, Grekin RJ, Vale WW. Acromegaly from ectopic growth hormone-releasing hormone secretion by a malignant carcinoid tumor. Successful treatment with long-acting somatostatin analogue SMS 201-995. Cancer. 1988;61:221–6.
45. Ghazi AA, Amirbaigloo A, Dezfooli AA, et al. Ectopic acromegaly due to growth hormone releasing hormone. Endocrine. 2013;43:293–302.
46. Weiss DE, Vogel H, Lopes MB, Chang SD, Katznelson L. Ectopic acromegaly due to a pancreatic neuroendocrine tumor producing growth hormone-releasing hormone. Endocr Pract. 2011;17:79–84.
47. Rick J, Jahangiri A, Flanigan PM, Chandra A, Kunwar S, Blevins L, Aghi MK. Growth hormone and prolactin-staining tumors causing acromegaly: a retrospective review of clinical presentations and surgical outcomes. J Neurosurg. 2018;131:147–53.
48. Amlashi FG, Tritos NA. Thyrotropin-secreting pituitary adenomas: epidemiology, diagnosis, and management. Endocrine. 2016;52:427–40.
49. Isidro ML, Iglesias Diaz P, Matias-Guiu X, Cordido F. Acromegaly due to a growth hormone-releasing hormone-secreting intracranial gangliocytoma. J Endocrinol Investig. 2005;28:162–5.
50. Hall WA, Luciano MG, Doppman JL, Patronas NJ, Oldfield EH. Pituitary magnetic resonance imaging in normal human volunteers: occult adenomas in the general population. Ann Intern Med. 1994;120:817–20.
51. Faje A, Tritos NA, Swearingen B, Klibanski A. Neuroendocrine disorders: pituitary imaging. Handb Clin Neurol. 2016;136:873–85.
52. Melmed S, Ezrin C, Kovacs K, Goodman RS, Frohman LA. Acromegaly due to secretion of growth hormone by an ectopic pancreatic islet-cell tumor. N Engl J Med. 1985;312:9–17.
53. Beuschlein F, Strasburger CJ, Siegerstetter V, et al. Acromegaly caused by secretion of growth hormone by a non-Hodgkin's lymphoma. N Engl J Med. 2000;342:1871–6.
54. Lonser RR, Kindzelski BA, Mehta GU, Jane JA Jr, Oldfield EH. Acromegaly without imaging evidence of pituitary adenoma. J Clin Endocrinol Metab. 2010;95:4192–6.
55. Muhammad A, Neggers SJ, van der Lely AJ. Pregnancy and acromegaly. Pituitary. 2017;20:179–84.

Chapter 4
Imaging in Acromegaly

Ian Mark and Javier Villanueva-Meyer

Anatomy

The sellar region can be affected by a variety of pathologies and intimate knowledge of sellar anatomy is critical for arriving at the appropriate diagnosis in a noninvasive fashion. For the purposes of this chapter, we will briefly review anatomy of the pituitary gland. The pituitary gland sits within a depression in the sphenoid bone, the sella turcica. Anterior and inferior to the gland sits the sphenoid sinus, through which the sella is accessed via the transsphenoidal approach commonly used in surgery for resection of pituitary lesions. Laterally are the cavernous sinuses through which the internal carotid artery and cranial nerves course. Posteriorly and anteriorly are the intercavernous sinuses linking the two cavernous sinuses. Superiorly is the sella turcica which is covered by dura known as the diaphragma sellae which has a central opening through which the pituitary stalk (or infundibulum) passes. Above the diaphragma sellae is the suprasellar cistern, a CSF containing space that the optic chiasm resides in.

The pituitary gland itself is divided into two components, the anterior lobe and posterior lobe. The anterior lobe is also called the adenohypophysis due to its glandular nature and can be further subdivided into three parts; the pars distalis, pars intermedia, and pars tuberalis. The pars distalis represents the majority of the gland itself. The pars intermedia sits between the pars distalis and the posterior lobe. The pars tuberalis is an upward extension from the pars distalis and extends to the pituitary stalk. The posterior lobe is also known as the neurohypophysis and is not glandular but consists of nervous tissue projecting from the hypothalamus.

I. Mark · J. Villanueva-Meyer (✉)
Department of Radiology and Biomedical Imaging, University of California San Francisco, San Francisco, CA, USA
e-mail: Ian.mark@ucsf.edu; Javier.villanueva-meyer@ucsf.edu

L. S. Blevins Jr., M. K. Aghi (eds.), *Acromegaly*, Contemporary Endocrinology,
https://doi.org/10.1007/978-3-031-16258-9_4

Imaging of the Pituitary Gland

Due to its superior soft tissue resolution and greater ability to inform on tissue characteristics, MRI is the preferred modality for imaging of the pituitary gland. CT is reserved for cases where a patient may have contraindications to MRI, although in modern times this scenario is becoming less common. Imaging the pituitary gland requires a dedicated MRI protocol. A typical "pituitary protocol" MRI involves small field of view sequences centered on the sellar region. These include spin echo T1-weighted images in the sagittal and coronal plane before and after the administration of intravenous gadolinium-based contrast agent. Post-contrast imaging should include a dynamic component for increased temporal resolution that is performed immediately after contrast injection and repeated in approximately 30-second intervals, as well as delayed post-contrast images (Fig. 4.1). Coronal T2-weighted images are also acquired. Diffusion-weighted imaging (DWI) is sometimes acquired as well. The added value of each of these sequences is listed in Table 4.1. Imaging can be obtained on clinically available 1.5 tesla (T) or 3 T

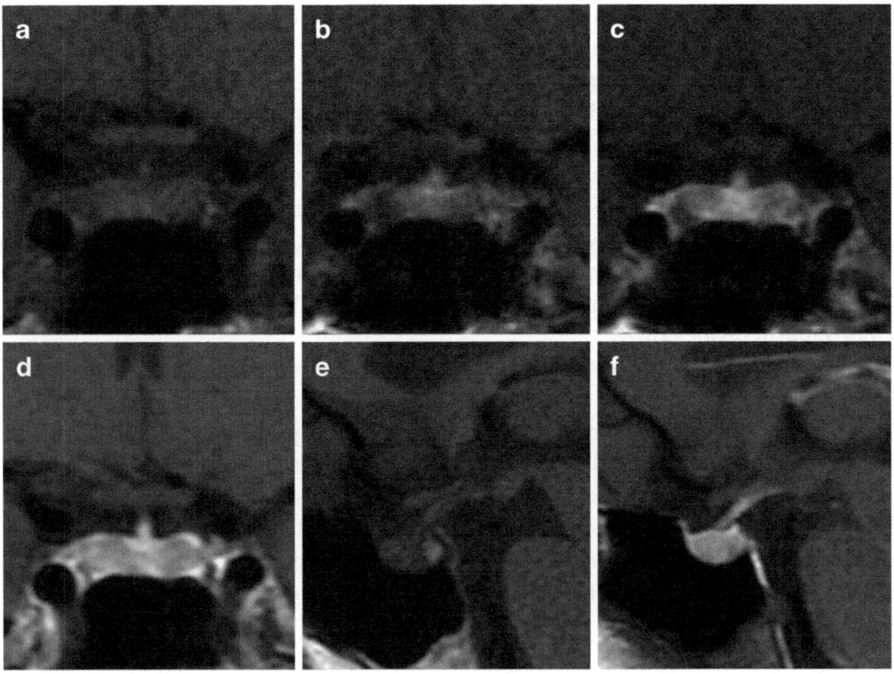

Fig. 4.1 Normal pituitary MRI with a small field of view. (**a–d**) Dynamic post-contrast T1-weighted coronal imaging shows progressive enhancement that begins with the infundibulum, and progressively fills the pituitary from central to peripheral. (**e**) Non-contrast T1-weighted sagittal imaging shows the normal appearance of the posterior pituitary bright spot. (**f**) Delayed post-contrast T1-weighted sagittal imaging shows homogeneous enhancement of the pituitary and infundibulum

Table 4.1 Standard pituitary MRI protocol and individual pulse sequence utility

Sequence	Utility
Sagittal T1	Intrinsic T1 hyperintensity of the normal neurohypophysis. Informs on signal characteristics of a lesion, intrinsic T1 hyperintensity seen in proteinaceous fluid, blood degradation products, and fat
Coronal T1	Informs on signal characteristics of a lesion, intrinsic T1 hyperintensity seen in proteinaceous fluid, blood degradation products, and fat
Coronal T2 with fat suppression	Informs on the consistency and cystic nature of a lesion. Helpful to evaluate cavernous sinuses. Helpful to evaluate the optic apparatus
Coronal diffusion-weighted imaging	Can inform on pyogenic infection/abscess
Dynamic post-contrast T1	Rapid and early contrast enhancement of the normal gland can be useful to differentiate a microadenoma, where more delayed enhancement ("hypoenhancement") is observed. Can be difficult to interpret in the post-operative setting
Sagittal T1 post-contrast with fat suppression	Delineates enhancing lesions including their invasion of adjacent structures. Macroadenomas and other larger lesions well seen
Coronal T1 post-contrast with fat suppression	Delineates enhancing lesions including their invasion of adjacent structures. Macroadenomas and other larger lesions well seen

scanners, with modern 3 T scanners permitting improved imaging by increased signal-to-noise ratio and reduced acquisition times.

The adenohypophysis is normally isointense to brain on T1- and T2-weighted images. The neurohypophysis is normally intrinsically T1 hyperintense. It should be noted that the expected enhancement pattern of the pituitary follows its blood supply, and consequentially enhancement begins with the infundibulum, followed by the central pituitary and lastly the lateral aspects of the pituitary. Understanding this is crucial to preventing misinterpretation of the normal enhancement pattern (Fig. 4.1c) as a lateral pituitary hypoenhancing lesion.

Angiography either by CTA or MRA can be of further utility to identify relationship of the circle of Willis vasculature to the lesion and inform on operative approach.

Newer techniques to image the pituitary gland are described in a subsequent section, "Advances in Imaging of the Pituitary Gland."

Imaging of Tumors in the Gland

Microadenoma (Fig. 4.2)

Contrast enhanced MRI is the mainstay for imaging diagnosis of a pituitary microadenoma. Highlighting the importance of appropriate imaging technique, a dedicated pituitary protocol will have several key differences compared to a standard

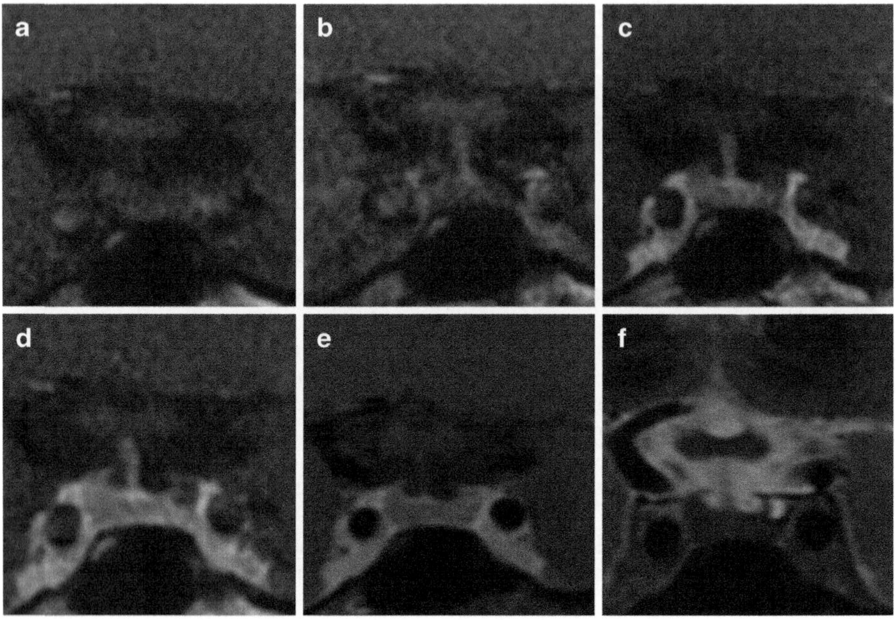

Fig. 4.2 MRI appearance of a pituitary microadenoma. (**a–d**) Dynamic post-contrast T1-weighted coronal imaging shows progressive enhancement of the pituitary with relative hypoenhancement of a small nodule in the left aspect of the pituitary, characteristic of a pituitary adenoma. (**e**) There is loss of visualization of the left-sided pituitary adenoma on delayed post-contrast T1-weighted coronal imaging. (**f**) T2-weighted coronal imaging shows associated T2 hyperintense signal

brain protocol that are imperative to making the diagnosis of a pituitary microadenoma, including thin slices, a small field of view, and dynamic post-contrast imaging. The classic imaging appearance of pituitary microadenomas will demonstrate a lesion that is hypoenhancing relative to the native pituitary gland on early post-contrast imaging but is isointense on delayed imaging. Dynamic T1-weighted post-contrast images improve the sensitivity of microadenoma detection but can yield false-positive findings. The T2 signal of pituitary microadenomas is quite variable; however, they can appear as T2 hyperintense relative to the pituitary. The small size of microadenomas results in difficulty using this sequence to define whether a tumor is densely or sparsely granulated.

In addition to the post-contrast findings, pituitary microadenomas can have subtle secondary signs from their mass effect. The superior boarder of the pituitary should be concave downward in all patients outside of women of childbearing age. A convex upward boarder should suggest that the pituitary is abnormally enlarged, possibly from an intrinsic pituitary mass such as an adenoma. Additionally, the normal infundibulum should be midline on coronal imaging. Therefore, a mass lesion such as a pituitary adenoma could deviate the infundibulum to the contralateral side.

Macroadenoma (Fig. 4.3)

As opposed to pituitary microadenomas, macroadenomas are more consistent in their enhancement pattern, often demonstrating heterogenous enhancement. The first challenge of interpreting the MR images in these cases is to determine if the mass lesion is originating from within the sella or, conversely, the suprasellar region with inferior extension into the sella. In this case, utilizing the coronal T2-weighted sequence to identify superior of inferior displacement of the diaphragma sellae can be helpful. A true sellar-based lesion will see upward tenting of the diaphragma sellae, which will appear as a thin hypointense line on coronal T2-weighted imaging (Fig. 4.3c). Additionally, MRI can be useful in assessing for hemorrhage and cystic degeneration, best appreciated on pre-contrast T1- and T2-weighted sequences, respectively.

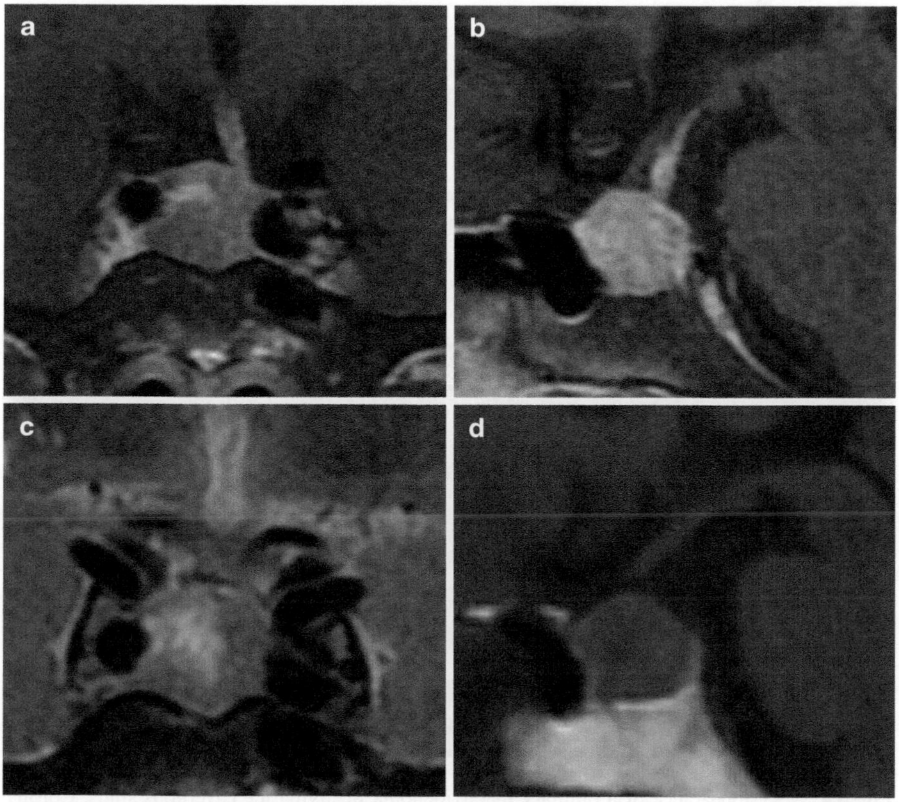

Fig. 4.3 MRI appearance of a pituitary macroadenoma. (**a, b**) Coronal and sagittal post-contrast T1-weighted imaging shows the characteristic heterogenous enhancement of a pituitary macroadenoma. The right-sided lesion causes leftward deviation of the pituitary infundibulum. (**c**) T2-weighted coronal imaging shows heterogeneously hyperintense signal in the mass. (**d**) Pre-contrast T1-weighted sagittal imaging shows loss of the normal posterior pituitary bright spot

In the setting of acromegaly, somatotropinomas with low T2 signal intensity are more likely to represent a densely granulated tumor and to respond to somatostatin analogs. Sparsely granulated tumors tend to be more T2 hyperintense and present with suprasellar and/or cavernous sinus invasion [1].

In addition to identifying the presence of a lesion, MR imaging of pituitary macroadenomas is crucial in determining the extent of local invasion. Laterally, sellar lesions can invade into the cavernous sinuses (Fig. 4.4). Several imaging criteria have been described to determine presence and degree of cavernous sinus invasion by macroadenoma; however, these are not universally accepted and may not reliably determine invasion. Of these imaging criteria, the Knosp classification (grades 0–4) is the most commonly used with a meta-analysis showing Knosp 3–4 as the best objective indicator of cavernous sinus invasion [2]. Superiorly, lesions can have suprasellar extension and exert mass effect on the optic chiasm or prechiasmatic optic nerves. Inferiorly and less commonly, pituitary adenomas can involve the sphenoid sinuses. Rarely do pituitary macroadenomas extend posteriorly into the prepontine cistern.

Mimics (Fig. 4.5)

While the imaging differential for sellar/suprasellar lesions is impressively extensive, one of the most common etiologies is a meningioma. This should be differentiated from a pituitary adenoma based on its epicenter outside of the sella, dural tail,

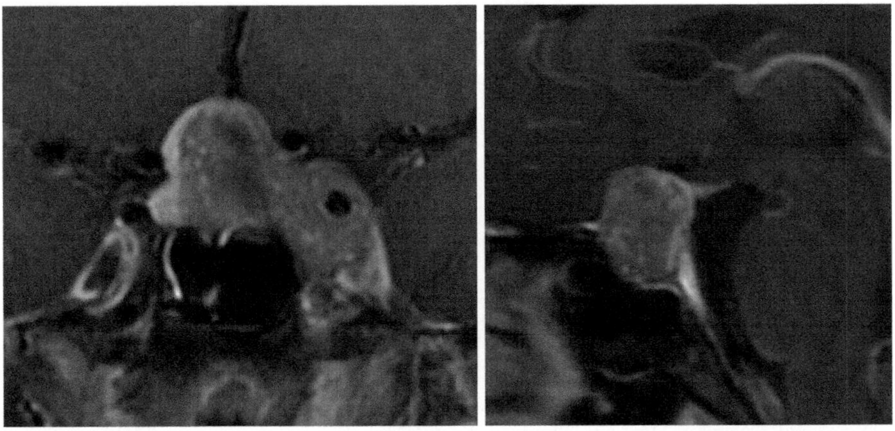

Fig. 4.4 MRI appearance of a pituitary macroadenoma involving the cavernous sinus. Coronal (left) and sagittal (right) T1-weighted post-contrast images show a large pituitary mass with heterogenous enhancement. There is both suprasellar extension and invasion into the left cavernous sinus that encases the left cavernous internal carotid artery, but does not narrow it

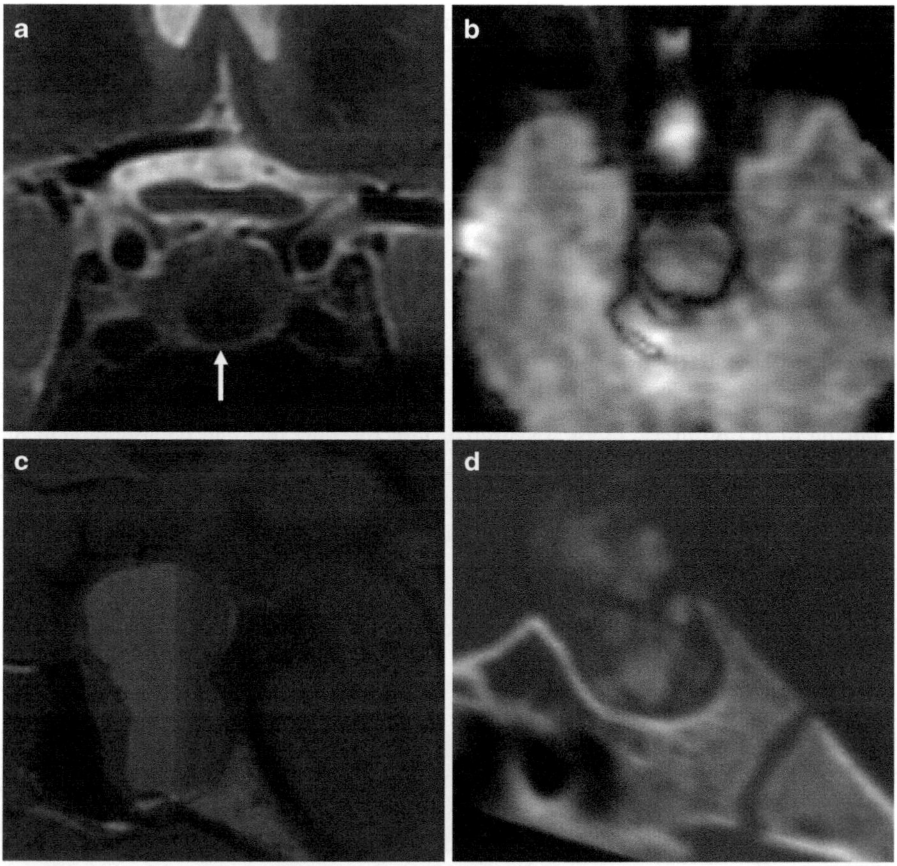

Fig. 4.5 Characteristic imaging findings of four different sellar lesions. (**a**) T2-weighted coronal imaging shows a T2 hypointense nodule (arrow), characteristic of a Rathke cleft cyst. (**b**) Axial diffuse weighted imaging shows restricted diffusion in a sellar mass, characteristic of a pituitary abscess. (**c**) Non-contrast T1-weighted sagittal image shows a blood fluid level in a large pituitary mass, seen in the setting of pituitary apoplexy. (**d**) Non-contrast sagittal CT shows a large calcified sellar mass, characteristic of an adamantinomatous craniopharyngioma. Note the non-fused spheno-occipital synchondrosis that does not fuse until adolescence

and homogeneous enhancement. If perfusion imaging is available, elevated perfusion would suggest a meningioma rather than a pituitary adenoma [3].

Of the many masses that can originate from within the sella, a common differential diagnosis includes a cystic adenoma versus a Rathke cleft cyst (RCC). While not always present, a pathognomonic finding of a RCC is a T2 hypointense nodule within the cyst representing an intracystic nodule of cellular debris [4].

Autoimmune hypophysitis, including both lymphocytic and granulomatous, can have an overlapping imaging appearance as a solidly enhancing adenoma. Extensive inflammatory changes including diffuse involvement of the pituitary, infundibular thickening, or adjacent dural inflammation would favor hypophysitis over an adenoma [5].

While diffusion-weighted imaging does not have significant utility in the identification of a pituitary adenoma, prominent restricted diffusion in the pituitary should raise concern for a pituitary abscess. On the post-contrast imaging, the lesion should have corresponding peripheral enhancement that would clearly distinguish it from an adenoma [6].

Systemic Findings of Acromegaly

Outside of the pituitary, there are multisystem findings that can be appreciated on standard radiographs (Fig. 4.6). Cranially, there can be marked calvarial thickening with frontal bossing, prognathism, enlarged frontal sinuses, and an enlarged sella turcica. In the spine, the increased risk of vertebral body fractures, particularly in the thoracic spine, provides evidence that spinal imaging should be included in routine follow-up for patients with acromegaly. In the extremities, findings can consistent of advanced degenerative joint disease, a spade appearance of the hypertrophied tufts, and increased heal pad thickness.

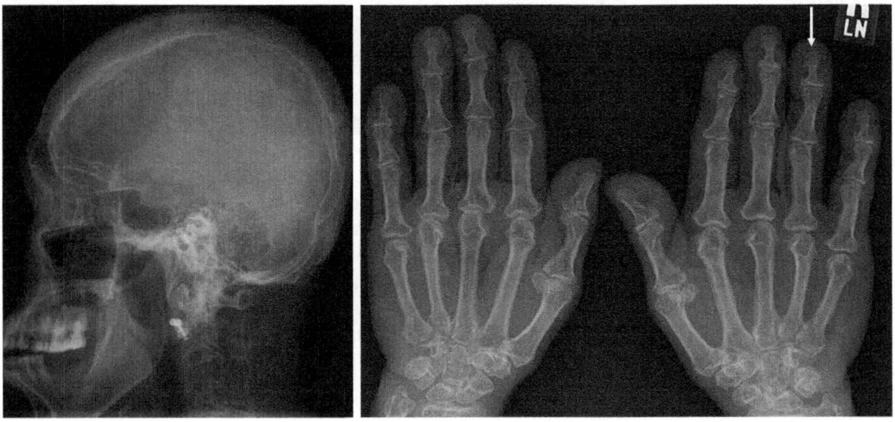

Fig. 4.6 Characteristic radiographic findings of acromegaly. Lateral skull radiograph shows an enlarged and thickened calvarium, frontal bossing, enlarged sella turcica, and enlarged mandible with prognathism. Hand radiograph shows hypertrophy of the phalangeal tufts with the characteristic "spade appearance" (arrow)

Advances in Imaging of the Pituitary Gland

While standard-of-care MRI of the pituitary gland is obtained using 2D pulse sequences, 3D gradient echo and fast spin echo sequences can play an important role in evaluating sellar lesions. 3D sequences are desirable as they enable superior soft tissue contrast, improved spatial resolution, and decrease partial volume effects compared to conventional 2D sequences. The main drawbacks of 3D sequences are longer scan times, particularly for fast spin echo sequences, and susceptibility artifact and high signal intensity from blood flow, commonly seen in gradient echo sequences. These are limiting factors in terms of potential patient motion and resultant artifact near the sphenoid sinus and cavernous internal carotid. Parallel imaging and compressed sensing are methods for accelerating MRI acquisition by acquiring less data, which can be used to mitigate some of these drawbacks. For the pituitary gland, these techniques have yielded improvements in overall image quality and a reduction in artifacts while maintaining anatomic and lesion conspicuity [7]. Studies have shown higher sensitivity for detection of microadenomas using 3D T1 and T2 post-contrast imaging compared with conventional 2D and dynamic imaging [8–10]. As MRI acceleration becomes more widely available, we will see increased adoption of 3D sequences in imaging of the pituitary gland.

Intraoperative MRI (iMRI) is an additional technique that can be used in the detection of unexpected residual tumor. The addition of image guidance during transsphenoidal tumor resection adds time and requires an iMRI that is readily accessible from the operating room. However, this can increase the likelihood of achieving gross total resection by up to 40%, benefitting patients with higher rates of disease-free survival and lower rates of radiation therapy [11]. Hardware and procedural technique can vary by site, with results favoring high volume centers with higher strength magnets.

Beyond 3 T, ultrahigh-field MRI using 7 T scanners is more possible than before due to clinically approved offerings from major MRI scanner manufacturers. MRI at 7 T permits higher signal-to-noise ratio, spatial resolution, and reduction in volume averaging to allow for better lesion detection and characterization. Ultrahigh-field MRI surpasses 3 T MRI for detection and delineation of pituitary microadenomas and correlates better with intraoperative findings [12]. The signal intensity and contrast resolution advantage conferred by 7 T MRI may provide valuable preoperative information regarding pituitary tumor consistency and therefore inform on surgical findings and physiology [13]. A potential application for ultrahigh-field MRI at 7 T could be its use in patients with hormone over-secretion and no discernable lesion using conventional 1.5 or 3 T MRI.

With advances in computational power, there has been a rapid increase in the use of artificial intelligence in medical imaging to enhance image quality. Artificial intelligence-based approaches use either raw MRI data or the images themselves to improve signal-to-noise ratios and provide sharper appearing images with scan time reductions [14]. This type of image enhancement is of particular interest in regions where smaller field of view may limit image appearance such as the sellar region. Studies have shown artificial intelligence enhanced images to provided higher sensitivity for the detection of pituitary adenoma and better delineation of normal pituitary anatomy compared to routine MRI [15, 16].

Beyond image enhancement, artificial intelligence is being applied to time-consuming tasks such as lesion segmentation and identification of surgically relevant anatomy. For example, automated adenoma delineation and cavernous sinus invasion have been performed using a deep learning model with high accuracy [17]. Further, artificial intelligence is driving a new field of imaging science, radiomics. Radiomics applies mathematical analyses to imaging based on the assumption that these images contain information of disease-specific processes that are imperceptible to the human eye [18]. Radiomic analysis of adenomas has been used to classify adenoma subtypes [19, 20] as well as predict tumor consistency [21], cavernous sinus invasion [22], and recurrence [23]. The coming years will see increasing use of artificial intelligence-based image analysis to aid in presurgical planning, prognostication, and postsurgical management.

Molecular imaging with positron emission tomography (PET) can provide complimentary functional information to MRI particularly in the postsurgical setting. The most used PET radiotracer, fluorodeoxyglucose – a glucose analog – has limited utility in pituitary imaging due to high background uptake in the normal brain and lack of specificity for adenoma [24]. Somatotropinomas avidly take up carbon-11 methionine, an amino acid radiotracer, which can be used to distinguish metabolically active residual or recurrent tumor from granulation tissue [25]. Practically, it is important to note that therapies, such as somatostatin analogues and dopamine agonists, can diminish PET radiotracer uptake [24]. PET imaging for acromegaly has the potential for greater adoption with the increased deployment of hybrid PET-MRI scanners.

References

1. Shih RY, Schroeder JW, Koeller KK. Primary tumors of the pituitary gland: radiologic-pathologic correlation. Radiographics. 2021;41(7):2029–46.
2. Dhandapani S, Singh H, Negm HM, Cohen S, Anand VK, Schwartz TH. Cavernous sinus invasion in pituitary adenomas: systematic review and pooled data meta-analysis of radiologic criteria and comparison of endoscopic and microscopic surgery. World Neurosurg. 2016;96:36–46.
3. Parikh D, Afshari FT, Sherlala K, Ahmed S, Shad A. Utility of arterial spin labeling magnetic resonance imaging in differentiating sellar region meningiomas from pituitary adenomas. World Neurosurg. 2020;142:e407–e12.
4. Park M, Lee SK, Choi J, Kim SH, Kim SH, Shin NY, et al. Differentiation between cystic pituitary adenomas and Rathke cleft cysts: a diagnostic model using MRI. AJNR Am J Neuroradiol. 2015;36(10):1866–73.
5. Imber BS, Lee HS, Kunwar S, Blevins LS, Aghi MK. Hypophysitis: a single-center case series. Pituitary. 2015;18(5):630–41.
6. Wang Z, Gao L, Zhou X, Guo X, Wang Q, Lian W, et al. Magnetic resonance imaging characteristics of pituitary abscess: a review of 51 cases. World Neurosurg. 2018;114:e900–e12.

7. Sartoretti T, Sartoretti E, Wyss M, Schwenk Á, van Smoorenburg L, Eichenberger B, et al. Compressed SENSE accelerated 3D T1w black blood turbo spin echo versus 2D T1w turbo spin echo sequence in pituitary magnetic resonance imaging. Eur J Radiol. 2019;120:108667.
8. Grober Y, Grober H, Wintermark M, Jane JA, Oldfield EH. Comparison of MRI techniques for detecting microadenomas in Cushing's disease. J Neurosurg. 2018;128(4):1051–7.
9. Wu Y, Cai Y, Rui W, Tang Y, Yang Z, He M, et al. Contrast-enhanced 3D-T2-weighted SPACE sequence for MRI detection and localization of adrenocorticotropin (ACTH)-secreting pituitary microadenomas. Clin Endocrinol. 2022;96(4):578–88.
10. Lonser RR, Kindzelski BA, Mehta GU, Jane JA Jr, Oldfield EH. Acromegaly without imaging evidence of pituitary adenoma. J Clin Endocrinol Metabol. 2010;95(9):4192–6.
11. Jones PS, Swearingen B. Intraoperative MRI for pituitary adenomas. Neurosurg Clin. 2019;30(4):413–20.
12. Eisenhut F, Schlaffer S-M, Hock S, Heynold E, Kremenevski N, Bluemcke I, et al. Ultra-high-field 7 T magnetic resonance imaging including dynamic and static contrast-enhanced T1-weighted imaging improves detection of secreting pituitary microadenomas. Investig Radiol. 2022;57(9):567–74. https://doi.org/10.1097/RLI.0000000000000872.
13. Yao A, Rutland JW, Verma G, Banihashemi A, Padormo F, Tsankova NM, et al. Pituitary adenoma consistency: direct correlation of ultrahigh field 7T MRI with histopathological analysis. Eur J Radiol. 2020;126:108931.
14. Knoll F, Hammernik K, Zhang C, Moeller S, Pock T, Sodickson DK, et al. Deep-learning methods for parallel magnetic resonance imaging reconstruction: a survey of the current approaches, trends, and issues. IEEE Signal Process Mag. 2020;37(1):128–40.
15. Lee DH, Park JE, Nam YK, Lee J, Kim S, Kim Y-H, et al. Deep learning-based thin-section MRI reconstruction improves tumour detection and delineation in pre- and post-treatment pituitary adenoma. Sci Rep. 2021;11(1):21302.
16. Kim M, Kim HS, Kim HJ, Park JE, Park SY, Kim Y-H, et al. Thin-slice pituitary MRI with deep learning–based reconstruction: diagnostic performance in a postoperative setting. Radiology. 2021;298(1):114–22.
17. Wang H, Zhang W, Li S, Fan Y, Feng M, Wang R. Development and evaluation of deep learning-based automated segmentation of pituitary adenoma in clinical task. J Clin Endocrinol Metabol. 2021;106(9):2535–46.
18. van Timmeren JE, Cester D, Tanadini-Lang S, Alkadhi H, Baessler B. Radiomics in medical imaging—"how-to" guide and critical reflection. Insights Imaging. 2020;11(1):91.
19. Peng A, Dai H, Duan H, Chen Y, Huang J, Zhou L, et al. A machine learning model to precisely immunohistochemically classify pituitary adenoma subtypes with radiomics based on preoperative magnetic resonance imaging. Eur J Radiol. 2020;125:108892.
20. Zhang S, Song G, Zang Y, Jia J, Wang C, Li C, et al. Non-invasive radiomics approach potentially predicts non-functioning pituitary adenomas subtypes before surgery. Eur Radiol. 2018;28(9):3692–701.
21. Cuocolo R, Ugga L, Solari D, Corvino S, D'Amico A, Russo D, et al. Prediction of pituitary adenoma surgical consistency: radiomic data mining and machine learning on T2-weighted MRI. Neuroradiology. 2020;62(12):1649–56.
22. Niu J, Zhang S, Ma S, Diao J, Zhou W, Tian J, et al. Preoperative prediction of cavernous sinus invasion by pituitary adenomas using a radiomics method based on magnetic resonance images. Eur Radiol. 2019;29(3):1625–34.
23. Zhang Y, Ko C-C, Chen J-H, Chang K-T, Chen T-Y, Lim S-W, et al. Radiomics approach for prediction of recurrence in non-functioning pituitary macroadenomas. Front Oncol. 2020;10:590083.
24. Bashari WA, Senanayake R, Fernández-Pombo A, Gillett D, Koulouri O, Powlson AS, et al. Modern imaging of pituitary adenomas. Best Pract Res Clin Endocrinol Metab. 2019;33(2):101278.
25. Rodriguez-Barcelo S, Gutierrez-Cardo A, Dominguez-Paez M, Medina-Imbroda J, Romero-Moreno L, Arraez-Sanchez M. Clinical usefulness of coregistered 11C-methionine positron emission tomography/3-T magnetic resonance imaging at the follow-up of acromegaly. World Neurosurg. 2014;82(3):468–73.

Chapter 5
The Clinical Presentation of Acromegaly

Lisa B. Nachtigall and Francisco J. Guarda

Background and Historical Perspective

Historical reports of patients suffering from acral enlargement date to as far as Ancient Egypt and even the Bible [1]. Throughout history, giants have been a matter of amazement among the public. Goliath's defeat by David in Judaic and Christian scriptures represents the most famous one to date. This exemplifies one of the first descriptions of a visual field defect present in acromegaly, as Goliath was killed after receiving an unseen strike with pebbles from his side by a much smaller opponent [1]. In Ancient Egypt, the Pharaoh Akenaten was believed to present with acromegalic features and hypogonadism, although scientists are conflicted regarding the actual diagnosis [1]. The study of historical cohorts of "giants" has led to important discoveries even in recent years. Genetic studies performed in the skeleton of the Irish giant, Charles Byrne, located in the Hunterian Museum in London, aided in determining the presence of aryl hydrocarbon receptor-interacting protein gene (AIP) and its relationship with the disease [2].

Several scientists, including Johanes Wier, Nicolas Saucerotte, Jean-Louis-Marc Alibert, Andre Verga, among many others, described cases of patients with gigantism, macroglossia, bone deformities, and dermatological and other clinical manifestations consistent with the diagnosis of acromegaly [2]. It was not until 1886

L. B. Nachtigall (✉)
Division of Endocrinology, Department of Medicine, The Neuroendocrine and Pituitary Tumor Clinical Center Massachusetts General Hospital/Harvard Medical School, Boston, MA, USA
e-mail: lnachtigall@partners.org

F. J. Guarda
Endocrinology Department, School of Medicine, Pontificia Universidad Católica de Chile, Santiago, Chile

Pituitary Tumor Program, Red de Salud UC-CHRISTUS, Santiago, Chile
e-mail: fjguarda@uc.cl

L. S. Blevins Jr., M. K. Aghi (eds.), *Acromegaly*, Contemporary Endocrinology,
https://doi.org/10.1007/978-3-031-16258-9_5

when Pierre Marie, a French neurologist trained by Charcot, introduced the term "acromegaly" in scientific literature with his classic report titled "Sur deux cas d'acromégalie; hypertrophie singulière non congénitale des extrémités supérieures, inférieures et céphalique" [3]. Although Pierre Marie did not initially associate the pituitary with the clinical features in acromegaly, Oscar Minkowski was the first to note this link in 1887, and, in 1892, Roberto Massalongo correlated features of acromegaly with a specific granulation pattern in pituitary specimens [2].

In popular culture, many individuals with acromegaly have participated in music, film, and TV, such as the American actor Richard Kiel who played a role in the James Bond saga. In television, Lurch, the butler from "the Addams Family," a 1960s series, was performed by Ted Cassidy, an actor with the diagnosis of acromegaly, who stood at 6 foot 9 inches and with his deep voice was also the vocalist for the Hulk on the television series, "the Incredible Hulk." Additionally, it is believed that Sergei Rachmaninov, a Russian musician, may have presented acromegaly due to coarse features and "big hands." In sports, the wrestler and actor Andre "the giant" Rousimoff and Gheorghe Muresan, a NBA basketball player, were known to have features of acromegaly [4].

Signs and Symptoms Prompting Diagnosis

A delay of 7–10 years between the time of initial symptoms and the diagnosis of acromegaly is reported [5]. Even though, in the last 2 decades, this has decreased, a diagnostic delay of 2.5–5.3 years persists [6–10]. This leads to several questions to consider regarding the diagnosis and presentation of acromegaly:

1. Why is there a prolonged delay in the diagnosis of acromegaly, given the typical uniform and recognizable clinical features of this disease?
2. What are the signs, symptoms, and/or reasons that ultimately lead to the diagnosis?
3. What signs and symptoms are present at the time of diagnosis of acromegaly?

Why Is There a Prolonged Delay in Diagnosis of Acromegaly, Given the Classic and Recognizable Clinical Features of this Disease?

Given that typical physical features of the disease are fairly common and plainly seen upon inspection of the face, hands, and feet [6, 7, 10], it may seem surprising that acromegaly remains undiagnosed for many years after it first occurs. There are many possible explanations for this:

1. The classical features that are easy to recognize are later manifestations of the disease. However, neither acral changes or facial changes appear to be later man-

ifestations of disease and have been reported to occur many years before the disease is recognized [11].
2. The disease is rare [7] so that general clinicians may not consider it.
3. The symptoms and signs change slowly over time [5, 6] so that the patient and the clinician do not notice the ongoing subtle changes.
4. The constellation of comorbidities that occur with growth hormone (GH) excess include many common medical problems such as hypertension, diabetes, cardiac disease, and sleep apnea [5, 6, 8–10], each of which in itself is not specific to acromegaly.
5. Finally, it is difficult to get perfectly accurate information on the time of the first sign or symptom of the disease, which occurred many years before, as it relies on patient's memory and self-reporting and thus recall bias which may be unreliable.
6. Photo review of facial changes may be a more accurate method to date the initial disease onset, but the use of photo analysis has rarely been reported [12]. Interestingly, the delay has been reportedly longer for women than men [8, 10], but it is unclear if this reflects the natural history of the disease, the difference in reporting between sexes, and/or the practioners' differences in management of women compared to men.

What Are the Signs, Symptoms, and/or Reasons That Ultimately Lead to the Diagnosis?

Facial features that changed were often reported by the patient or noticed incidentally as the initial sign leading to diagnosis in 15–22% [6, 8, 9], and acral enlargement was the other major sign leading to in diagnosis in 13–24% [6, 8, 9]. Other presenting signs included headache (8–18%) [8, 9] and sleep apnea in <2.0% [6, 8, 9]. In 8–13% of female patients, menstrual disturbances were among the symptoms prompting the diagnosis of acromegaly [5, 8, 9]. The type of physician or medical professional who made the diagnosis is shown in Table 5.1.

Table 5.1 Types of professionals who make the diagnosis of acromegaly

Type of professional	Nachtigall et al. (2008) ($N = 100$) [9]	Petrossians et al. (2017) ($N = 3173$) [8]
Endocrinologist	13	45
Primary care physician	44	31
Emergency room staff	10	–
Patient (self-referred)	7	2
Neurologist	6	3
Dentist	3	1
Ophthalmologist	3	2
Others	14	16

What Signs and Symptoms Are Present at the Time of Diagnosis of Acromegaly?

Acromegaly is typically diagnosed in the fifth decade [5, 6, 8, 9, 13, 14], affecting a relatively even proportion of men and women, although a slight female predominance has been reported in several cohorts [8–10, 13]. Once diagnosed, most patients exhibit changes in their facial features [6, 10, 11, 15] compared to before the onset of GH excess. This includes coarsening of features, enlargement of the brow, thickening of the nasal bridge, growth of the jaw, new spaces between the teeth, malocclusion of the jaw due to prognathism, and enlargement of the tongue [16] (Fig. 5.1; Table 5.2). Some of these changes can cause difficulty chewing and speaking. The vast majority of patients will also have acral enlargement at the time of diagnosis [6, 10, 11, 14, 15]. The hands will typically appear swollen and doughlike (Fig. 5.2), and many will report an increase in hat size, foot size, or ring size. Many patients will report having to resize their rings, sometimes more than once. Interestingly, these features of acral and/or facial changes are present in most patients but only serve as the sign that prompts the diagnosis in approximately 20% of patients [8]. However,

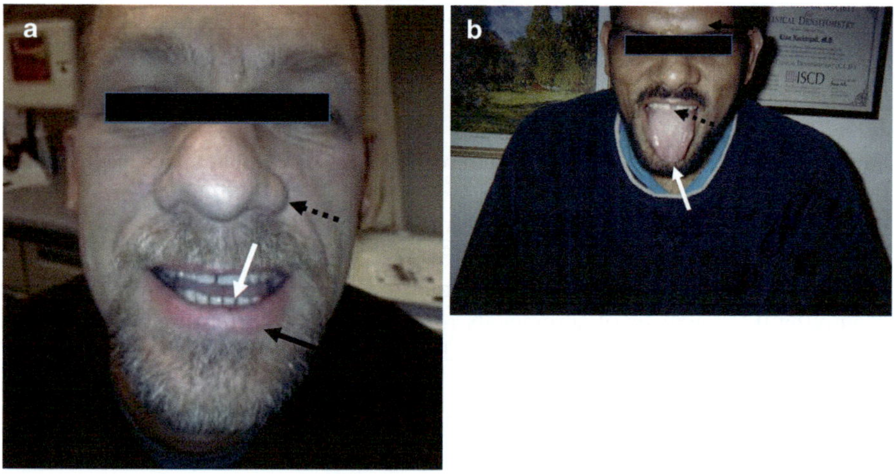

Fig. 5.1 Facial features of acromegaly at diagnosis. Figures (**a**, **b**) are photographs of patients with acromegaly at the time of diagnosis, who granted permission to share the image. (**a**) Dashed arrow indicates widened, enlarged nose. White arrow indicates space between lower teeth. Black arrow indicates thickening of lower lip. (**b**) White arrow indicates macroglossia. Dashed arrow indicates space between upper teeth. Black arrow indicates thickening. Photos from Lisa Nachtigall MD

Table 5.2 Clinical manifestations associated with acromegaly

Organ system	Clinical manifestations
Skin and soft tissue	Skin thickening and skin tags
	Hyperhidrosis
	Cutis verticis gyrata (increased skin folds in scalp)
	Peripheral edema
	Macroglossia
	Hypertrichosis
	Gingival hyperplasia
	Coarse features
Bone and cartilage	Acral enlargement
	Increased fracture risk
	Kyphoscoliosis
	Hypercalcemia and hyperphosphatemia
	Elevated 1,25-dihydroxyvitamin D
	Hypercalciuria
	Degenerative joint disease (acromegalic arthropathy)
	Maxillary and jaw overgrowth (prognathism) and increased space between teeth
Central and peripheral nervous system	Visual loss
	Carpal tunnel syndrome
	Increased risk factors for cerebrovascular disease
	Headache
Respiratory	Sleep apnea
	Respiratory insufficiency
Cardiovascular	Increased risk factors for ischemic heart disease
	Valvular disease (mitral and aortic regurgitation)
	Left ventricular hypertrophy/diastolic dysfunction
	Arterial hypertension
Gastrointestinal	Colon polyps and colon cancer
	Fatty liver disease
Female gonadal function	Menstrual irregularities
	Hyperandrogenism (PCOS-like)
	Infertility
	Hypogonadism
Male gonadal function	Infertility
	Hypogonadism and sexual dysfunction
Metabolic	Diabetes mellitus
	Glucose intolerance and insulin resistance
	Hyperlipidemia (high triglycerides and low HDL cholesterol)
Endocrine	Thyroid nodules
	Goiter
	Hyperthyroidism (co-secretion of TSH or toxic multinodular goiter)
	Hyperprolactinemia
	Hypopituitarism

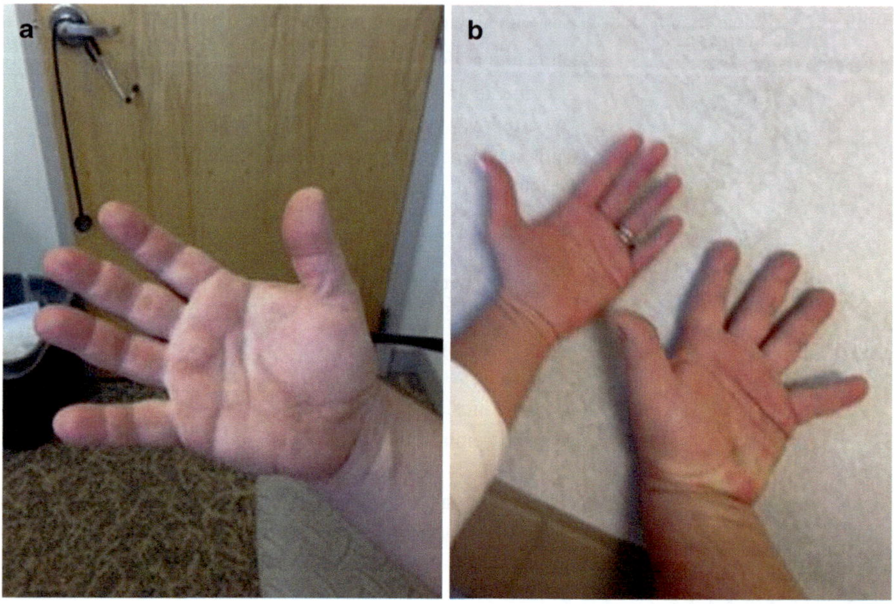

Fig. 5.2 Acral enlargement. (**a**) Hand of patient with acromegaly at time of diagnosis. (**b**) Hand of the patient compared to an unaffected person's hand

these features are typically recognized and are present once the diagnosis has been made (Table 5.3).

While hypertension, diabetes, and sleep apnea are common in the general population, in acromegaly these may cluster. When several of these comorbidities are present along with other manifestations of acromegaly and/or other complications, such as carpal tunnel, colon polyps, and skeletal abnormalities (such as arthropathy and kyphoscoliosis), acromegaly should be considered [12]. Hyperhidrosis is another highly prevalent feature at baseline [5, 6, 10, 11, 14, 15]. Menstrual disorders in women and male hypogonadism may also be present at baseline [1, 2, 6, 7, 10] (Table 5.3). The diagnosis of sleep apnea is underreported if sleep tests are not done. For example, 69% of patients tested with sleep tests vs. 26% of all patients with acromegaly had sleep apnea at baseline [8], and this explains the very low rate in studies, in which sleep tests were not routinely performed or results were not available at diagnosis [9]. Cardiac effects of excess GH and IGF-1 will commonly cause myocardial hypertrophy and less frequently severe ischemia and myocardial infarction [5, 8].

Table 5.3 Prevalence of clinical features of acromegaly at diagnosis

Author (recruitment years)	Site *N* (% female)	Facial coarsening	Acral enlargement	Hyperhidrosis	Gonadal dysfunction	HA	HTN	DM	Cardiac disease	SA
Nabarro 1966–1986 [5]	England 256 (48%)	100% acral and/or facial changes		50%	44% amenorrhea 36% male sexual dysfunction	37%	31%	19%	11% severe CAD	NA
Jadresic et al. Before 1982 [14]	USA 155 (51%)	NA	100%	65%	NA	55%	32%	27%	34% "cardiac problems"	NA
Reid et al. 1981–2006 [6]	USA 324 (49%)[a]	84%	86%	55%	33%	47%	37%	16%	NA	24%
Nachtigall et al. 1985–2005 [9]	USA 100 (55%)	NA	NA	NA	NA	NA	25%	15%	5% CAD	1%
Petrossians et al. 1990–2010 [8]	Europe 3173 (54%)	NA	NA	NA	NA	NA	29%	28%	15.5% hypertrophy, 3.5% ischemia, 1.6% HF	26% (69% among tested)
Guo et al. 1996–2019 [10]	China 473 (59%)	90%	92%	55%	23% (66% women with menstrual dysfunction)	57%	NA	NA	NA	25%
Dutta et al. 2000–2014 [26]	India 271 (51%)	14%	89%	NA	20% amenorrhea12% erectile dysfunction or loss of libido	49%	18%	16%	4% cardiac dysfunction	10%
Al Dhamani et al. 2000–2018 [27]	United Arab Emirates 75 (40%)	82%	80%	31%	NA	82%	36%	45%	NA	NA

(continued)

Table 5.3 (continued)

Author (recruitment years)	Site *N* (% female)	Facial coarsening	Acral enlargement	Hyperhidrosis	Gonadal dysfunction	HA	HTN	DM	Cardiac disease	SA
Lawrence et al. 2003–2018 [28]	USA136 (54%)	90% (“musculoskeletal manifestations”)		NA	45% hypogonadism	NA	57%	44%	17% CAD or HF or CM	48%
Kamseh et al.[b] 2014–2016 [29]	Iran 85 (45%)	NA	81%	NA	68% hypogonadal symptoms	64%	NA	NA	NA	NA
Total		14–100%	80–100%	31–65%	Variable	37–82%	18–37%	15–45%	Variable definitions	1–48%

HA headache, *HTN* hypertension, *DM* diabetes mellitus, *SA* sleep apnea, *NA* not available, *HF* heart failure, *CAD* coronary artery disease, *CM* cardiomyopathy

[a]In this study, patients were divided into an early group ($n = 108$, 56% female) and a late group ($n = 216$, 45% female). The percentages shown across this row are calculated from the original data by a weighted average

[b]Study included all types of pituitary tumors, but data was extracted from patients with acromegaly

Severity of the Disease

The slow-onset and gradual changes in physical features may make the diagnosis challenging in many cases. Most patients do not notice these subtle variations in their physical appearance through time and may be diagnosed when the disease is already established and systemic complications are evident and severe [5, 6, 9]. Several studies have reported an increased risk of neoplasms among patients with acromegaly and an excess mortality due to cancer and cardiovascular and respiratory diseases [8, 17, 18]. Nevertheless, some recent studies have shown a significant reduction in this excess mortality due to improvement in therapies and increased rate of disease control [18, 19]. Although acromegaly is associated with increased risk factors for cardiovascular and cerebrovascular disease, such as hypertension, dyslipidemia, and diabetes mellitus, recent studies have shown a lower incidence of stroke or myocardial infarction than prior reports [12, 18]. Signs and symptoms of heart disease should be evaluated according to risk stratification but may not be present explicitly by the time of diagnosis [18]. The delay in diagnosis and treatment may lead to more severe manifestations and, therefore, increased risk of complications and mortality. Due to the myriad of effects of the GH/IGF-1 axis, the clinical manifestations involve almost all systems. Table 5.2 shows a summary of the most prominent features [18, 20–22].

Diseases or Conditions with Clinical Overlap That May Mimic Acromegaly

In rare cases, clinical manifestations suggestive of acromegaly may be mimicked by other conditions. Several genetic, metabolic, endocrine, and neoplastic diseases have been associated with an acromegaly-like phenotype, which has been termed as "pseudoacromegaly" or "acromegaloidism" [23]. In these cases, biochemical testing excludes excess GH and IGF-1. Some drugs have also been associated with the phenotype [23]. The diagnosis of pseudoacromegaly is difficult, given that the differential diagnosis is extensive and there are no widely available workup panels.

Although rare, there are some common conditions that can produce the phenotype. Severe primary hypothyroidism can be associated with signs and symptoms suggestive of acromegaly, especially macroglossia [23, 24]. Also, non-islet cell tumor-induced hypoglycemia, which is associated with excess IGF-2, can generate features of acromegaly due to activation of the IGF-1 receptor. Severe hyperinsulinism and insulin resistance, usually explained by genetic variants that increase the mitogenic pathways of insulin signaling, can be also associated with clinical features that may mimic GH excess [23, 25]. Among the more infrequent conditions associated with the disease, pachydermoperiostosis or primary hypertrophic osteoarthropathy is a genetic disease characterized by skin thickening, digital clubbing, arthralgias, and coarse facial features caused by a defect in prostaglandin E2 metabolism [23].

Interestingly, the use of minoxidil, a vasodilator usually prescribed for hair loss, may also generate a phenotype masquerading as acromegaly. The pathophysiological mechanism is a phenocopy of Cantú syndrome, which is associated with a persistent activation of an ATP-sensitive potassium channel or a gain-of-function mutation of *ABCC9*. Phenytoin has also been described as a cause of a pseudoacromegaly. Other conditions associated with pseudoacromegaly are beyond the scope of this chapter but include Beckwith-Wiedemann syndrome, Sotos syndrome, Marfan syndrome, among many others [23].

Conclusions

Despite advances in acromegaly and a minor decrease in time to recognition of the disease, diagnosis remains delayed largely because classic features occur slowly and are underrecognized. Once the diagnosis is made, most patients manifest typical physical signs of acral and facial changes. Signs and symptoms of acromegaly affect almost every organ system; hence, multiple subspecialists are involved in making this diagnosis. There is a spectrum of severity in the clinical manifestations of acromegaly and several rare conditions that may mimic it.

Others include orthopedists, gastrointestinal disease specialists, pulmonologists, ENT, and gynecologists.

References

1. Sheaves R. A history of acromegaly. Pituitary. 1999;2(1):7–28.
2. de Herder WW. The history of acromegaly. Neuroendocrinology. 2016;103(1):7–17.
3. Mammis A, Eloy JA, Liu JK. Early descriptions of acromegaly and gigantism and their historical evolution as clinical entities. Neurosurg Focus. 2010;29(4):E1.
4. Kumar P, Simcic KJ, McDermott MT. Chapter 61 - famous people with endocrine disorders. In: Endocrine secrets; 2013. p. 516–20.
5. Nabarro JDN. Acromegaly. Clin Endocrinol. 1987;26(4):481–512.
6. Reid TJ, Post KD, Bruce JN, Nabi Kanibir M, Reyes-Vidal CM, Freda PU. Features at diagnosis of 324 patients with acromegaly did not change from 1981 to 2006: acromegaly remains under-recognized and under-diagnosed. Clin Endocrinol. 2010;72(2):203–8.
7. Lavrentaki A, Paluzzi A, Wass JA, Karavitaki N. Epidemiology of acromegaly: review of population studies. Pituitary. 2017;20(1):4–9.
8. Petrossians P, Daly AF, Natchev E, Maione L, Blijdorp K, Sahnoun-Fathallah M, et al. Acromegaly at diagnosis in 3173 patients from the Liège Acromegaly Survey (LAS) database. Endocr Relat Cancer. 2017;24(10):505–18.
9. Nachtigall L, Delgado A, Swearingen B, Lee H, Zerikly R, Klibanski A. Extensive clinical experience: changing patterns in diagnosis and therapy of acromegaly over two decades. J Clin Endocrinol Metabol. 2008;93(6):2035–41.
10. Guo X, Wang K, Yu S, Gao L, Wang Z, Zhu H, et al. Patient characteristics, diagnostic delays, treatment patterns, treatment outcomes, comorbidities, and treatment costs of acromegaly in China: a nationwide study. Front Endocrinol. 2020;11:610519.

11. Caron P, Brue T, Raverot G, Tabarin A, Cailleux A, Delemer B, et al. Signs and symptoms of acromegaly at diagnosis: the physician's and the patient's perspectives in the ACRO-POLIS study. Endocrine. 2019;63(1):120–9.
12. Colao A, Grasso LFS, Giustina A, Melmed S, Chanson P, Pereira AM, et al. Acromegaly. Nat Rev Dis Primers. 2019;5(1):20.
13. Ghajar A, Jones PS, Guarda FJ, Faje A, Tritos NA, Miller KK, et al. Biochemical control in acromegaly with multimodality therapies: outcomes from a pituitary center and changes over time. J Clin Endocrinol Metabol. 2019;105(3):e532–43.
14. Jadresic A, Banks LM, Child DF, Diamant L, Doyle FH, Fraser TR, et al. The acromegaly syndrome. Relation between clinical features, growth hormone values and radiological characteristics of the pituitary tumours. Q J Med. 1982;51(202):189–204.
15. Clemmons DR, Chihara K, Freda PU, Ho KK, Klibanski A, Melmed S, et al. Optimizing control of acromegaly: integrating a growth hormone receptor antagonist into the treatment algorithm. J Clin Endocrinol Metab. 2003;88(10):4759–67.
16. Ben-Shlomo A, Melmed S. Acromegaly. Endocrinol Metab Clin N Am. 2008;37(1): 101–22, viii.
17. Wu JC, Huang WC, Chang HK, Ko CC, Lirng JF, Chen YC. Natural history of acromegaly: incidences, re-operations, cancers, and mortality rates in a national cohort. Neuroendocrinology. 2020;110(11–12):977–87.
18. Gadelha MR, Kasuki L, Lim DST, Fleseriu M. Systemic complications of acromegaly and the impact of the current treatment landscape: an update. Endocr Rev. 2019;40(1):268–332.
19. Swearingen B, Barker FG 2nd, Katznelson L, Biller BM, Grinspoon S, Klibanski A, et al. Long-term mortality after transsphenoidal surgery and adjunctive therapy for acromegaly. J Clin Endocrinol Metab. 1998;83(10):3419–26.
20. Lause M, Kamboj A, Fernandez Faith E. Dermatologic manifestations of endocrine disorders. Transl Pediatr. 2017;6(4):300–12.
21. Colao A, Ferone D, Marzullo P, Lombardi G. Systemic complications of acromegaly: epidemiology, pathogenesis, and management. Endocr Rev. 2004;25(1):102–52.
22. Grynberg M, Salenave S, Young J, Chanson P. Female gonadal function before and after treatment of acromegaly. J Clin Endocrinol Metab. 2010;95(10):4518–25.
23. Marques P, Korbonits M. Pseudoacromegaly. Front Neuroendocrinol. 2019;52:113–43.
24. Kumar KV, Shaikh A, Anwar I, Prusty P. Primary hypothyroidism presenting as pseudoacromegaly. Pituitary. 2012;15(Suppl 1):S49–52.
25. Stone SI, Wegner DJ, Wambach JA, Cole FS, Urano F, Ornitz DM. Digenic variants in the FGF21 signaling pathway associated with severe insulin resistance and pseudoacromegaly. J Endocr Soc. 2020;4(12):bvaa138.
26. Dutta P, Hajela A, Pathak A, Bhansali A, Radotra BD, Vashishta RK, et al. Clinical profile and outcome of patients with acromegaly according to the 2014 consensus guidelines: impact of a multi-disciplinary team. Neurol India. 2015;63(3):360–8.
27. Al Dahmani K, Afandi B, Elhouni A, Dinwal D, Philip J, Bashier A, et al. Clinical presentation, treatment, and outcome of acromegaly in the United Arab Emirates. Oman Med J. 2020;35(5):e172.
28. Lawrence L, Alkwatli K, Bena J, Prayson R, Kshettry V, Recinos P, et al. Acromegaly: a clinical perspective. Clin Diabetes Endocrinol. 2020;6:15.
29. Khamseh ME, Mohajeri Tehrani MR, Mousavi Z, Malek M, Imani M, Hoshangian Tehrani N, et al. Iran pituitary tumor registry: description of the program and initial results. Arch Iran Med. 2017;20(12):746–51.

Chapter 6
Sleep-Disordered Breathing in Acromegaly

Diane Donegan and Stephanie M. Stahl

Introduction

Acromegaly is a multisystem disease due to excess growth hormone (GH) secretion and consequently insulin-like growth factor (IGF)-1, most commonly due to a pituitary adenoma [1]. Chronic unregulated GH release, direct effect of the tumor itself, and/or adverse effects of treatment (surgery, medication and radiation treatment) contribute to the development of comorbidities in patients with acromegaly [2, 3]. Given the ubiquitous distribution of GH and IGF-1 receptors, systemic complications associated with acromegaly are diverse and include metabolic effects (e.g., insulin resistance, hyperlipidemia, and obesity), cardiovascular and cerebrovascular disease, neoplasia, arthropathy, decreased quality of life (QOL), and respiratory disease necessitating treatment [4, 5].

Untreated or persistent acromegaly is associated with increased mortality [6–8]. The leading cause of death has been attributed to cancer, cardiovascular, cerebrovascular, and respiratory disorders [9, 10]. With effective treatment, a reduction in GH and normalization of IGF-1 can reduce mortality to that of the general population [11, 12]. Although many complications may improve with acromegaly treatment, some continue and may contribute to the persistent decrease in health-related

D. Donegan (✉)
Division of Endocrinology, Diabetes and Metabolism, Indiana University School of Medicine, Indianapolis, IN, USA
e-mail: diadoneg@iu.edu

S. M. Stahl
Division of Pulmonary, Critical Care, Sleep and Occupational Medicine, Department of Medicine, Indiana University School of Medicine, Indianapolis, IN, USA

Department of Neurology, Indiana University School of Medicine, Indianapolis, IN, USA
e-mail: smtieken@iu.edu

L. S. Blevins Jr., M. K. Aghi (eds.), *Acromegaly*, Contemporary Endocrinology,
https://doi.org/10.1007/978-3-031-16258-9_6

QOL demonstrated in several studies [13–15]. Thus, identifying and adequately treating comorbidities associated with acromegaly is important.

Sleep-disordered breathing (SDB) is common in patients with acromegaly. SDB is categorized into obstructive sleep apnea (OSA), central sleep apnea (CSA) syndromes, sleep-related hypoxemia, and sleep-related hypoventilation disorders. OSA is the most commonly reported SDB condition in the general population as well as in patients with acromegaly. OSA has known negative health effects, including those observed in morbidity and mortality in acromegaly, and therefore, awareness and treatment of OSA are important in the holistic management of patients with acromegaly.

Obstructive Sleep Apnea

Definition and Diagnosis

OSA is characterized by repetitive full or partial obstructions in the upper airway during sleep. The most common site of obstruction is the retropalatal region but also frequently includes collapse at the retroglossal and hypopharyngeal areas [16]. OSA is diagnosed by either in-laboratory polysomnography (PSG) or by home sleep apnea testing (HSAT; also referred to as portable monitoring or out-of-center testing). PSG is the gold standard for diagnosis. During PSG, several physiologic parameters are continuously recorded, including electroencephalogram (EEG), electrooculogram (EOG), electromyogram (EMG), electrocardiogram (ECG), snoring, respiratory flow and effort, body position, oxygen saturation, and often continuous carbon dioxide levels measured typically by end-tidal carbon dioxide. HSAT parameters are often limited to oxygen saturation and some measurement of limited respiratory effort and flow but do not commonly include EEG, EOG, EMG, ECG, or carbon dioxide monitoring. HSAT may be considered for patients at high risk for OSA who do not have comorbidities that would place them at risk for other SDB conditions, such as CSA, hypoventilation, or hypoxemia. Such excluding conditions include congestive heart failure, opiate use, chronic obstructive pulmonary disease, neuromuscular conditions, and atrial fibrillation [17]. CSA is reported in up to 33% of patients with acromegaly as detailed later in this chapter [18, 19]; therefore, in-laboratory PSG rather than HSAT should be considered.

Diagnostic testing for OSA evaluates for the presence, frequency, and type of respiratory events referred to as apneas and hypopneas. An apnea is defined as complete or near-complete cessation of airflow for at least 10 s. A hypopnea is defined as a reduction in airflow by ≥30% of pre-event baseline for at least 10 s and associated with (1) a ≥4% oxygen desaturation from pre-event baseline ("acceptable" definition) or (2) a ≥3% oxygen desaturation from pre-event baseline or an arousal ("recommended" definition) [20]. A respiratory event is defined as obstructive if respiratory effort is present, central if no respiratory effort is present, and mixed if initially no respiratory effort is present followed by respiratory effort in the latter portion of the event. Depending on the sleep laboratory in which testing occurs, respiratory effort-related arousals (RERAs) may also be reported. A RERA is defined by a change in the airflow lasting for at least 10 s leading to an arousal from sleep that does not meet the criteria for an apnea or hypopnea [20].

The International Classification of Sleep Disorders, 3rd Edition, provides the current diagnostic criteria for OSA, which differs for adults and children. The diagnosis of adult OSA requires the presence of either (1) ≥15 predominantly obstructive respiratory events per hour of sleep during PSG or per hour of monitoring during an HSAT or (2) ≥5 predominantly obstructive respiratory events per hour of sleep during a PSG or per hour of monitoring during an HSAT with symptoms (i.e., snoring, witnessed apneas, sleepiness, fatigue, nonrestorative sleep, insomnia, or waking with gasping or choking) or comorbidities (i.e., congestive heart failure, coronary artery disease, atrial fibrillation, stroke, hypertension, cognitive dysfunction, mood disorder, or type 2 diabetes mellitus) [21].

The severity of OSA is defined by the apnea-hypopnea index (AHI; number of apneas and hypopneas per hour of sleep on PSG), respiratory event index (REI; number of apneas and hypopneas per hour of recording on HSAT), or respiratory disturbance index (RDI; number of apneas, hypopneas, and RERAs per hour of sleep on PSG). The terms AHI, REI, and RDI are often used synonymously, and for simplicity, these terms will collectively be referred to as the AHI in this chapter unless otherwise stated. Severity of OSA is defined as mild when the AHI is 5 to <15/hour (h), moderate when 15 to <30/h, and severe when ≥30/h. Other variables important to consider in the severity of sleep apnea are the degree and duration of oxygen desaturation, severity of daytime sleepiness, and amount of sleep fragmentation, which can be determined by the arousal index, sleep efficiency (total time asleep divided by the total recording time), and percentage of time spent in the various stages of sleep.

Night-to-night variations in the AHI along with differences in testing and the definition of respiratory events lead to variable reporting of sleep apnea prevalence and severity. Currently, the Centers for Medicare and Medicaid Services uses only the "acceptable" definition for hypopneas (i.e., ≥4% oxygen desaturation) and do not consider RERAs, leading many sleep centers to report only this definition of hypopneas and not reporting RERAs. Thus, variance can be present from one center to another. If the recommended definition of hypopneas and scoring of RERAs are used, the prevalence and severity of OSA would increase. Additionally, HSAT often underestimates the REI. Therefore, an understanding of the parameters reported and recognition of their limits are crucial when reviewing the sleep study report for the diagnosis and management of patients. Due to these variances if the patient receives a negative test result, but a high index of suspicion for OSA is present, repeat sleep testing is recommended.

Epidemiology

The prevalence of OSA in the general population has varied over time. This variance is in part due to the different definitions of respiratory events and criteria used for diagnosis. It is also likely due to an increase in diseases such as obesity. In 2013, the Wisconsin Sleep Cohort Study estimated the prevalence of OSA using the ≥4% desaturation rule for hypopneas to be 26% of adults 30–70 years old. Additionally, at least 1 in 10 adults have moderate or severe OSA (i.e., AHI ≥15/h) [22]. This prevalence, however, varies widely with population characteristics [23].

In patients with acromegaly, the prevalence of OSA is reported to be as high as 100%; however, the prevalence range is wide and likely related to subject selection, study design, and diagnostic criteria. In studies where all patients with acromegaly are evaluated by PSG, 37–100% were diagnosed with OSA (Table 6.1) [18, 19, 24–42]. In population or multicenter-based studies, such as the French, Spanish, or Belgian (AcroBel) acromegaly registries, 13–26% of patients were diagnosed with OSA [43–47]. Two cross-sectional examinations of major claims databases in the United States noted a diagnosis of OSA in 11.5–29.6% of patients with acromegaly [48, 49]. Only one study has attempted to assess the incidence of OSA in those with acromegaly, which was calculated to be 1.3/10,000 person years based on the administrative claims of 949 health plan enrollees [49]. These lower percentages reported in acromegaly registries and the claims databases highlight the underdiagnosis of OSA, as not all patients were systematically assessed for sleep apnea. Moreover, the method of evaluation and diagnostic criteria were not outlined.

The variance in OSA reported in patients with acromegaly may also be due to differences in study populations assessed (treatment naive vs prior treatment or both; active disease vs disease remission or both), although a recent meta-analysis did not show a difference in the prevalence of OSA in those with active compared to controlled acromegaly [50]. Alternatively, selection bias may contribute to higher prevalence rates and may be more likely when patients were selected for OSA assessment when screened using the Epworth Sleepiness Scale (ESS) or were consecutively recruited from sleep medicine clinics [18, 38, 40]. When taken altogether the prevalence of OSA in patients with acromegaly is estimated to be approximately 68.8% (range 37–100%).

Given that acromegaly is rare with a prevalence that ranges between 2.8 and 13.7 cases per 100,000 [51], one would expect the prevalence of acromegaly in those with OSA to be low. Indeed, three studies, which screened for acromegaly using IGF-1 alone or IGF-1 in those with at least 1 acral enlargement symptom followed by confirmatory oral glucose GH suppression testing, found the prevalence of acromegaly in those with OSA to be 0.004–0.35% [52–54]. Whether screening of all patients with OSA for acromegaly would be cost-effective is to be determined.

Table 6.1 Prevalence of sleep apnea in patients with acromegaly and effects of treatment

Authors	Year	Single or multicenter	Country	Total (female)	Average age, years	Treatment naive	Active acromegaly at enrollment (yes/no/both)	Interven-tion adminis-tered	Type of intervention	Prevalence of sleep apnea (*N*/total), %	Severity of sleep apnea			AHI at start (SD)	AHI at follow-up (SD)
											Mild	Moderate	Severe		
Grunstein et al. [18]	1991	Multicenter	Australia	53 (14)	54 ± 2 in those with sleep apnea and 40 ± 4 without	20 naive and 33 received some form of therapy	Both	No	NA	43/53, 81%	NR	NR	NR	NR	NR
Grunstein et al. [19]	1994	Single	Australia	19 (5)	50 ± 2	12 naive and 6 previously treated	Yes	Yes	Octreotide 6 months	19/29, 65.5%	5	0	14	39	19
Ip et al. [24]	2001	Multicenter	Hong Kong	14 (3)	42 ± 8.1	No	Yes	Yes	Octreotide LAR 6 months	8/14, 57%	NR	NR	NR	29.4 (22.6)	13.4 (11.12)
Hermann et al. [25]	2004	Single	Germany	14 (8)	57 ± 4	Yes	Yes	Yes	Octreotide 6 months	14/14, 100% (100% OSA, 0% CSA)	NR	NR	NR	NR	NR
Sze et al. [26]	2007	Single	Switzerland	13 (7)	women, aged 33–77 years men, aged 25–72 years	Yes	Yes	Yes	Surgery	6/13, 46% (17% CSA)	NR	NR	NR	41 (20.5)	11.3 (13.3)
Davi et al. [27]	2008	Single	Italy	36 (18)	52.11 ± 13.1	No	Both (19 active and 19 controlled)	No	NA	17/36, 47%	6	6	5	31.2 (16.4)	21.3 (18.2)

(continued)

Table 6.1 (continued)

Authors	Year	Single or multicenter	Country	Total (female)	Average age, years	Treatment naive	Active acromegaly at enrollment (yes/no/both)	Interven-tion adminis-tered	Type of intervention	Prevalence of sleep apnea (*N*/total), %	Severity of sleep apnea			AHI at start (SD)	AHI at follow-up (SD)
											Mild	Moderate	Severe		
Van Haute et al. [28]	2008	Single	Brazil	24 (12)	Median 50 (2–75)	No	Yes	No	NA	21/24, 87.5% (83% OSA, 4% CSA)	6	3	12	35 (5.5–79)	NR
Berg et al. [29]	2009	Single	Germany	12 (6)	57 ± 15	No	Yes	Yes	Pegvisomant 6 months	10/12, 83%	2	5	3	2 (22)	18 (18)
Attal et al. [30]	2010	Single	France	18 (NR)	NR	No	NR	No	NA	12/18, 66%	NR	NR	NR	22.5 (6.5)	19.5 (5.6)
Roemmler et al. [31]	2012	Single	Germany	52 (25)	Median 51 (19–82)	17 treatment naive	Both (29 active, 9 controlled)	No	NA	30/52, 58% (52% OSA, 6% CSA)	14	7	9	NR	NR
Hernandez-Gordillo et al. [32]	2012	Single	Mexico	35 (20)	51 (39–63)[a]	No	Both (7 active, 28 controlled)	No	NA	34/35, 97% (100% OSA, 0% CSA)	7	6	21	34 (22–57)[a]	NR
Annamalai et al. [33]	2013	Single	UK	30 (15)	54.3 (23–78)	Yes	Yes	Yes	Lanreotide ATG 24 weeks	23/29, 79%	9	5	9	NR	NR
Akkoyunlu et al. [34]	2013	Single	Turkey	42 (25)	41 (35–41)	15 naive, rest had received treatment	Both (20 active 22 controlled)	No	NA	22/42, 52%	7	4	11	31.5 (14.4-38.3)	24.6 (12.4-31.4)
Chemla et al. [35]	2014	Single	France	16 (4)	43 ± 12	Yes	Yes	Yes	Surgery in all, further treatment in 9	7/16, 43.7%	NR	NR	NR	33 (21)	NR
Kuhn et al. [36]	2015	Single	Germany	12 (NR)	6 (15–64)	No	No	Yes	Pegvisomant	9/12, 75%	4	2	3	NR	NR

Castellani et al. [37]	2016	Single	Italy	58 (26)	52.9 (13.7)	No	Both (33 active, 25 controlled, multimodal)	No	NA	34/58, 58.6%, (in those with active acromegaly 21/33, 63.6)	18	7	9	NR	NR
Tasbakan et al. [38]	2017	Single	Turkey	28 (11)	48.7 ± 10.1	No	No	No	NA	25/28, 89.3%	NR	NR	NR	7.7 (28.8)	NA
Guo et al. [39]	2018	Single	China	25 (9)	41.3 ± 10.7	Yes	Yes	Yes	Surgery	13/25, 52%	NR	10 had >15	NR	15.3	NR
Vouzouneraki et al. [40]	2018	Multicenter	Sweden	259 (127)	57 ± 13	No	Both (controlled in 177, 9%)	No	NA	95/259, 37%	NR	NR	NR	NR	NR
Zhang et al. [42]	2018	Single	China	24 (7)[b]	43.79 ± 12.22	Yes	Yes	Yes	Surgery	21/22, 95.5%	NR	NR	NR	26	18
Wolters et al. [41]	2020	Single	Netherlands	27 (15)	51.3 ± 13.5	Yes	Yes	Yes	6 months SSA if persistent surgery or additional medical therapy	20/27, 74%	5	6	9	14.2 (0.5–64.6)[c]	4 (0–23.6)

Severity of sleep apnea: mild (AHI 5 to <15/h), moderate (AHI 15 to <30/h), severe (AHI ≥30/h). *AHI* apnea-hypopnea index, *CSA* central sleep apnea, *NA* not applicable, *NR* not reported, *OSA* obstructive sleep apnea, *SD* standard deviation, *SSA* somatostatin analogue

[a]Interquartile range

[b]Total was 48, but assessed only those who achieved remission

[c]AHI for all 27 patients

Symptoms and Risk Factors

Symptoms of OSA include loud or frequent snoring, witnessed pauses in breathing during sleep, daytime sleepiness or fatigue, unrefreshing sleep, night sweats, nocturia, morning headaches, memory impairment, frequent nocturnal awakenings, irritability, and nocturnal gastroesophageal reflux (Table 6.2) [55]. While one or more of these symptoms may prompt the patients to discuss concerns with their healthcare provider, many patients may not recognize the importance of or experience significant symptoms. In such patients, recognizing risk factors for those who should be screened for OSA is important. Several screening questionnaires, such as the STOP-BANG or Berlin Questionnaire, are validated screening tools for OSA in the general population; however, these tools have not been validated in patients with acromegaly [56, 57]. Given the high frequency of OSA in acromegaly, all patients with acromegaly should be screened for symptoms of OSA and PSG considered. Additionally, screening for OSA prior to and after surgical treatment of those with acromegaly is recommended [2].

Many factors play a role in upper airway patency during sleep. Any feature that can cause narrowing or collapse in the pharyngeal airway can increase the risk of OSA. Risk factors for OSA include male gender, age, body habitus, abnormal neuromuscular control, and craniofacial and upper airway abnormalities or features [22, 58]. Men are twice as likely to have OSA. In the United States, approximately 34% of men compared to 17.4% of women ages 30–70 years old have OSA [22]. OSA risk also increases with age. For example, the prevalence of OSA in men and women 30–49 years old is approximately 26.6% and 8.7%, respectively, compared to 43.2% of men and 27.8% of women ages 50–70 years old [22]. Certain body habitus features, such as obesity, central body fat distribution, and large neck size,

Table 6.2 Symptoms of obstructive sleep apnea

Loud or frequent snoring
Witnessed pauses in breathing during sleep
Daytime sleepiness
Unrefreshing sleep
Fatigue
Night sweats
Dry mouth upon awakening
Nocturia
Waking with gasping or choking
Morning headaches
Poor concentration
Memory impairment
Frequent nocturnal awakenings
Insomnia
Decreased libido
Irritability
Nocturnal gastroesophageal reflux

are strong risk factors for OSA [58]. In men ages 30–49 a BMI of <25 is associated with about a 7% prevalence of OSA compared to 18.3% for BMI 25–29.9 (overweight category), 44.6% for BMI 30–39.9 (obesity category), and 79.5% for BMI ≥40 (morbid obesity category) [22].

Generally, risk factors for the development of OSA in those with acromegaly are similar to those of the general population. OSA is more likely in men [41] and in those with a large neck circumference or older age [28, 59, 60]. While some studies noted a higher risk of OSA with increasing BMI, diabetes and hypertension, these risk factors are not noted in all [61]. OSA is more common in those with active acromegaly compared to those without. Additionally, positive correlations between AHI and IGF-1 and/or GH have been observed; however, not all studies have demonstrated such correlations [28, 61, 62].

Abnormalities or enlargement of craniofacial and upper airway structures is important in the development of OSA. Alterations in structures that increase the risk of OSA include tongue enlargement, retrognathia, micrognathia, tonsillar hypertrophy, and uvula enlargement [16]. Such structural changes can be a result of genetics, developmental abnormalities, or from other causes, such as endocrine disorders including acromegaly [63]. In patients with acromegaly, excess GH is associated with both osseous and soft-tissue changes in the upper airway, which contribute to the increased risk of OSA. Increased deposition of collagen and glycosaminoglycan [64, 65], in addition to increased extracellular fluid [66, 67], leads to enlargement of soft-tissue structures. Moreover, bone growth of all parts of the neurocranium and orofacial bones (except maxilla), due to abnormal modeling and remodeling, leads to the craniofacial features that typify acromegaly [68–70].

Studies have used a variety of different radiological techniques to identify the level of greatest impact for the development of OSA and its association to acromegaly disease activity. Based on morphological studies using X-rays, patients with acromegaly develop enlargement of most bones, but notable growth is seen in the mandible as well as narrowing of the pharyngeal airspace [29, 70–72]. High-resolution computed tomography of the upper airway typically demonstrates thickening or enlargement of the tongue, soft plate, and posterior pharyngeal soft tissues in those with acromegaly who have OSA [24, 39, 60]. Similar findings using magnetic resonance imaging (MRI) have been noted with tongue and soft palate enlargement most commonly seen [25, 28]. Endoscopic evaluation of those with acromegaly demonstrates macroglossia and hypertrophy of the laryngeal mucosa, aryepiglottic and ventricular folds as well as false vocal cords [73, 74].

In general, the severity of OSA, as measured by AHI, is associated with aforementioned changes that occur in the upper airways in acromegaly. In particular, the AHI has correlated positively with soft palate as well as pharyngeal enlargement and negatively with airway narrowing [24, 75]. Moreover, the typical risk factors associated with OSA, such as increasing age and BMI as well as male sex, are associated with a higher AHI [27]. Although the prevalence of OSA is higher in those with acromegaly compared to the general population, hormonal levels (GH and IGF-1) have not always correlated positively with the severity of the AHI [18, 28]. Some studies have noted that higher GH levels are associated with increased MRI signal intensity, reflective of soft-tissue edema, correlated with IGF-1 levels [24]. Higher IGF-1 and GH levels have been associated with increased post-pharyngeal thickness and vallecular tongue length [25].

Complications of Untreated Obstructive Sleep Apnea

Obstructive respiratory events can cause intermittent hypoxemia and elevations in carbon dioxide levels. These changes induce sympathetic activation and chemoreflexive arousals from sleep to stimulate return of ventilation. Consequently, a number of effects can result, including sleep fragmentation with a reduction in the deeper and more restful stages of sleep, metabolic dysregulation including insulin resistance, endothelial dysfunction, systemic inflammation, oxidative stress, and hypercoagulability [76]. Intrathoracic pressure changes with attempted respirations against a closed or narrowed airway can also increase transmural gradients of the heart, leading to increased left atrial size and impaired diastolic function [77].

With a number of systemic effects, untreated OSA is associated with many negative health consequences including increased risk of cardiovascular and cerebrovascular disease, neurologic disorders, endocrine dysfunction, ocular manifestations, mood disorders, poor daytime functioning, and mortality (Table 6.3). The presence of OSA is associated with a number of cardiovascular disorders, including increased risk of systemic hypertension, heart failure, stroke, bradyarrhythmias, atrial fibrillation, ventricular arrhythmias, myocardial ischemia and infarction, and pulmonary arterial hypertension [76]. OSA is also associated with many neurologic disorders, including increased risk of neurodegenerative conditions, such as dementia [78] and Parkinson disease [79], stroke [80], headaches, and poor seizure control [81]. Neurocognitive function is also impacted, causing deficits in attention, vigilance, executive function, and long-term and possibly short-term memory [82]. OSA affects glucose metabolism and is associated with increased risk of type 1 and 2 diabetes mellitus as well as gestational diabetes [83]. Ocular manifestations and vision-threatening conditions associated with OSA include floppy eyelid syndrome, nonarteritic anterior ischemic optic neuropathy, central serous retinopathy, retinal vein occlusion, and glaucoma [84]. Other conditions in which OSA has been reported to be associated with include depression [85], post-traumatic stress disorder [85], cancer [86], and gastro-esophageal reflux [87]. Individuals with OSA also have a higher risk of motor vehicle accidents, work-related accidents, and poorer work performance [88]. Consequently, mortality rate is increased in patients with OSA with untreated sleep apnea associated with about a fourfold increased all-cause mortality risk after adjusting for confounders [55]. Cardiovascular events are a common cause of mortality in patients with OSA, accounting for approximately 40% of deaths in patients with severe sleep apnea [55].

Until recently, the leading cause of mortality in those with untreated or persistent acromegaly was cardiovascular disease. In a study by Orme et al., where 366 deaths occurred among 1362 acromegaly patients, 40% of deaths were due to

Table 6.3 Negative health effects associated with untreated obstructive sleep apnea

Cardiovascular disease
Hypertension
Heart Failure
Arrhythmias
Myocardial infarction
Pulmonary arterial hypertension
Neurologic disorders
Stroke
Dementia
Parkinson disease
Headaches
Poor seizure control
Deficits in attention, vigilance, and executive function
Impaired long- and short-term memory
Endocrine dysfunction
Type 1 and 2 diabetes mellitus
Gestational diabetes
Ocular manifestations
Floppy eyelid syndrome
Nonarteritic anterior ischemic optic neuropathy
Central serous retinopathy
Retinal vein occlusion
Glaucoma
Depression
Post-traumatic stress disorder
Cancer
Gastroesophageal reflux
Mortality

cardiovascular disease, and in 11% the cause of death was respiratory-related [89]. Previously, respiratory disorders accounted for up to 25% of mortality in patients with acromegaly, which was a two to threefold higher risk than the general population [90]. Metabolic complications seen in OSA are also present in acromegaly. However, with advances in treatment and resultant normalization in hormonal parameters, mortality has declined to levels similar to the general population with cancer, now emerging as the leading cause of death as life expectancy increases [9]. Acromegaly has also been associated with cardiomyopathy, hypertension, arrythmias, and endothelial dysfunction [53]; therefore, the presence of untreated OSA likely confers additional cardiovascular risk if overlooked and contributes to morbidity.

Treatment of Obstructive Sleep Apnea

Decision to treat OSA depends on the severity as well as symptoms and comorbidities. Treatment is indicated for patients with moderate or severe OSA and for patients with mild OSA who have symptoms or associated comorbidities [91]. Since one of the leading causes of death in patients with acromegaly is cardiovascular in nature, recognition and treatment of OSA are of importance.

Several OSA treatments are available. The first-line treatment for OSA, especially if moderate or severe, is positive airway pressure (PAP) therapy. PAP therapy is delivered by continuous, bilevel, or auto-titrating modes typically through a nasal or oronasal interface. Continuous or auto-titrating PAP modes are typically used first line; however, bilevel PAP may be considered for patients with hypoventilation or difficulties tolerating continuous modes. Hernandez-Gordillo et al. demonstrated that bilevel PAP had no advantages over CPAP in sleep architecture, residual AHI, tolerance, or gas exchange in a group of patients with acromegaly [32]. Little data is available on PAP adherence in patients with acromegaly, but one group reported PAP adherence (defined as usage of PAP for >4 h for at least 70% of nights) to be 50% [38].

Other OSA treatments include an oral appliance, surgery, behavioral modifications, and other adjunctive treatments. Surgical options include upper airway stimulation, uvulopalatopharyngoplasty, tongue advancement or stabilization, maxillomandibular advancement, tracheostomy, and bariatric surgery. In adults, several factors affect surgical success, and most sleep apnea surgeries are uncommonly curative. Adjunctive treatments and behavioral modifications, including weight loss, exercise, positional therapy (i.e., prevention of sleeping supine), and avoidance of alcohol and other respiratory depressants, may also lead to improvements in OSA [91].

In acromegaly, evidence suggests that treatment of the underlying condition may be associated with improvement or, in some cases, resolution of sleep apnea. Response to therapy, however, is variable. In treatment-naive patients with active acromegaly who had surgery as first-line therapy, Zhang et al. noted that among those who achieved biochemical remission, OSA had improved in 55% of patients at 6 months with the percentage of severe OSA falling from 45.8% to 28%. Additionally, in the same study, a significant reduction in AHI was seen at 1- and 3-months following surgery after which it stabilized [42]. Sze et al. reported a more dramatic effect of transsphenoidal tumor resection with a statistically significant reduction in AHI (41.0 ± 20.5 pretreatment vs 11.3 ± 13.3 posttreatment, $P \leq 0.05$) and ESS (12.7 ± 3.2 vs 8.2 ± 3.1, $P \leq 0.05$). In 33% of patients, sleep apnea resolved with an AHI of <5/h [26].

The use of somatostatin analogues (SSA) in treatment-naive patients with active acromegaly may also lead to improvement in OSA in some patients as demonstrated in several studies [24, 25, 33]. In a study of eight patients with acromegaly and OSA, the AHI improved from 29.4 ± 22.6 pretreatment to 13.4 ± 11.1 ($P = 0.025$) posttreatment with 6 months of octreotide [24]. In another study, the AHI decreased in 64%, and 8% had resolution of sleep apnea after 6 months of treatment with octreotide [25]. Another study with 24 weeks of lanreotide autogel demonstrated that 61% of patients with OSA at baseline had an improvement in the AHI with 2/23 patients having resolution of OSA. The patients that had a resolution of OSA had mild OSA at baseline. While the majority of patients had improvements, 30.4% had a significant worsening in OSA, and one patient with no OSA at baseline developed mild OSA despite improvements in IGF-1 and GH levels. The authors, however, identified a >4.5 kg weight gain in five of the seven patients who had worsening of OSA, which may have contributed to this deterioration as AHI correlated with weight ($R^2 = 0.43$, $P = 0.0001$) [33]. This finding highlights the importance of controlling for other OSA risk factors.

The use of pegvisomant and its impact on OSA in those with acromegaly have also been assessed. In 12 patients with active acromegaly despite surgery and octreotide, 6 months of pegvisomant use successfully lowered IGF-1 levels with a resultant decrease in tongue volume and a decrease in AHI in 75% of patients. The pretreatment AHI was 23 ± 22/h and reduced to 18 ± 18/h posttreatment ($P = 0.007$) [29]. While this change was statistically significant, the clinical significance is in question as the posttreatment AHI for the group remained in the moderate OSA category and resolution of sleep apnea to an AHI <5/h occurred in none of the patients diagnosed with OSA prior to treatment. In a retrospective study assessing the use of pegvisomant of varying duration among patients with OSA and active acromegaly despite treatment, pegvisomant use resulted in significant decrease in IGF-1 levels and normalized in 10/12 patients with a resultant overall statistically significant improvement in AHI ($P < 0.05$) and resolution of OSA in two patients. In this study, patients with a higher AHI at baseline had less clinically significant improvements in OSA with pegvisomant. Three patients at baseline had severe OSA, and after pegvisomant, one patient continued to have severe OSA and two had reduced to moderate OSA [36].

No head-to-head comparisons are available to assess the efficacy of acromegaly treatments, including transsphenoidal surgery and medical therapies, in the improvement of OSA. Differing definitions of OSA and its severity used in studies also make comparisons of studies and treatments difficult. Studies have evaluated those with multimodal acromegaly therapy (i.e., combination of medical, surgical, and/or radiotherapy). Overall, as observed in a recent meta-analysis, any form of treatment was associated with a decrease in the AHI with no difference noted between varying treatment modalities ($P = 0.26$) [35]. Similar to monotherapies, resolution of OSA does not always occur with acromegaly remission despite multimodal therapies [29, 35]; however, after 2.5 years of follow-up, resolution of OSA (defined as an AHI <5/h in this study) has been reported in up to 68.8% of patients treated [41].

Although changes in OSA do not always correlate with IGF-1 or GH levels, improvements in AHI are often seen irrespective of the form of treatment utilized. However, complete resolution of sleep apnea with acromegaly treatment alone is less frequently observed, and some patients develop OSA over the course of acromegaly treatment. The documented varying OSA response to acromegaly therapy may be due to the duration of acromegaly disease prior to intervention and severity of OSA at baseline as well as differing patient characteristics or comorbidities. Irreversible factors, as a consequence of acromegaly, likely contribute to the persistence of OSA seen in some. Additionally, other risk factors known to contribute to OSA, such as increased weight, may remain or increase following treatment (e.g., in the setting of hypopituitarism). Therefore, ongoing assessment with sleep medicine is crucial in the comprehensive care of patients with acromegaly.

Central Sleep Apnea

CSA has also been reported in up to 33% of individuals with acromegaly. Higher prevalence of CSA was reported in older studies, whereas more recent studies report the prevalence of CSA in patients with acromegaly around 0–6% [18, 19, 24, 27, 28, 31, 42, 60, 92]. The reason for reduction in CSA prevalence in patients with acromegaly is not known and may be related to the earlier recognition and treatment of acromegaly or advancements in technology used in SDB diagnosis in that some patients diagnosed with CSA actually had OSA.

The cause of CSA in acromegaly is less well-known but may be due to alterations in the central respiratory center either by reflex inhibition secondary to narrowing of the upper airways or change in ventilatory response in relation to carbon dioxide levels [90, 93]. Studies have demonstrated that CSA was associated with higher levels of GH and IGF-1 [18, 31] as well as lower carbon dioxide levels upon waking compared to those with OSA [18]. One study noted that the single patient diagnosed with CSA out of the 24 patients in the study had congestive heart failure, which is a condition in the general population associated with CSA and highlights that comorbidities aside from acromegaly itself can be the cause of SDB [28].

The consequences of untreated CSA are less well understood, and currently unknown is whether treatment of CSA leads to improved outcomes. Similar to patients with OSA, some studies have demonstrated that treatment of acromegaly led to improvement in CSA [19, 26]. Treatment of CSA differs from OSA treatment and may include advanced PAP therapy such as adaptive servo-ventilation [94]. Referral to a sleep medicine specialist for further evaluation and management is recommended.

Conclusion

SDB is common in acromegaly. Given the potential complications associated with OSA, all patients with acromegaly should be assessed for sleep apnea. Questionnaires can be used in clinic to screen for sleep apnea, but polysomnography is required for confirmation. Given that SDB improves in some following acromegaly treatment and, in others, may develop over the course of treatment, patients should be reevaluated to assess ongoing needs for SDB treatment. In the majority, however, SDB persists, requiring long-term management. Risk factors for the development or persistence of sleep apnea should be addressed, including obesity, smoking, optimal hormonal replacement, and ensuring appropriate disease control.

References

1. Melmed S. Medical progress: acromegaly. N Engl J Med. 2006;355(24):2558–73.
2. Giustina A, Barkan A, Beckers A, Biermasz N, Biller BMK, Boguszewski C, et al. A consensus on the diagnosis and treatment of acromegaly comorbidities: an update. J Clin Endocrinol Metab. 2020;105(4):dgz096.
3. McCabe J, Ayuk J, Sherlock M. Treatment factors that influence mortality in acromegaly. Neuroendocrinology. 2016;103(1):66–74.
4. Gadelha MR, Kasuki L, Lim DST, Fleseriu M. Systemic complications of acromegaly and the impact of the current treatment landscape: an update. Endocr Rev. 2019;40(1):268–332.
5. Pivonello R, Auriemma RS, Grasso LF, Pivonello C, Simeoli C, Patalano R, et al. Complications of acromegaly: cardiovascular, respiratory and metabolic comorbidities. Pituitary. 2017;20(1):46–62.
6. Ritvonen E, Loyttyniemi E, Jaatinen P, Ebeling T, Moilanen L, Nuutila P, et al. Mortality in acromegaly: a 20-year follow-up study. Endocr Relat Cancer. 2016;23(6):469–80.
7. Dekkers OM, Biermasz NR, Pereira AM, Romijn JA, Vandenbroucke JP. Mortality in acromegaly: a metaanalysis. J Clin Endocrinol Metab. 2008;93(1):61–7.
8. Holdaway IM. Excess mortality in acromegaly. Horm Res. 2007;68(Suppl 5):166–72.
9. Bolfi F, Neves AF, Boguszewski CL, Nunes-Nogueira VS. Mortality in acromegaly decreased in the last decade: a systematic review and meta-analysis. Eur J Endocrinol. 2018;179(1):59–71.
10. Kasuki L, Rocha PDS, Lamback EB, Gadelha MR. Determinants of morbidities and mortality in acromegaly. Arch Endocrinol Metab. 2019;63(6):630–7.
11. Mercado M, Gonzalez B, Vargas G, Ramirez C, de los Monteros AL, Sosa E, et al. Successful mortality reduction and control of comorbidities in patients with acromegaly followed at a highly specialized multidisciplinary clinic. J Clin Endocrinol Metab. 2014;99(12):4438–46.
12. Bolfi F, Neves AF, Boguszewski CL, Nunes-Nogueira VS. Mortality in acromegaly decreased in the last decade: a systematic review and meta-analysis. Eur J Endocrinol. 2019;181(5):L5–6.
13. Ben-Shlomo A, Sheppard MC, Stephens JM, Pulgar S, Melmed S. Clinical, quality of life, and economic value of acromegaly disease control. Pituitary. 2011;14(3):284–94.
14. Biermasz NR, Pereira AM, Smit JW, Romijn JA, Roelfsema F. Morbidity after long-term remission for acromegaly: persisting joint-related complaints cause reduced quality of life. J Clin Endocrinol Metab. 2005;90(5):2731–9.
15. Biermasz NR, van Thiel SW, Pereira AM, Hoftijzer HC, van Hemert AM, Smit JW, et al. Decreased quality of life in patients with acromegaly despite long-term cure of growth hormone excess. J Clin Endocrinol Metab. 2004;89(11):5369–76.
16. Dempsey JA, Veasey SC, Morgan BJ, O'Donnell CP. Pathophysiology of sleep apnea. Physiol Rev. 2010;90(1):47–112.
17. Kapur VK, Auckley DH, Chowdhuri S, Kuhlmann DC, Mehra R, Ramar K, et al. Clinical practice guideline for diagnostic testing for adult obstructive sleep apnea: an American Academy of Sleep Medicine clinical practice guideline. J Clin Sleep Med. 2017;13(3):479–504.
18. Grunstein RR, Ho KY, Sullivan CE. Sleep apnea in acromegaly. Ann Intern Med. 1991;115(7):527–32.
19. Grunstein RR, Ho KK, Sullivan CE. Effect of octreotide, a somatostatin analog, on sleep apnea in patients with acromegaly. Ann Intern Med. 1994;121(7):478–83.
20. Berry R. The AASM manual for the scoring of sleep and associated events: rules, terminology and technical specifications. Illinois: Darien; 2020.
21. Medicine AAoS. International classification of sleep disorders. 3rd ed. Illinois: Darien; 2014.
22. Peppard PE, Young T, Barnet JH, Palta M, Hagen EW, Hla KM. Increased prevalence of sleep-disordered breathing in adults. Am J Epidemiol. 2013;177(9):1006–14.
23. Chen X, Wang R, Zee P, Lutsey PL, Javaheri S, Alcantara C, et al. Racial/ethnic differences in sleep disturbances: the Multi-Ethnic Study of Atherosclerosis (MESA). Sleep. 2015;38(6):877–88.

24. Ip MS, Tan KC, Peh WC, Lam KS. Effect of Sandostatin LAR on sleep apnoea in acromegaly: correlation with computerized tomographic cephalometry and hormonal activity. Clin Endocrinol (Oxf). 2001;55(4):477–83.
25. Herrmann BL, Wessendorf TE, Ajaj W, Kahlke S, Teschler H, Mann K. Effects of octreotide on sleep apnoea and tongue volume (magnetic resonance imaging) in patients with acromegaly. Eur J Endocrinol. 2004;151(3):309–15.
26. Sze L, Schmid C, Bloch KE, Bernays R, Brandle M. Effect of transsphenoidal surgery on sleep apnoea in acromegaly. Eur J Endocrinol. 2007;156(3):321–9.
27. Davi MV, Dalle Carbonare L, Giustina A, Ferrari M, Frigo A, Lo Cascio V, et al. Sleep apnoea syndrome is highly prevalent in acromegaly and only partially reversible after biochemical control of the disease. Eur J Endocrinol. 2008;159(5):533–40.
28. van Haute FR, Taboada GF, Correa LL, Lima GA, Fontes R, Riello AP, et al. Prevalence of sleep apnea and metabolic abnormalities in patients with acromegaly and analysis of cephalometric parameters by magnetic resonance imaging. Eur J Endocrinol. 2008;158(4):459–65.
29. Berg C, Wessendorf TE, Mortsch F, Forsting M, Teschler H, Weischer T, et al. Influence of disease control with pegvisomant on sleep apnoea and tongue volume in patients with active acromegaly. Eur J Endocrinol. 2009;161(6):829–35.
30. Attal P, Chanson P. Endocrine aspects of obstructive sleep apnea. J Clin Endocrinol Metab. 2010;95(2):483–95.
31. Roemmler J, Gutt B, Fischer R, Vay S, Wiesmeth A, Bidlingmaier M, et al. Elevated incidence of sleep apnoea in acromegaly-correlation to disease activity. Sleep Breath. 2012;16(4):1247–53.
32. Hernandez-Gordillo D, Ortega-Gomez Mdel R, Galicia-Polo L, Castorena-Maldonado A, Vergara-Lopez A, Guillen-Gonzalez MA, et al. Sleep apnea in patients with acromegaly. Frequency, characterization and positive pressure titration. Open Respir Med J. 2012;6:28–33.
33. Annamalai AK, Webb A, Kandasamy N, Elkhawad M, Moir S, Khan F, et al. A comprehensive study of clinical, biochemical, radiological, vascular, cardiac, and sleep parameters in an unselected cohort of patients with acromegaly undergoing presurgical somatostatin receptor ligand therapy. J Clin Endocrinol Metab. 2013;98(3):1040–50.
34. Akkoyunlu ME, Ilhan MM, Bayram M, Tasan E, Yakar F, Ozcelik HK, et al. Does hormonal control obviate positive airway pressure therapy in acromegaly with sleep-disordered breathing? Respir Med. 2013;107(11):1803–9.
35. Chemla D, Attal P, Maione L, Veyer AS, Mroue G, Baud D, et al. Impact of successful treatment of acromegaly on overnight heart rate variability and sleep apnea. J Clin Endocrinol Metab. 2014;99(8):2925–31.
36. Kuhn E, Maione L, Bouchachi A, Roziere M, Salenave S, Brailly-Tabard S, et al. Long-term effects of pegvisomant on comorbidities in patients with acromegaly: a retrospective single-center study. Eur J Endocrinol. 2015;173(5):693–702.
37. Castellani C, Francia G, Dalle Carbonare L, Ferrari M, Viva E, Cerini R, et al. Morphological study of upper airways and long-term follow-up of obstructive sleep apnea syndrome in acromegalic patients. Endocrine. 2016;51(2):308–16.
38. Tasbakan MS, Kacmaz Basoglu O, Yildirim Simsir I, Saygili F. Obstructive sleep apnea characteristics in patients with well-controlled acromegaly and their compliance with positive airway pressure therapy. Turk J Med Sci. 2017;47(5):1348–53.
39. Guo X, Zhao Y, Wang M, Gao L, Wang Z, Zhang Z, et al. The posterior pharyngeal wall thickness is associated with OSAHS in patients with acromegaly and correlates with IGF-1 levels. Endocrine. 2018;61(3):526–32.
40. Vouzouneraki K, Franklin KA, Forsgren M, Warn M, Persson JT, Wik H, et al. Temporal relationship of sleep apnea and acromegaly: a nationwide study. Endocrine. 2018;62(2):456–63.
41. Wolters TLC, Roerink S, Drenthen LCA, van Haren-Willems J, Wagenmakers M, Smit JWA, et al. The course of obstructive sleep apnea syndrome in patients with acromegaly during treatment. J Clin Endocrinol Metab. 2020;105(1):290–304.
42. Zhang Z, Li Q, He W, Qiu H, Ye H, Wang Y, et al. The comprehensive impact on human body induced by resolution of growth hormone excess. Eur J Endocrinol. 2018;178(4):365–75.

43. Bex M, Abs R, T'Sjoen G, Mockel J, Velkeniers B, Muermans K, et al. AcroBel—the Belgian registry on acromegaly: a survey of the 'real-life' outcome in 418 acromegalic subjects. Eur J Endocrinol. 2007;157(4):399–409.
44. Mestron A, Webb SM, Astorga R, Benito P, Catala M, Gaztambide S, et al. Epidemiology, clinical characteristics, outcome, morbidity and mortality in acromegaly based on the Spanish Acromegaly Registry (Registro Espanol de Acromegalia, REA). Eur J Endocrinol. 2004;151(4):439–46.
45. Maione L, Brue T, Beckers A, Delemer B, Petrossians P, Borson-Chazot F, et al. Changes in the management and comorbidities of acromegaly over three decades: the French Acromegaly Registry. Eur J Endocrinol. 2017;176(5):645–55.
46. Lesen E, Granfeldt D, Houchard A, Dinet J, Berthon A, Olsson DS, et al. Comorbidities, treatment patterns and cost-of-illness of acromegaly in Sweden: a register-linkage population-based study. Eur J Endocrinol. 2017;176(2):203–12.
47. Petrossians P, Daly AF, Natchev E, Maione L, Blijdorp K, Sahnoun-Fathallah M, et al. Acromegaly at diagnosis in 3173 patients from the Liege Acromegaly Survey (LAS) Database. Endocr Relat Cancer. 2017;24(10):505–18.
48. Broder MS, Neary MP, Chang E, Cherepanov D, Katznelson L. Treatments, complications, and healthcare utilization associated with acromegaly: a study in two large United States databases. Pituitary. 2014;17(4):333–41.
49. Burton T, Le Nestour E, Bancroft T, Neary M. Real-world comorbidities and treatment patterns of patients with acromegaly in two large US health plan databases. Pituitary. 2013;16(3):354–62.
50. Parolin M, Dassie F, Alessio L, Wennberg A, Rossato M, Vettor R, et al. Obstructive sleep apnea in acromegaly and the effect of treatment: a systematic review and meta-analysis. J Clin Endocrinol Metab. 2020;105(3):dgz116.
51. Lavrentaki A, Paluzzi A, Wass JA, Karavitaki N. Epidemiology of acromegaly: review of population studies. Pituitary. 2017;20(1):4–9.
52. Heinrich DA, Reinholz C, Bauer M, Tufman A, Frohner R, Schopohl J, et al. IGF-1-based screening reveals a low prevalence of acromegaly in patients with obstructive sleep apnea. Endocrine. 2018;60(2):317–22.
53. Galerneau LM, Pepin JL, Borel AL, Chabre O, Sapene M, Stach B, et al. Acromegaly in sleep apnoea patients: a large observational study of 755 patients. Eur Respir J. 2016;48(5):1489–92.
54. Sesmilo G, Resmini E, Sambo M, Blanco C, Calvo F, Pazos F, et al. Prevalence of acromegaly in patients with symptoms of sleep apnea. PLoS One. 2017;12(9):e0183539.
55. Young T, Finn L, Peppard PE, Szklo-Coxe M, Austin D, Nieto FJ, et al. Sleep disordered breathing and mortality: eighteen-year follow-up of the Wisconsin sleep cohort. Sleep. 2008;31(8):1071–8.
56. Nagappa M, Liao P, Wong J, Auckley D, Ramachandran SK, Memtsoudis S, et al. Validation of the STOP-Bang Questionnaire as a screening tool for obstructive sleep apnea among different populations: a systematic review and meta-analysis. PLoS One. 2015;10(12):e0143697.
57. Netzer NC, Stoohs RA, Netzer CM, Clark K, Strohl KP. Using the Berlin Questionnaire to identify patients at risk for the sleep apnea syndrome. Ann Intern Med. 1999;131(7):485–91.
58. Young T, Skatrud J, Peppard PE. Risk factors for obstructive sleep apnea in adults. JAMA. 2004;291(16):2013–6.
59. Rosenow F, Reuter S, Deuss U, Szelies B, Hilgers RD, Winkelmann W, et al. Sleep apnoea in treated acromegaly: relative frequency and predisposing factors. Clin Endocrinol (Oxf). 1996;45(5):563–9.
60. Turan O, Akinci B, Ikiz AO, Itil O, Oztura I, Ada E, et al. Airway and sleep disorders in patients with acromegaly. Clin Respir J. 2018;12(3):1003–10.
61. Kashine S, Kishida K, Funahashi T, Shimomura I. Characteristics of sleep-disordered breathing in Japanese patients with acromegaly. Endocr J. 2012;59(1):31–8.

62. Kovaleva YA, Dreval AV, Kulakov NV, Fedorova SI, Ilovayskaya IA. Prevalence and risk factors of sleep breathing disorders in patients with acromegaly from Moscow region. Ter Arkh. 2018;90(10):65–70.
63. Lavrentaki A, Ali A, Cooper B, Tahrani A. Mechanisms of disease: the endocrinology of obstructive sleep apnoea. Eur J Endocrinol. 2019;180(3):R91–125.
64. Addy TM, Hafler J, Galerneau F. Faculty development for fostering clinical reasoning skills in early medical students using a modified bayesian approach. Teach Learn Med. 2016;28(4):415–23.
65. Centurion SA, Schwartz RA. Cutaneous signs of acromegaly. Int J Dermatol. 2002;41(10):631–4.
66. Kamenicky P, Blanchard A, Frank M, Salenave S, Letierce A, Azizi M, et al. Body fluid expansion in acromegaly is related to enhanced epithelial sodium channel (ENaC) activity. J Clin Endocrinol Metab. 2011;96(7):2127–35.
67. Moller J. Growth hormone and fluid homeostasis. Front Horm Res. 2005;33:161–84.
68. Vilar L, Vilar CF, Lyra R, Lyra R, Naves LA. Acromegaly: clinical features at diagnosis. Pituitary. 2017;20(1):22–32.
69. Mazziotti G, Lania AGA, Canalis E. Management of endocrine disease: bone disorders associated with acromegaly: mechanisms and treatment. Eur J Endocrinol. 2019;181(2):R45–56.
70. Dostalova S, Sonka K, Smahel Z, Weiss V, Marek J. Cephalometric assessment of cranial abnormalities in patients with acromegaly. J Craniomaxillofac Surg. 2003;31(2):80–7.
71. Herrmann BL, Mortsch F, Berg C, Weischer T, Mohr C, Mann K. Acromegaly: a cross-sectional analysis of the oral and maxillofacial pathologies. Exp Clin Endocrinol Diabetes. 2011;119(1):9–14.
72. Hochban W, Ehlenz K, Conradt R, Brandenburg U. Obstructive sleep apnoea in acromegaly: the role of craniofacial changes. Eur Respir J. 1999;14(1):196–202.
73. Cadieux RJ, Kales A, Santen RJ, Bixler EO, Gordon R. Endoscopic findings in sleep apnea associated with acromegaly. J Clin Endocrinol Metab. 1982;55(1):18–22.
74. Pelttari L, Polo O, Rauhala E, Vuoriluoto J, Aitasalo K, Hyyppa MT, et al. Nocturnal breathing abnormalities in acromegaly after adenomectomy. Clin Endocrinol (Oxf). 1995;43(2):175–82.
75. Guo X, Gao L, Zhao Y, Wang M, Jiang B, Wang Q, et al. Characteristics of the upper respiratory tract in patients with acromegaly and correlations with obstructive sleep apnoea/hypopnea syndrome. Sleep Med. 2018;48:27–34.
76. Somers VK, White DP, Amin R, Abraham WT, Costa F, Culebras A, et al. Sleep apnea and cardiovascular disease: an American Heart Association/american College Of Cardiology Foundation Scientific Statement from the American Heart Association Council for High Blood Pressure Research Professional Education Committee, Council on Clinical Cardiology, Stroke Council, and Council On Cardiovascular Nursing. In collaboration with the National Heart, Lung, and Blood Institute National Center on Sleep Disorders Research (National Institutes of Health). Circulation. 2008;118(10):1080–111.
77. Otto ME, Belohlavek M, Romero-Corral A, Gami AS, Gilman G, Svatikova A, et al. Comparison of cardiac structural and functional changes in obese otherwise healthy adults with versus without obstructive sleep apnea. Am J Cardiol. 2007;99(9):1298–302.
78. Yaffe K, Laffan AM, Harrison SL, Redline S, Spira AP, Ensrud KE, et al. Sleep-disordered breathing, hypoxia, and risk of mild cognitive impairment and dementia in older women. JAMA. 2011;306(6):613–9.
79. Yeh NC, Tien KJ, Yang CM, Wang JJ, Weng SF. Increased risk of Parkinson's disease in patients with obstructive sleep apnea: a population-based, propensity score-matched, longitudinal follow-up study. Medicine (Baltimore). 2016;95(2):e2293.
80. Yaggi HK, Concato J, Kernan WN, Lichtman JH, Brass LM, Mohsenin V. Obstructive sleep apnea as a risk factor for stroke and death. N Engl J Med. 2005;353(19):2034–41.
81. Lin Z, Si Q, Xiaoyi Z. Obstructive sleep apnoea in patients with epilepsy: a meta-analysis. Sleep Breath. 2017;21(2):263–70.
82. Bucks RS, Olaithe M, Eastwood P. Neurocognitive function in obstructive sleep apnoea: a meta-review. Respirology. 2013;18(1):61–70.

83. Reutrakul S, Mokhlesi B. Obstructive sleep apnea and diabetes: a state of the art review. Chest. 2017;152(5):1070–86.
84. Santos M, Hofmann RJ. Ocular Manifestations of Obstructive Sleep Apnea. J Clin Sleep Med. 2017;13(11):1345–8.
85. Gupta MA, Simpson FC. Obstructive sleep apnea and psychiatric disorders: a systematic review. J Clin Sleep Med. 2015;11(2):165–75.
86. Martinez-Garcia MA, Campos-Rodriguez F, Barbe F. Cancer and OSA: current evidence from human studies. Chest. 2016;150(2):451–63.
87. Shepherd KL, James AL, Musk AW, Hunter ML, Hillman DR, Eastwood PR. Gastro-oesophageal reflux symptoms are related to the presence and severity of obstructive sleep apnoea. J Sleep Res. 2011;20(1 Pt 2):241–9.
88. Sanna A. Obstructive sleep apnoea, motor vehicle accidents, and work performance. Chron Respir Dis. 2013;10(1):29–33.
89. Orme SM, McNally RJ, Cartwright RA, Belchetz PE. Mortality and cancer incidence in acromegaly: a retrospective cohort study. United Kingdom Acromegaly Study Group. J Clin Endocrinol Metab. 1998;83(8):2730–4.
90. Fatti LM, Scacchi M, Pincelli AI, Lavezzi E, Cavagnini F. Prevalence and pathogenesis of sleep apnea and lung disease in acromegaly. Pituitary. 2001;4(4):259–62.
91. Epstein LJ, Kristo D, Strollo PJ Jr, Friedman N, Malhotra A, Patil SP, et al. Clinical guideline for the evaluation, management and long-term care of obstructive sleep apnea in adults. J Clin Sleep Med. 2009;5(3):263–76.
92. Vannucci L, Luciani P, Gagliardi E, Paiano S, Duranti R, Forti G, et al. Assessment of sleep apnea syndrome in treated acromegalic patients and correlation of its severity with clinical and laboratory parameters. J Endocrinol Invest. 2013;36(4):237–42.
93. Grunstein RR, Ho KY, Berthon-Jones M, Stewart D, Sullivan CE. Central sleep apnea is associated with increased ventilatory response to carbon dioxide and hypersecretion of growth hormone in patients with acromegaly. Am J Respir Crit Care Med. 1994;150(2):496–502.
94. Badr MS, Dingell JD, Javaheri S. Central sleep apnea: a brief review. Curr Pulmonol Rep. 2019;8(1):14–21.

Chapter 7
Cardiovascular Pathology in Acromegaly

Adnan Ajmal

Background

Excess of growth hormone [GH] and insulin-like growth factor [IGF-1] exerts regulatory effects on the cardiovascular system [CV] through autocrine and paracrine mechanisms, leading to structural and functional abnormalities in the heart and causing impairment of the vascular system [1]. Acromegaly is associated with increased cardiovascular morbidity and mortality [2] through the complex interplay of elevated GH/IGF-1 levels, which exerts direct effects on the heart via GH and IGF-1 receptors on the cardiac myocytes and indirectly through increasing the prevalence of traditional CV risks, like hypertension [HTN], insulin resistance, and hyperlipidemia. This interaction between direct affect and traditional CV risks manifests itself as cardiomyopathy especially left ventricular [LV] hypertrophy and diastolic dysfunction, valvular heart defects especially mitral and aortic regurgitation, arrythmias, atherosclerotic arterial disease including coronary artery disease [CAD], and cerebrovascular disease [CVD].

Acromegalic cardiomyopathy, defined as hyperkinetic syndrome followed by concentric biventricular hypertrophy, diastolic dysfunction, and eventually diastolic heart failure with preserved systolic function, is the classic initial presentation. Its prevalence increases with age and long-standing disease but even shorter exposure to GH and IGF-1 excess leads to structural heart changes [1]. Cardiomyopathy is aggravated by concomitant presence of hypertension, which has a prevalence of almost 50% in acromegaly patients, but acromegalic cardiomyopathy is also seen without hypertension [1, 3]. Diastolic dysfunction, in the context of cardiomyopathy, is also very prevalent in acromegaly patients and progresses to diastolic heart failure, if mitigation strategies are not implemented early enough to control

A. Ajmal (✉)
Department of Endocrinology, Cleveland Clinic Abu Dhabi, Abu Dhabi,
United Arab Emirates
e-mail: ajmala@clevelandclinicabudhabi.ae

L. S. Blevins Jr., M. K. Aghi (eds.), *Acromegaly*, Contemporary Endocrinology,
https://doi.org/10.1007/978-3-031-16258-9_7

coexisting hypertension and valvular heart disease. This is a vicious cycle in which ventricular remodeling aggravates valvular regurgitation, which in turn worsens ventricular hypertrophy [2]. This is worth mentioning that the prevalence of CAD reaches almost 100% in patients with hypertension and diabetes mellitus [1]. Cardiomyopathy, ischemic cardiac disease and higher prevalence of hypertension, diabetes mellitus, hyperlipidemia, and obstructive sleep apnea [OSA] account for almost 60% of deaths in this cohort [3]. Autopsy studies have confirmed the presence of increased LV mass, myocardial fibrosis, and myocardial ischemia [4].

The pathogenesis of CAD in acromegaly is very complex, and the fundamental question remains unanswered that either it is excess GH/IGF per se, contributing to development of atherosclerotic arterial disease, or it is the increased prevalence of classic risk factors like HTN, DM, or hyperlipidemia, which we see in acromegaly. Acromegaly patients stratified based on Framingham's score [FS] and Agatston score [AS] have shown that 41% of these patients have increased atherosclerosis risk, but control of acromegaly did not decrease this high risk [5]. It is also not very clear if increased prevalence of atherosclerotic arterial disease increases mortality in acromegaly. Animal studies have shown higher mortality in acromegaly is due to cardiomyopathy rather than CAD [2]. Studies have shown that cardiovascular mortality is improved with effective control of GH/IGF excess and associated CV risk factors, like diabetes mellitus, hypertension, and hyperlipidemia, but its effect on morbidity remains unclear. Moreover, it is also not very clear who is at higher risk to get severe ischemic CV events and should be stratified, as one prospective study has shown low CAD risk in acromegaly with no one getting severe ischemic events, but other study predicted an increased risk of lethal ischemic event when AS was >400, though overall incidence of lethal events remained low [6].

Pathogenesis

Acromegalic Cardiomyopathy

Left ventricular hypertrophy with a prevalence of 36–80% and diastolic dysfunction with prevalence of 29–40% are the most common morphologic and functional manifestations of acromegalic cardiomyopathy, respectively [7], with age, basal metabolic index [BMI], and disease duration being the biggest predictors [8] of acromegaly cardiomyopathy.

Myocyte growth and function, cardiac contractility, and vascular function are effected in acromegaly [9]. On cellular level, the milieu of excess GH and increased IGF-1 expression causes increased amino-acid/protein synthesis, increase in myocyte size, and expression of cardiac muscle contractile gene [9]. Intracellular calcium concentrations rise with an increase in calcium sensitivity of cardiac myofilaments by the upregulation of GH/IGF receptors on cardiomyocytes altering cardiac contractility, leading to concentric hypertrophy and positive ionotropic affect in the early phase of this process [1, 3]. A pro-inflammatory and proatherogenic environment is created through GH-mediated increase in LDL-C, oxidized LDL, and endothelin I expression, leading to insulin resistance causing endothelial injury [2]. Cardiac fibrosis is a very peculiar feature of this cardiomyopathy. Underlying histology is consistent with interstitial fibrosis, which happens through deposition of extracellular collagen matrix, myofibrillary derangements, infiltration of lymphomononuclear cells, and necrosis. Focal fibrosis gives rise to slow and nonhomogeneous conduction pathways [1, 3], eventually leading to diastolic dysfunction and heart failure with preserved ejection fraction. Progression to systolic dysfunction and clinical heart failure are rarely seen in acromegaly [~2–10%]. Though cardiomyopathy is more prevalent in older patients with longer duration of disease younger patients with short-term exposure are also not immune to it.

Classic acromegalic cardiomyopathy has a prevalence of 70–90% and consists of three distinct phases. (1) Hyperkinetic phase presents early in the course of disease process after initial exposure to high IGF-1/GH concentrations, leading to concentric hypertrophy, increase myocardial contractility, and higher heart rate with increase cardiac output. (2) As ventricular hypertrophy worsens, there is decrease in diastolic filling and shortening of LV ejection period, leading to systolic dysfunction with exercise. (3) The last phase is mostly seen in patients who remain undiagnosed for an extended period of time or have uncontrolled disease [3]. In this scenario, there is significant systolic and diastolic dysfunction at rest with low cardiac output and finally development of congestive heart failure [CHF]. Though both ventricles are affected, LV and interventricular septal hypertrophy are more pronounced. Left ventricular mass is shown to increase from young to older acromegalics overtime [1], and the presence of HTN and other classic cardiac risk factors aggravate this process. Concomitant presence of HTN significantly increases the prevalence of LV hypertrophy but later can happen without the presence of HTN [10]. Decrease in GH/IGF levels leads to improvement in diastolic dysfunction, but improvement in systolic dysfunction and exercise tolerance is variable and depends on associated risk factors like the presence of HTN and duration of disease [2].

In addition to ventricular hypertrophy, we also see dysregulation of cardiac water balance leading to cardiac edema [3] consequently seen as higher T2 values on cardiac MRI. Cardiac edema has an important prognostic value, and as it improves promptly during the treatment of acromegaly, it ascribes itself higher sensitivity than left ventricular mass index in detecting early reversal of cardiomyopathy [11].

The underlying extensive interstitial fibrosis due to myocardial necrosis is unique to acromegalic cardiomyopathy, which leads to abnormal ventricular relaxation times. As isovolumetric relaxation is prolonged, we see decrease in transvalvular flow velocities with a 19% risk of developing regurgitant valvular disease per year [9].

Hypertension

Hypertension is the most prevalent cardiovascular comorbidity found in acromegaly patients with metanalysis of several studies showing a mean prevalence of 35% with a range of 18–60% [3, 12]. Difference in prevalence is likely related to various methods of measurement, which range from conventional sphygmomanometer measurement of blood pressure [BP] to 24-h ambulatory blood pressure measurement [ABPM] and various cutoffs used for systolic and diastolic BP [3, 12]. In one study, a difference in prevalence of 42.5% vs. 17.5% was observed between clinical measurement and 24-h ABPM, respectively [13]. In addition to the difference in measurement techniques and criteria used, several other factors, like age, gender, age at diagnosis, and pituitary hormone status, and additional CV risk factors, like insulin resistance, obesity, and smoking, affect the prevalence of HTN in acromegaly [12, 14]. Though there is no direct correlation found between HTN and GH/IGF-1 levels, control of disease by surgical, medical, and radiologic approach has shown to significantly improve systolic and diastolic BP, suggesting the role of chronic GH/IGF-1 exposure [12]. Interestingly, a pooled study has shown a positive relationship between HTN and high IGF-1 levels in uncontrolled disease [15]. Concurrent presence of HTN increases the risk of LVH as compared to patients with uncomplicated acromegaly [75% vs. 37.2%] [12].

As far as pathogenesis of hypertension is concerned, several mechanisms could be responsible, including plasma volume expansion, direct GH/IGF-1 action on vascular system, renin-angiotensin-aldosterone system [RAAS] activation, reduction of atrial natriuretic peptide secretion, increased sympathetic tone, hyperinsulinemia, and cardiac dyskinesia (Fig. 7.1) [12].

As cardiac output increases in the initial phase of acromegalic cardiomyopathy, two other concomitant processes likely contribute to the development of hypertension, including activation of renal and extrarenal epithelial sodium channels, causing volume expansion and increased peripheral resistance due to endothelial dysfunction [3, 16]. Endothelial dysfunction is assessed by some of the invasive techniques showing increased arterial pulse wave velocity, which is a surrogate marker of arterial stiffness, and decreased volume-mediated dilation of brachial artery, which signals endothelial dysfunction from hypertrophic remodeling of the arteries [17]. Multiple studies have shown vascular dysfunction in acromegaly and report increased intima-media thickness and decreased cardio-ankle vascular index [2].

GH and IGF receptors are also expressed in kidneys. IGF-1 increases Na absorption through distal tubular Na channels, and GH increases GFR and renal plasma flow, leading to increased total and exchangeable Na levels in the body causing plasma expansion [12, 18]. Exchangeable Na is correlated positively with GH/IGF-1 level and HTN. Treatment has shown to reduce Na levels as GH/IGF-1 level

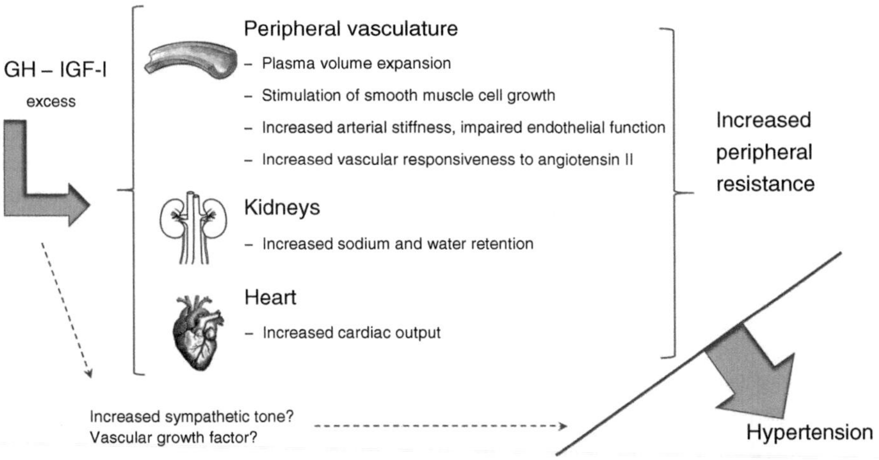

Fig. 7.1 Mechanisms involved in development of hypertension. ([Used with permission from Springer Nature]. *Ramos-Leví AM, Marazuela M. Cardiovascular comorbidities in acromegaly: an update on their diagnosis and management. Endocrine. 2017 Feb;55(2):346–359. https://doi.org/10.1007/s12020-016-1191-3. Epub 2017 Jan 2. PMID: 28042644)*

decrease [19]. As far as activation of RAAS is concerned, it seems to be related to acromegaly-related changes in plasma volume rather than an independent event, though there is evidence of direct GH-related secretion of aldosterone through its effect on adrenal cortex [12, 20].

Homeostatic model assessment for insulin resistance [HOMA-IR] studies have shown decrease insulin sensitivity in acromegaly leading to hyperinsulinemia [21]. How hyperinsulinemia contributes to the development of HTN is not fully understood. Hyperinsulinemia can cause activation of RAAS, vascular hypertrophy, endothelial dysfunction, and increased peripheral resistance, but it is increased sympathetic tone that likely plays a dominant role [12, 22].

Circadian catecholamine rhythm is disturbed in acromegaly. One study has shown lack of normal circadian norepinephrine rhythm and flat BP and norepinephrine profiles in untreated acromegaly with restoration of normal rhythm and BP profiles in cured patients [23]. An increased prevalence of OSA in acromegaly, which is reported to be around 60–75%, also leads to increased urinary catecholamine metabolites, and there is "non-dipper" pattern seen in acromegalics, where there is lack of nocturnal fall in BP contributing to insulin resistance, in turn altering sympathetic tone [24, 25]. Taken together, increase plasma volume, insulin resistance, and OSA contribute to the development of HTN, by altering the 24-h catecholamine profile [12].

During the early phase of increased GH/IGF-1 exposure, there is an increase in plasma flow, which contributes to cardiac hyperkinesia and eventually leads to the development of HTN [12].

Coronary Arterial Disease

Development of atherosclerotic arterial disease in acromegaly, causing CAD and CVD, is complex, and data is limited and mix. Different national registries have shown a prevalence of 5–12% [3]. Then, there is the presence of traditional CV risk factors, like impaired glucose tolerance, hypertension, and hyperlipidemia, and direct effects of GH/IGF-1 excess on function and morphology of vascular system, which play a role [26]. Risk stratification based on FS and AS has shown an increased risk of atherosclerosis of 40–50% in acromegaly patients, but prospective studies have shown lower CV risk with none of the patients having major CV events in 5 years of follow-up [5, 26]. Similar findings are reported in another study where low AS were noted in acromegaly patients as compared to the general population with risk not changing over 5 years of follow-up [27]. The German Acromegaly Registry found that incidence of MI and stroke is not higher in acromegaly patients as compared to the general population but found higher prevalence of HTN and DM in patients who suffered MI and stroke [26]. There is no relationship found between radiation treatment and risk of stroke [28].

One study looked at the relationship between major adverse cardiac events [MACE] and traditional risk factors in acromegaly. Uncontrolled disease is strongly associated with the development of DM, but the prevalence of MACE and HTN is increased in older patients with smoking having a positive significant correlation [29]. A MACE prevalence of 8.5% at baseline and incidence of 11.8% during study period was found [29]. We would have expected DM to lead to a higher incidence of atherosclerosis in acromegaly, but we are not seeing it, and one possible mechanism is that acromegaly patients develop impaired glucose tolerance at a younger age and low BMI, as compared to the general population, and presumably the relationship between DM and atherosclerotic arterial disease is different in acromegaly patients in comparison to the general population [26].

Difference in these findings could be related to various study populations used with treatment-naïve, resistant, and untreated patients and treated patients with various modalities, where some of the traditional risks are expected to improve. To overcome this heterogeneity, one study looked at treatment-naïve patients with 7 years of disease and found CV risk to be low based on the Systemic Coronary Risk Evaluation project of the European Society of Cardiology [ESC] classification in majority of the patients [5]. AS correlated with ESC, and majority of the patients have no detectable calcium. AS was higher in patients with strong FH of CAD, suggesting transitional risks playing a role rather than excess GH/IGF-1 per se [5]. Authors went on to propose that GH/IGF-1 might have a protective role rather than promoting atherosclerosis, and indirect evidence comes from GHD patients, who have adverse CV risk profile and early atherosclerosis [5].

Arrythmias

Acromegaly patients have an increased risk to develop arrhythmias with a prevalence of 7–40%, and especially important is increased QT dispersion in this group, leading to malignant ventricular arrythmias [30]. Additionally, supraventricular tachycardia, atrial fibrillation, sick sinus syndrome, bundle branch block, and complex ventricular arrhythmias are also common and mostly occur during physical exercise [3, 31] and increase risk for sudden cardiac death in acromegaly [30]. Pathogenesis of these rhythm abnormalities is multifactor, as acromegaly causes cardiac autonomic nervous system dysfunction, leading to increased heart rate variability, and this affect is compounded by the presence of OSA which leads to arrythmias [32]. Complex ventricular arrythmias are related to the duration of disease and LVH with a prevalence of 48% [31]. As acromegaly induced cardiomyopathy sets in and areas of myocardial necrosis and eventually fibrosis develop risk of slowing and inhomogeneous conduction in cardiac circuits increases. Moreover, we see the development of late potentials, with a prevalence of 56% which increases risk for ventricular tachyarrhythmias [1, 3]. There is prolongation of QT interval, which creates an arrhythmogenic environment [33], along with direct effects of excess GH/IGF-1 on cardiac synchronicity, leading to left ventricular dyssynchrony, and it is independent of other risk factors ,like age of onset or duration of disease [3].

Valvular Heart Disease

Almost 20% of the acromegaly patients have some degree of valvular involvement, with mitral and aortic valve dysfunction being the most common. Valvular disease worsens with disease duration, and a case-control study has shown 19% increase in odds every year [34]. GH regulates extracellular matrix, and chronic excess leads to ring fragility and leaflet disarray by way of increased metalloproteinases expression, proteoglycans synthesis, and collagen deposition. Valvular regurgitations further worsen LVH, arrythmias, and heart failure [3].

Diagnostic Evaluation

There is no consensus on timing and sequence of diagnostic modalities used in the evaluation of cardiovascular complications of acromegaly, but prompt diagnosis is of paramount importance in reversing the course of cardiovascular morbidity and decreasing mortality. In this section, we will address individual complications and risk factors with corresponding diagnostic workup (Table 7.1).

Table 7.1 Cardiovascular comorbidities/risk factors and diagnostic workup ([Used with permission from Springer Nature]. *Ramos-Leví AM, Marazuela M. Cardiovascular comorbidities in acromegaly: an update on their diagnosis and management. Endocrine. 2017 Feb;55(2):346–359. https://doi.org/10.1007/s12020-016-1191-3. Epub 2017 Jan 2. PMID: 28042644)*

Hypertension	• Office manual blood pressure measurement
	• Repeated home blood pressure measurement
	• 24 h Ambulatory BP Monitoring
	• Automated Office BP measurement
Cardiomyopathy	• Single clinic 12-lead ECG
	• 24 h Holter ECG monitoring
	• Exercise, treadmill, or stress tolerance test
	• Echocardiography
	• Cardiac magnetic resonance imaging
Heart valve disease	• Exercise or stress tolerance test
	• Echocardiography
	• Cardiac magnetic resonance imaging
Arrhythmias	• Single clinic 12-lead ECG
	• 24 h Holter ECG monitoring
	• Exercise, treadmill, or stress tolerance test
Atherosclerosis and coronary artery disease	• Exercise, treadmill, or stress tolerance test
	• Ultrasound and duplex study of carotid and supraaortic trunk
	• Intima-media thickness measurement
	• Quantification of internal carotid stenosis
	• Number, morphology, and surface characteristics of carotid plaques
	• Other specific baseline and dynamic tests (computed tomography angiography, coronary catheterization, positron-emitted tomography)

HTN

As HTN is very prevalent in acromegaly and aggravates cardiomyopathy, early detection and aggressive management could be very beneficial. It can simply start with office measurement of BP during clinic visit, followed by either advising patients to keep a home log of BP or arranging for 24-h ABPM [3] because office measurement can overestimate HTN due to "white coat" phenomenon. In one study, elevated BP diagnosed by ABPM was positively associated with cardiomyopathy on echocardiogram [35].

Cardiomyopathy

An early noninvasive echocardiography will reveal the extent of cardiomyopathy along with state of cardiac fibrosis, valvular dysfunction, and diastolic function [3]. Interventricular septum and posterior wall thickness, LV ejection fraction, and LV mass index can be measured [10]. Dopplers studies can assess the functional status by measuring ventricular filling by measuring isovolumetric relaxation times [IVRT] and ratio of maximal early-to-late diastolic flow velocities across the mitral valve [E/A] [10].

As concomitant presence of HTN and IGT/DM significantly increases prevalence of LVH, impaired diastolic filling and systolic function only at rest and it can go undetected initially. Pulse tissue Doppler can help detect subclinical biventricular systolic dysfunction [3].

Echocardiography is noninvasive and readily available, but it has its limitations in measuring cardiac function due to intra- and interobserver variability and has low sensitivity in calculating LV ejection fraction. In such scenarios where suspicion is high, radionuclide angiography can be used to assess cardiac performance [36]. Radionuclide angiography has shown significant decrease in LV systolic function and diastolic filing with increased duration of acromegaly especially in older patients [36].

Gadolinium-enhanced MRI is gold standard in assessment of acromegalic cardiomyopathy giving a superior estimate of cardiac structure and function due to its higher accuracy and reproducibility [37]. Myocardial fibrosis is another typical feature of acromegalic cardiomyopathy, and myocardial T1 mapping gives an estimate of extracellular volume fraction, which is a marker of interstitial fibrosis [37]. Myocardial transverse relaxation time gives more accurate assessment of direct effects of GH/IGF-1 on myocardial tissue by measuring cardiac edema, which improves early during treatment [3]. As we mentioned above, myocardial transverse relaxation time is more sensitive than LV mass index in the assessment of efficacy of acromegaly treatment [3].

Arrythmias

Though most of the arrythmias in acromegaly can be of low clinical significance, a baseline ECG and subsequent 24-h Holter monitoring in select cases can prevent future complications. Prolongation in QT interval and development of late potentials increase risk of clinically significant arrythmias, but there are currently no guidelines to register them as their prognostic importance is not well-known [3].

Atherosclerotic Arterial Disease

Currently, there are no guidelines to develop a special assessment and surveillance program to look at CV status of acromegaly patients apart from what is needed in the presence of traditional cardiac risk factors [3], as development of atherosclerotic disease is complex and multifactor in acromegaly. In special circumstances, it is helpful to identify vascular dysfunction by measuring carotid intima-media thickness, flow-mediated dilatation of brachial A, cardio-ankle flow index, CT angiography, and cardiac catheterization [3].

Treatment of Cardiovascular Complications in Acromegaly

Aims of acromegaly therapy go beyond biochemical control of hormone hypersecretion and include amelioration of cardiovascular dysfunction along with improving traditional cardiovascular risks, like HTN, glucose intolerance, and hyperlipidemia. As we mentioned earlier LV hypertrophy and diastolic dysfunction are the most prevalent manifestations of acromegaly cardiomyopathy, response to therapy can be assessed by LV mass index and ventricular filling capacity with later measured by E/A ratio and isovolumetric relaxation time [38].

Acromegaly is associated with increased mortality rate due to cardiovascular and cerebrovascular factors. Historically, standardized mortality ratio [SMR] of 2–3 were reported, but with multimodal therapy with surgery, medications, and radiation treatment, SMR of 0.7–1.7 is now noticed in recent studies [7]. In spite of this reduction in SMR, risk of death is still higher than the general population, and cardiovascular events remain the main cause of death [39]. Control of acromegaly achieving GH <1 and normalization of IGF-1 has shown to arrest progression of cardiovascular complications, both morphologic and functional [3]. Improvement in survival curves comparable to the general population was achieved with control of excess GH and IGF-1, where before disease control higher mortality was reported. In another study, uncontrolled acromegaly was associated with higher prevalence of DM and HTN, which in term lead to higher morbidity and mortality [29]. It is imperative that in addition to controlling GH hypersecretion, traditional CV risks are also addressed.

Now it is worth mentioning that in an apparent paradox, not all cardiovascular complications uniformly improve with normalization of hormone hypersecretion, and some comorbidities get better with treatment of acromegaly without normalization of GH/IGF. HTN is the most prevalent cardiovascular risk and does not always improve with treatment of acromegaly, in which case it is treated as conventionally as in patients without acromegaly. Acromegaly cardiomyopathy worsens with disease duration and increasing age, and early intervention has shown better outcomes. Valvular heart disease seems to be irreversible, and optimal control of acromegaly only prevents progression.

When we compare outcomes of various therapies, it becomes apparent that there is heterogeneity in results. Transsphenoidal surgery improves LV mass index along with diastolic dysfunction and ejection fraction. Somatostatin analogs [SSA] also improve LV mass index and diastolic dysfunction, but the effect on BP is not profound. Addition of GH receptor antagonist in patients with resistance to SSA shows more profound effect ameliorating various manifestations of cardiovascular dysfunction, including LV mass index, systolic and diastolic functions, BP, and improvement in FS [7].

Acromegaly patients have a higher prevalence of DM [20–35%] and HTN [30–40%] when compared to the general population [40]. There is some evidence that chronic exposure to elevated GH/IGF leads to permanent changes in insulin production and sensitivity and irreversible damage to endothelial function [40].

Though surgical cure or pharmacologic control offers improvement in comparison to uncontrolled disease, the prevalence of DM and HTN stays higher than the general population [40–42]. Pharmacotherapy with SSA has a more complex effect on metabolic function in comparison to surgery. Growth hormone/IGF-1 excess increases insulin resistance, leading to impaired glucose tolerance, impaired fasting glucose, and frank DM. Somatostatin analog therapy is reported to have a mild net deteriorating effect on glucose homeostasis, as, on one hand, it improves sensitivity by lowering GH/IGF-1 levels but, on the other hand, it has a inhibitory effect on insulin release [43, 44]. It is important to mention that in spite of this overall outcome, patients are at increased risk of hypoglycemia with SSA therapy, especially if DM is treated with secretagogues or insulin [43, 45].

Transsphenoidal Surgery

As first-line treatment, transsphenoidal surgery offers biochemical remission in 45–80% patients with acromegaly. One study showed that in well-controlled patients, LV mass index and diastolic indices like E/A and IVRT improved and systolic BP decreased significantly [46]. This benefit on LV hypertrophy and diastolic filling is present in patients who receive only transsphenoidal surgery and is independent of direct effects of SSA therapy [47]. Surgery has also shown to improve cardiac performance measured by radionuclide angiography as LV ejection fraction at peak exercise [36].

Somatostatin Analogs

SSA therapy is shown to rapidly improve LV hypertrophy. Slow-release octreotide [OCT-LAR] significantly reduced LV mass index, interventricular septal thickness, and LV posterior wall thickness in all patients treated for 3–6 months, with more than 50% patients showing normalizing of LV hypertrophy [48]. Diastolic dysfunction also improves, as measured by decrease ratio of E-wave and A-waves of peak velocities across the mitral valve [E/A] [49]. These effects are maintained in long-term treatment, and 5 years of primary SSA therapy with octreotide LAR or lanreotide has shown significant improvements in the prevalence of HTN, arrythmias, LV hypertrophy, and diastolic and systolic dysfunctions [50].

Improvement in BP is not as uniform as improvement in acromegaly cardiomyopathy. There is likely an independent SSA effect on cardiac morphology, as some studies have not shown significant lowering of BP [49].

Twelve months of SSA therapy improved LV hypertrophy in 100% of young and 50% of middle age patients with improvement in EF in 80% young and 50% middle-aged patients [38, 51]. Young participant also showed improvements in exercise capacity and duration [51]. In patients who have partial response to SSA therapy, there is still improvement in LVH and diastolic dysfunction, but interestingly the prevalence of these disorders doesn't decrease highlighting a couple of points: one being likely direct effect on cardiac myocytes through GH/IGF receptors and second through decrease in GH/IGF-1 level [38]. As far as insulin and glucose metabolism is concerned, results from various studies are discordant with dominant effect being the modest negative affect. One large study has shown that in comparison with surgery, SSA therapy also improves metabolic parameters, including A1c and fasting glucose, as long as disease control is achieved [52]. This observation brings home the issue of long-term biochemical control of acromegaly with SSA therapy.

GHR Antagonists

Acromegalics have a higher prevalence of cardiac arrythmias, mostly ventricular arrythmias, and these complex ventricular arrythmias are related to duration of disease and LV hypertrophy [31]. Though SSA therapy is shown to decrease HR by lowering IGF-1 levels and its affect is more pronounced than surgery, likely from the direct effect on cardiac myocytes SA node, native somatostatin is known to increase the QT interval. It is important to know that GH receptor antagonist pegvisomant is not arrhythmogenic and decreases HR measured by Holter monitoring [31]. Pegvisomant has more potent effect on IGF-1 excess and subsequently causes decrease in LV mass, which is correlated with minimal, maximal, and mean HR in short term and long term [31]. Literature also shows that GHR antagonist-mediated normalization of IGF-1 also decreases the prevalence of rhythm abnormalities.

In addition to the benefits on cardiac rhythm problems, using GH receptor antagonist therapy in SSA-resistant patients improves the LV mass index and cardiac performance. In spite of the initial response to SSA therapy, ~25% patients develop a partial to complete resistance, and in such cases, addition of pegvisomant has shown to improve the CV and metabolic outcomes, and likely there is a role for direct affect through GH receptors on cardiomyocytes [38]. One study has shown that combined therapy for 60 months has shown to decrease the prevalence of metabolic syndrome and significantly improved LV mass index, ejection fraction, E/A ratio, and IVRT [38].

Summary

Early detection and treatment of cardiovascular risk factors and comorbidities in acromegaly patients prevent irreversible cardiac morphologic and functional changes and help decrease CV mortality directly by cardiac remodeling and indirectly by lowering GH and normalizing IGF-1 levels [53, 54] (Table 7.2). Somatostatin analogs have the unique ability to induce cardiac remodeling through direct effects on cardiomyocytes. Before therapy is considered, either surgery or pharmacotherapy, baseline parameters can be established. For metabolic

Table 7.2 Cardiovascular outcomes after treatment ([Used with permission from Springer Nature]. *Ramos-Leví AM, Marazuela M. Cardiovascular comorbidities in acromegaly: an update on their diagnosis and management. Endocrine. 2017 Feb;55(2):346–359. https://doi.org/10.1007/s12020-016-1191-3. Epub 2017 Jan 2. PMID: 28042644)*

↓ Blood pressure
↓ Left ventricular mass
↑ Diastolic function
↑ Left ventricular ejection fraction
↓ Heart rate
↓ Ventricular ectopic beats
↓ QT interval duration
↓ Intima-media thickness
Improvement of obstructive sleep apnea, improvement of lipid profile, change in glucose status (SSA have double effect, pegvisomant improves, cabergoline is neutral)

↓ decrease; ↑ increase

parameters, glucose tolerance, hemoglobin A1c, insulin levels, and HOMA-IR should be measured. Cardiac morphology and function can be estimated by measuring LV mass index, E/A, and valvular dysfunction. Blood pressure and heart rate should be assessed at rest and with exercise. After surgery with and without somatostatin analog therapy, all metabolic and cardiac parameters improve except valvular regurgitation and morphology. Glucose tolerance mostly remains unchanged.

References

1. Lombardi G, Galdiero M, Auriemma RS, Pivonello R, Colao A. Acromegaly and the cardiovascular system. Neuroendocrinology. 2006;83(3–4):211–7.
2. Fleseriu M. Insight into cardiovascular risk factors in patients with acromegaly. Endocrine. 2014;47(1):1–2.
3. Ramos-Levi AM, Marazuela M. Cardiovascular comorbidities in acromegaly: an update on their diagnosis and management. Endocrine. 2017;55(2):346–59.
4. Gadelha MR, Kasuki L, Lim DST, Fleseriu M. Systemic complications of acromegaly and the impact of the current treatment landscape: an update. Endocr Rev. 2019;40(1):268–332.
5. Akutsu H, Kreutzer J, Wasmeier G, Ropers D, Rost C, Mohlig M, et al. Acromegaly per se does not increase the risk for coronary artery disease. Eur J Endocrinol. 2010;162(5):879–86.
6. Ragonese M, Alibrandi A, Di Bella G, Salamone I, Puglisi S, Cotta OR, et al. Cardiovascular events in acromegaly: distinct role of Agatston and Framingham score in the 5-year prediction. Endocrine. 2014;47(1):206–12.
7. Ioachimescu AG. Impact of acromegaly treatment on cardiovascular complications. Endocrine. 2017;55(3):659–61.
8. Guo X, Gao L, Zhang S, Li Y, Wu Y, Fang L, et al. Cardiovascular system changes and related risk factors in acromegaly patients: a case-control study. Int J Endocrinol. 2015;2015:573643.
9. Sharma AN, Tan M, Amsterdam EA, Singh GD. Acromegalic cardiomyopathy: epidemiology, diagnosis, and management. Clin Cardiol. 2018;41(3):419–25.
10. Colao A, Baldelli R, Marzullo P, Ferretti E, Ferone D, Gargiulo P, et al. Systemic hypertension and impaired glucose tolerance are independently correlated to the severity of the acromegalic cardiomyopathy. J Clin Endocrinol Metab. 2000;85(1):193–9.

11. Gouya H, Vignaux O, Le Roux P, Chanson P, Bertherat J, Bertagna X, et al. Rapidly reversible myocardial edema in patients with acromegaly: assessment with ultrafast T2 mapping in a single-breath-hold MRI sequence. AJR Am J Roentgenol. 2008;190(6):1576–82.
12. Bondanelli M, Ambrosio MR, degli Uberti EC. Pathogenesis and prevalence of hypertension in acromegaly. Pituitary. 2001;4(4):239–49.
13. Minniti G, Moroni C, Jaffrain-Rea ML, Bondanini F, Gulino A, Cassone R, et al. Prevalence of hypertension in acromegalic patients: clinical measurement versus 24-hour ambulatory blood pressure monitoring. Clin Endocrinol (Oxf). 1998;48(2):149–52.
14. Ezzat S, Forster MJ, Berchtold P, Redelmeier DA, Boerlin V, Harris AG. Acromegaly. Clinical and biochemical features in 500 patients. Medicine (Baltimore). 1994;73(5):233–40.
15. Schutte AE, Volpe M, Tocci G, Conti E. Revisiting the relationship between blood pressure and insulin-like growth factor-1. Hypertension. 2014;63(5):1070–7.
16. Kamenicky P, Viengchareun S, Blanchard A, Meduri G, Zizzari P, Imbert-Teboul M, et al. Epithelial sodium channel is a key mediator of growth hormone-induced sodium retention in acromegaly. Endocrinology. 2008;149(7):3294–305.
17. Rizzoni D, Porteri E, Giustina A, De Ciuceis C, Sleiman I, Boari GE, et al. Acromegalic patients show the presence of hypertrophic remodeling of subcutaneous small resistance arteries. Hypertension. 2004;43(3):561–5.
18. Hansen TK, Moller J, Thomsen K, Frandsen E, Dall R, Jorgensen JO, et al. Effects of growth hormone on renal tubular handling of sodium in healthy humans. Am J Physiol Endocrinol Metab. 2001;281(6):E1326–32.
19. Davies DL, Beastall GH, Connell JM, Fraser R, McCruden D, Teasdale GM. Body composition, blood pressure and the renin-angiotensin system in acromegaly before and after treatment. J Hypertens Suppl. 1985;3(3):S413–5.
20. Lin CJ, Mendonca BB, Lucon AM, Guazzelli IC, Nicolau W, Villares SM. Growth hormone receptor messenger ribonucleic acid in normal and pathologic human adrenocortical tissues—an analysis by quantitative polymerase chain reaction technique. J Clin Endocrinol Metab. 1997;82(8):2671–6.
21. Kasayama S, Otsuki M, Takagi M, Saito H, Sumitani S, Kouhara H, et al. Impaired beta-cell function in the presence of reduced insulin sensitivity determines glucose tolerance status in acromegalic patients. Clin Endocrinol (Oxf). 2000;52(5):549–55.
22. Ikeda T, Terasawa H, Ishimura M, Ochi H, Ohtani I, Fujiyama K, et al. Correlation between blood pressure and plasma insulin in acromegaly. J Intern Med. 1993;234(1):61–3.
23. Bondanelli M, Ambrosio MR, Franceschetti P, Margutti A, Trasforini G, Degli Uberti EC. Diurnal rhythm of plasma catecholamines in acromegaly. J Clin Endocrinol Metab. 1999;84(7):2458–67.
24. Elmasry A, Lindberg E, Hedner J, Janson C, Boman G. Obstructive sleep apnoea and urine catecholamines in hypertensive males: a population-based study. Eur Respir J. 2002;19(3):511–7.
25. Grunstein RR, Ho KY, Sullivan CE. Sleep apnea in acromegaly. Ann Intern Med. 1991;115(7):527–32.
26. Schofl C, Petroff D, Tonjes A, Grussendorf M, Droste M, Stalla G, et al. Incidence of myocardial infarction and stroke in acromegaly patients: results from the German Acromegaly Registry. Pituitary. 2017;20(6):635–42.
27. Bogazzi F, Battolla L, Spinelli C, Rossi G, Gavioli S, Di Bello V, et al. Risk factors for development of coronary heart disease in patients with acromegaly: a five-year prospective study. J Clin Endocrinol Metab. 2007;92(11):4271–7.
28. Flickinger JC, Nelson PB, Taylor FH, Robinson A. Incidence of cerebral infarction after radiotherapy for pituitary adenoma. Cancer. 1989;63(12):2404–8.
29. Sardella C, Cappellani D, Urbani C, Manetti L, Marconcini G, Tomisti L, et al. Disease activity and lifestyle influence comorbidities and cardiovascular events in patients with acromegaly. Eur J Endocrinol. 2016;175(5):443–53.
30. Unubol M, Eryilmaz U, Guney E, Ture M, Akgullu C. QT dispersion in patients with acromegaly. Endocrine. 2013;43(2):419–23.

31. Auriemma RS, Pivonello R, De Martino MC, Cudemo G, Grasso LF, Galdiero M, et al. Treatment with GH receptor antagonist in acromegaly: effect on cardiac arrhythmias. Eur J Endocrinol. 2013;168(1):15–22.
32. Chemla D, Attal P, Maione L, Veyer AS, Mroue G, Baud D, et al. Impact of successful treatment of acromegaly on overnight heart rate variability and sleep apnea. J Clin Endocrinol Metab. 2014;99(8):2925–31.
33. Breitschaft A, Hu K, Darstein C, Ligueros-Saylan M, Jordaan P, Song D, et al. Effects of subcutaneous pasireotide on cardiac repolarization in healthy volunteers: a single-center, phase I, randomized, four-way crossover study. J Clin Pharmacol. 2014;54(1):75–86.
34. Pereira AM, van Thiel SW, Lindner JR, Roelfsema F, van der Wall EE, Morreau H, et al. Increased prevalence of regurgitant valvular heart disease in acromegaly. J Clin Endocrinol Metab. 2004;89(1):71–5.
35. Costenaro F, Martin A, Horn RF, Czepielewski MA, Rodrigues TC. Role of ambulatory blood pressure monitoring in patients with acromegaly. J Hypertens. 2016;34(7):1357–63.
36. Colao A, Cuocolo A, Marzullo P, Nicolai E, Ferone D, Della Morte AM, et al. Is the acromegalic cardiomyopathy reversible? Effect of 5-year normalization of growth hormone and insulin-like growth factor I levels on cardiac performance. J Clin Endocrinol Metab. 2001;86(4):1551–7.
37. dos Santos Silva CM, Gottlieb I, Volschan I, Kasuki L, Warszawski L, Balarini Lima GA, et al. Low frequency of cardiomyopathy using cardiac magnetic resonance imaging in an acromegaly contemporary cohort. J Clin Endocrinol Metab. 2015;100(12):4447–55.
38. Auriemma RS, Grasso LF, Galdiero M, Galderisi M, Pivonello C, Simeoli C, et al. Effects of long-term combined treatment with somatostatin analogues and pegvisomant on cardiac structure and performance in acromegaly. Endocrine. 2017;55(3):872–84.
39. Mercado M, Gonzalez B, Vargas G, Ramirez C, de los Monteros AL, Sosa E, et al. Successful mortality reduction and control of comorbidities in patients with acromegaly followed at a highly specialized multidisciplinary clinic. J Clin Endocrinol Metab. 2014;99(12):4438–46.
40. Gonzalez B, Vargas G, de Los Monteros ALE, Mendoza V, Mercado M. Persistence of diabetes and hypertension after multimodal treatment of acromegaly. J Clin Endocrinol Metab. 2018;103(6):2369–75.
41. Carmichael JD, Broder MS, Cherepanov D, Chang E, Mamelak A, Said Q, et al. The association between biochemical control and cardiovascular risk factors in acromegaly. BMC Endocr Disord. 2017;17(1):15.
42. Jonas C, Maiter D, Alexopoulou O. Evolution of glucose tolerance after treatment of acromegaly: a study in 57 patients. Horm Metab Res. 2016;48(5):299–305.
43. Tolis G, Angelopoulos NG, Katounda E, Rombopoulos G, Kaltzidou V, Kaltsas D, et al. Medical treatment of acromegaly: comorbidities and their reversibility by somatostatin analogs. Neuroendocrinology. 2006;83(3–4):249–57.
44. Gerich JE. Role of somatostatin and its analogues in the pathogenesis and treatment of diabetes mellitus. Metabolism. 1990;39(9 Suppl 2):52–4.
45. Lehnert H, Beyer J, Weber P, Krause U, Schrezenmeir J. Treatment of severe reactive hypoglycemia with a somatostatin analogue (SMS 201-995). Arch Intern Med. 1990;150(11):2401–2.
46. Minniti G, Moroni C, Jaffrain-Rea ML, Esposito V, Santoro A, Affricano C, et al. Marked improvement in cardiovascular function after successful transsphenoidal surgery in acromegalic patients. Clin Endocrinol (Oxf). 2001;55(3):307–13.
47. Colao A, Pivonello R, Galderisi M, Cappabianca P, Auriemma RS, Galdiero M, et al. Impact of treating acromegaly first with surgery or somatostatin analogs on cardiomyopathy. J Clin Endocrinol Metab. 2008;93(7):2639–46.
48. Colao A, Marzullo P, Ferone D, Spinelli L, Cuocolo A, Bonaduce D, et al. Cardiovascular effects of depot long-acting somatostatin analog Sandostatin LAR in acromegaly. J Clin Endocrinol Metab. 2000;85(9):3132–40.
49. Maison P, Tropeano AI, Macquin-Mavier I, Giustina A, Chanson P. Impact of somatostatin analogs on the heart in acromegaly: a metaanalysis. J Clin Endocrinol Metab. 2007;92(5):1743–7.

50. Colao A, Auriemma RS, Galdiero M, Lombardi G, Pivonello R. Effects of initial therapy for five years with somatostatin analogs for acromegaly on growth hormone and insulin-like growth factor-I levels, tumor shrinkage, and cardiovascular disease: a prospective study. J Clin Endocrinol Metab. 2009;94(10):3746–56.
51. Colao A, Ferone D, Marzullo P, Cappabianca P, Cirillo S, Boerlin V, et al. Long-term effects of depot long-acting somatostatin analog octreotide on hormone levels and tumor mass in acromegaly. J Clin Endocrinol Metab. 2001;86(6):2779–86.
52. Giordano C, Ciresi A, Amato MC, Pivonello R, Auriemma RS, Grasso LF, et al. Clinical and metabolic effects of first-line treatment with somatostatin analogues or surgery in acromegaly: a retrospective and comparative study. Pituitary. 2012;15(4):539–51.
53. Colao A. 5 Long-term acromegaly and associated cardiovascular complications: a case-based review. Best Pract Res Clin Endocrinol Metab. 2009;23(Suppl 1):S31–8.
54. Colao A, Marzullo P, Cuocolo A, Spinelli L, Pivonello R, Bonaduce D, et al. Reversal of acromegalic cardiomyopathy in young but not in middle-aged patients after 12 months of treatment with the depot long-acting somatostatin analogue octreotide. Clin Endocrinol (Oxf). 2003;58(2):169–76.

Chapter 8
Diabetes Mellitus in Acromegaly

Samina Afreen

Epidemiology

Disorders of glucose metabolism are frequently associated with acromegaly [1]. The prevalence of glucose intolerance in acromegaly has been reported to range between 19% and 56% in various studies, and up to 20% may have diabetes at diagnosis [1].

Glucose homeostasis is related to disease activity in acromegaly, as higher insulin-like growth factor-1 (IGF-I) concentrations were found associated with lower insulin sensitivity [2]. Age and positive family history for diabetes mellitus were found to be independently associated with impairment of glucose metabolism in acromegaly [2].

Pathogenesis of Diabetes in Acromegaly

Insulin resistance is the state whereby the cells of the liver, muscle, and adipose tissue fail to respond to insulin, thereby leading to increased glucose synthesis and decreased glucose uptake and metabolism. Excess growth hormone (GH) leads to insulin resistance in the liver, muscle, and the adipose tissues. The main driving factor for the increased insulin resistance in acromegaly is the increased lipolysis induced by the excess GH in the circulation [2]. The increased free fatty acids (FFA) in the cells leads to post-receptor defect in insulin signaling cascade [3–5].

S. Afreen (✉)
Center for Diabetes and Endocrine Health, Allegheny Clinic, Erie, PA, USA

L. S. Blevins Jr., M. K. Aghi (eds.), *Acromegaly*, Contemporary Endocrinology,
https://doi.org/10.1007/978-3-031-16258-9_8

Excess Growth Hormone Leads to Increased Lipolysis

In adipocytes, lipolysis is a highly regulated process involving hormonal signals, lipid droplet-associated proteins, and lipases. Complete hydrolysis of triglycerides (TG) to FFAs and glycerol requires three consecutive steps that involve different enzymes: adipose triglyceride lipase (ATGL), hormone-sensitive lipase (HSL), and monoacylglycerol lipase. ATGL is the rate-limiting enzyme for lipolysis in adipocytes, catalyzing the first step of hydrolysis of TG to diacylglycerol and FFA, [6–11].

Interaction of GH with its receptor (GHR) results in dimerization of GHR, followed by tyrosine phosphorylation of GHR and Janus activating kinase 2 (JAK2). Activated JAK2 leads to the activation of several signaling pathways, including the signal transducer and activator of transcription (STATs), extracellular signal-regulated kinases (ERK)1/2, and phosphatidylinositol 3-kinase (PI3K)/Akt pathways [12].

The activation of the MEK–ERK pathway causes phosphorylation of peroxisome proliferator-activated receptor-γ (PPARγ), resulting in PPARγ inactivation. PPARγ inactivation leads to the downregulation of fat-specific protein 27 (FSP27) in adipocytes [13].

FSP27 is a protein present in adipocytes, which interacts with ATGL and inhibits ATGL-mediated lipolysis. FSP27 downregulation, caused by PPARγ inactivation, increases lipolysis [6].

Parallel to the above pathway, GH binding to its receptors also activates signal transducer and activator of transcription 5 (STAT5), which is a positive regulator of PPARγ, but the MEK–ERK activation pathway predominates to inactivate PPARγ [13].

In addition, GH induces lipolysis by activating HSL and by increasing the de novo expression of HSL mRNA via the activation of protein kinase C and ERK [13].

Increased Free Fatty Acids Interfere with Insulin Signaling Pathway

Insulin normally binds to the insulin receptor and activates PI3K and, subsequently, AKT. AKT then inhibits GSK-3β by phosphorylation [14]. GSK-3β normally phosphorylates and inactivates glycogen synthase (GS). Inhibition of GSK-3β activates glycogen synthase [14].

Excess FFAs interfere with the insulin signaling pathway. They inhibit insulin receptor substrate (IRS-1) and PI3K in the skeletal muscle and liver, thereby leading to inhibition of AKT and subsequently inactivation of glycogen synthase, thereby decreasing glycogen synthesis [15].

But the inhibition of AKT in the skeletal muscle and liver also leads to reduced GLUT4 translocation [16, 17]. In adipose tissue, negative regulation of

PI3K-dependent insulin signaling leads to decreased expression of the GLUT1 and GLUT4 as well [16–18]. Inhibition of GLUTs in muscle, liver, and adipose tissues leads to decrease in uptake of glucose by the peripheral tissues.

Increased Free Fatty Acids Promote Gluconeogenesis and Inhibit Glycolysis

GH by stimulating lipolysis provides FFAs and glycerol to serve as metabolic substrates for gluconeogenesis [19]. In the hepatocytes, the increase in GH-induced FFA uptake leads to an increase in lipid oxidation and accumulation of acetyl coenzyme A. Acetyl coenzyme A stimulates enzymes that participate in gluconeogenesis, such as pyruvate carboxylase and phosphoenolpyruvate carboxykinase. Acetyl coenzyme A also stimulates the glucose 6 phosphatase, which increases the release of glucose in the liver [15, 20]. Additionally, GH inhibits insulin-induced suppression of hepatic gluconeogenesis [21].

FFAs released from fat stores compete with pyruvate substrates, to serve as energy source, thereby inhibiting the glycolytic pathway and inhibiting glucose disposal in peripheral tissues [2].

Increased Expression of Pro-inflammatory Adipokines and Cytokines

Acromegaly is also associated with decreased expression of the insulin-sensitizing adipokine, adiponectin, and increased circulating concentrations of the pro-inflammatory adipokine, visfatin [2]. In addition, GH excess in acromegaly increases the expression of pro-inflammatory cytokines within the adipose tissue. These are linked to enhanced inflammation and insulin resistance [2].

β-Cell Dysfunction

GH-induced insulin resistance is followed by compensatory hyperfunction of β cells, which aims at maintaining euglycemia [2, 20, 22].

Over time, chronic insulin resistance and fatty acid-induced lipotocixity eventually lead to β-cell dysfunction with failure to fully counterbalance the increased needs for insulin secretion [2, 20, 22].

Abnormal glucose tolerance develops in patients with acromegaly with concomitant β-cell insufficiency [23], and a proportion of patients (19–38%) develop overt diabetes mellitus [23].

Treatment

The risk of diabetes mellitus is higher in biochemically uncontrolled patients compared to their controlled counterparts [24]. Surgical cure of acromegaly improves insulin sensitivity and lowers circulating glucose and insulin concentrations [2].

However, unlike other comorbidities associated with acromegaly, glucose disorders are higher in acromegaly patients even after treatment, in comparison to the general population. Hence, glucose disorders should be monitored closely on a long-term basis after the control of GH hypersecretion [25].

Choice of Therapy for Acromegaly

Transsphenoidal surgical adenomectomy establishes "safe" GH levels in less than 50% of patients with a macroadenoma [26–29]. External beam pituitary irradiation, although an effective adjunctive treatment, works slowly [26–29]. Hence, many patients, who are not cured by surgery or who are awaiting the effects of pituitary irradiation, require medical therapy to control the GH/IGF-I axis. Current options for medical therapy include dopamine agonists (cabergoline) and somatostatin analogs (SSA), (octreotide, lanreotide, pasireotide) and GH receptor antagonist, pegvisomant (PEGV) [29].

SSAs bind to somatostatin receptors in the pituitary adenoma, leading to decrease in GH secretion and consequently improvement in insulin sensitivity [30]. However, they also exert a concomitant nonspecific inhibitory effect on insulin, glucagon, and gastrointestinal hormone secretion, with a net balance leaning toward a deterioration in glucose homeostasis [30, 31].

As a result, insulin secretagogues (and/or insulin) should probably be preferred to insulin sensitizers in patients with acromegaly developing diabetes while on somatostatin analogs [30].

Among the SSAs, the affinity with which octreotide and lanreotide bind to the somatostatin (sst) receptors differs as compared to pasireotide. Octreotide and lanreotide bind with high affinity to sst2 only, have moderate affinity to sst3 and sst5, and show very low or absent binding to sst1 and sst4 [32]. Pasireotide binds with high affinity to all somatostatin receptors, except sst4 [33]. In contrast to octreotide, pasireotide exhibits particular high affinity to sst5 [34].

Sst2 receptors are expressed mainly on pancreatic α cells, and sst5 are expressed mainly on β cells [35, 36].

The higher incidence and greater degree of severity of hyperglycemia and diabetes with pasireotide as compared to octreotide and lanreotide are due to the greater affinity of pasireotide to sst5 receptors that are present on pancreatic β cells. Thus, the greater increase in blood glucose levels during pasireotide treatment appears to result from greater suppression of insulin secretion.

Unlike SSAs that target the pituitary gland, PEGV works peripherally by blocking the GH receptor, thereby decreasing IGF-I [31]. A key difference between SSAs and PEGV is their effect on glycemic control. PEGV improves insulin sensitivity by blocking the effects of excess GH on insulin action [31]. This may be an important consideration in selecting medical therapy in patients with glucose intolerance or type 2 diabetes mellitus, in whom PEGV might be a better choice.

Treatment of Diabetes in Patients with Acromegaly

Cases of euglycemic diabetic ketoacidosis (EuDKA) with sodium glucose cotransporter 2 inhibitors (SGLT2is) used for accompanying diabetes mellitus have been reported in patients with unrecognized acromegaly [37].

A suggested potential mechanism for SGLTis induction of EuDKA is that renal glucose losses due to SGLT2is result in decreased insulin secretion, which is followed by decreased paracrine intraislet insulin inhibition of glucagon secretion. Glucagon secretion is further stimulated by decreased α-cell glucose uptake resulting from SGLT2 inhibition [35]. Increased glucagon-to-insulin ratio leads to increase in ketogenesis through enhanced fat oxidation [36]. In addition to increased production, diminished renal ketone-body elimination occurs during SGLT2 inhibition [38–40].

If SGLT2i are started in mildly ketonemic state such as is present in uncontrolled acromegaly, mild ketonemia may rapidly progress to ketoacidosis within a few days. Owing to ongoing renal glucose wasting, this progression occurs in the presence of only mildly elevated glucose levels [41].

Interestingly, a reciprocal positive interaction is achieved with SGLT2is in combination with SSAs and PEGV in patients with acromegaly complicated with diabetes [35].

Hyperinsulinemia has a negative effect upon normalizing IGF-I levels [35]. Higher normalization rates of IGF-I levels were achieved in patients without diabetes as compared to those with diabetes, when treated with SSAs, alone or in combination with PEGV [42]. The German cohort of the ACROSTUDY showed that patients with acromegaly and diabetes achieved lower response with PEGV and required a higher dose of PEGV for IGF-I normalization, especially in those treated with insulin [43].

The use of SGLT2is results in significant fall in insulin levels. This fall in insulin level might promote an additive effect by decreasing hepatic GH receptor expression and further suppression of IGF-I levels in patients already under treatment with long-acting somatostatin analogs (LA-SSAs), with or without PEGV [35].

On the one hand, SGLT-2is attenuate the hyperglycemic effect induced by decreased insulin secretion due to SSA therapy; on the other hand, SSAs in combination with PEGV attenuate the hyperglucagonemia induced by SGLT2is [35]. PEGV via peripheral (extrahepatic) suppression of GHR in different tissues decreases lipid oxidation [44]. These mechanisms of action are supposed to minimize the appearance of EuDKA [35].

Hence, SGLT-2is can be recommended for the management of uncontrolled diabetes mellitus in patients with acromegaly already under treatment with PEGV monotherapy or in combination with SSAs [35]. Treatment with SGLT2is in this group of patients can be initiated after metformin monotherapy or metformin in combination with dipeptidyl peptidase inhibitors (DDP-4is) or glucagon-like peptide-1 receptor (GLP-1R) agonists [35].

Treatment with SGLT2is is contraindicated in patients with acromegaly with type 1 diabetes mellitus and in patients with secondary diabetes due to unrecognized acromegaly [35].

Precautions should be taken in patients with long duration of diabetes and acromegaly. SGLT2is might be considered in this category after laboratory evaluation for β-cell reserve including C-peptide levels and islets cell antibodies for those with suspected latent autoimmune diabetes in adults (LADA) [35].

The appearance of EuDKA in patients with already diagnosed and treated acromegaly, using SGLT2is, seems to be rare, particularly in patients treated with PEGV as monotherapy or in combination with LA-SSAs, where the potential mechanisms for this complication are attenuated [35].

Control of GH excess usually results in improved glucose metabolism, and insulin therapy could be withdrawn during follow-up in most patients with an initial ketoacidotic presentation [45].

References

1. Shekhawat VS, Bhansali S, Dutta P, Mukherjee KK, Vaiphei K, Kochhar R, et al. Glucose-dependent insulinotropic polypeptide resistance and beta cell dysfunction contribute to hyperglycaemia in acromegaly. Sci Rep. 2019;9:5646.
2. Vila G, Jørgensen JOL, Luger A, Stalla GK. Insulin resistance in patients with acromegaly. Front Endocrinol (Lausanne). 2019;10:509.
3. Muggeo M, Saviolakis GA, Businaro V, Valerio A, Moghetti P, Crepaldi G. Insulin receptor on monocytes from patients with acromegaly and fasting hyperglycemia. J Clin Endocrinol Metab. 1983;56:733–8.
4. Hansen I, Tsalikian E, Beaufrere B, Gerich J, Haymond M, Rizza R. Insulin resistance in acromegaly: defects in both hepatic and extrahepatic insulin action. Am J Physiol. 1986;250:E269–73.
5. Popovic V, Korbonits M, editors. Metabolic syndrome consequent to endocrine disorders. Front Horm Res, vol. 49. Basel: Karger; 2018. p. 20–8.
6. Grahn THM, Kaur R, Yin R, Schweiger M, Sharma VM, Lee MJ, et al. Fat-specific protein 27 (FSP27) interacts with adipose triglyceride lipase (ATGL) to regulate lipolysis and insulin sensitivity in human adipocytes. J Biol Chem. 2014;289(17):12029–39.
7. Zechner R, Zimmermann R, Eichmann TO, Kohlwein SD, Haemmerle G, Lass A, et al. Fat signals—lipases and lipolysis in lipid metabolism and signaling. Cell Metab. 2012;15:279–91.
8. Villena JA, Roy S, Sarkadi-Nagy E, Kim KH, Sul HS. Desnutrin, an adipocyte gene encoding a novel patatin domain-containing protein, is induced by fasting and glucocorticoids: ectopic expression of desnutrin increases triglyceride hydrolysis. J Biol Chem. 2004;279:47066–75.

9. Zimmermann R, Strauss JG, Haemmerle G, Schoiswohl G, Birner-Gruenberger R, Riederer M, et al. Fat mobilization in adipose tissue is promoted by adipose triglyceride lipase. Science. 2004;306:1383–6.
10. Ahmadian M, Wang Y, Sul HS. Lipolysis in adipocytes. Int J Biochem Cell Biol. 2010;42:555–9.
11. Jenkins CM, Mancuso DJ, Yan W, Sims HF, Gibson B, Gross RW. Identification, cloning, expression, and purification of three novel human calcium independent phospholipase A2 family members possessing triacylglycerol lipase and acylglycerol transacylase activities. J Biol Chem. 2004;279:48968–75.
12. Xu J, Keeton AB, Franklin JL, Li X, Venable DY, Frank SJ, et al. Insulin enhances growth hormone induction of the MEK/ERK signaling pathway. J Biol. 2006;281:982–92.
13. Kopchick JJ, Berryman DE, Puri V, Kevin YL, Jorgensen JOL. The effects of growth hormone on adipose tissue: old observations, new mechanisms. Nat Rev Endocrinol. 2010;16:135–46.
14. Arneth B, Arneth R, Shams M. Metabolomics of type 1 and type 2 diabetes. Int J Mol Sci. 2019;20(10):2467.
15. Garmes HM, Castillo AR. Insulin signaling in the whole spectrum of GH deficiency. Arch Endocrinol Metab. 2019;63(6):582–91.
16. Dresner A, Laurent D, Marcucci M, Griffin ME, Dufour S, Cline GW, et al. Effects of free fatty acids on glucose transport and IRS-1-associated phosphatidylinositol 3-kinase activity. J Clin Invest. 1999;103:253–9.
17. Aguirre V, Uchida T, Yenush L, Davis R, White MF. The c-Jun NH2-terminal kinase promotes insulin resistance during association with insulin receptor substrate-1 and phosphorylation of Ser307. J Biol Chem. 2000;275:9047–54.
18. Kilgour E, Baldwin SA, Flint DJ. Divergent regulation of rat adipocyte GLUT1 and GLUT4 glucose transporters by GH. J Endocrinol. 1995;145:27–33.
19. Barkan AL, Burman P, Clemmons DR, Drake WM, Gagel RF, Harris PE, et al. Glucose homeostasis and safety in patients with acromegaly converted from long-acting octreotide to pegvisomant. J Clin Endocrinol Metab. 2005;90(10):5684–91.
20. Kovacs P, Stumvoll M. Fatty acids and insulin resistance in muscle and liver. Best Pract Res Clin Endocrinol Metab. 2005;19:625–35.
21. Clemmons DR. The relative roles of growth hormone and IGF-1 in controlling insulin sensitivity. J Clin Invest. 2004;113:25–7.
22. Defronzo RA, Banting lecture. From the triumvirate to the ominous octet: a new paradigm for the treatment of type 2 diabetes mellitus. Diabetes. 2009;58:773–95.
23. Kasayama S, Otsuki M, Takagi M, Saito H, Sumitani S, Kouhara H, et al. Impaired beta-cell function in the presence of reduced insulin sensitivity determines glucose tolerance status in acromegalic patients. Clin Endocrinol. 2000;52:549–55.
24. Carmichael JD, Broder MS, Cherepanov D, Chang E, Mamelak A, Said Q, et al. The association between biochemical control and cardiovascular risk factors in acromegaly. BMC Endocr Disord. 2017;17(1):15.
25. Rochelle C, Graillon T, Albarel F, Morange I, Dufour H, Brue T, et al. Increased risk of persistent glucose disorders after control of acromegaly. J Endocr Soc. 2017;1(12):1531–9.
26. Freda PU, Wardlaw SL, Post KD. Long-term endocrinological follow-up evaluation in 115 patients who underwent transsphenoidal surgery for acromegaly. J Neurosurg. 1998;89:353–8.
27. Eastman RC, Gorden P, Roth J. Conventional supervoltage irradiation is an effective treatment for acromegaly. J Clin Endocrinol Metab. 1979;48:931–40.
28. Biermasz NR, van Dulken H, Roelfsema F. Long-term follow-up results of postoperative radiotherapy in 36 patients with acromegaly. J Clin Endocrinol Metab. 2000;85:2476–82.
29. Drake WM, Rowles SV, Roberts ME, et al. Insulin sensitivity and glucose tolerance improve in patients with acromegaly converted from depot octreotide to pegvisomant. Eur J Endocrinol. 2003;149:521–7.
30. Tolis G, Angelopoulos NG, Katounda E, Rombopoulos G, Kaltzidou V, Kaltsas D, et al. Medical treatment of acromegaly: comorbidities and their reversibility by somatostatin analogs. Neuroendocrinology. 2006;83:249–57.

31. Ghigo E, Biller BMK, Colao A, Kourides IA, Rajicic N, Hutson RK, et al. Comparison of pegvisomant and long-acting octreotide in patients with acromegaly naïve to radiation and medical therapy. J Endocrinol Invest. 2009;32(11):924–33.
32. Lesche S, Lehmann D, Nagel F, Schmid HA, Schulz S. Differential effects of octreotide and pasireotide on somatostatin receptor internalization and trafficking in vitro. J Clin Endocrinol Metab. 2009;94(2):654–61.
33. Lewis I, Bauer W, Albert R, Chandramouli N, Pless J, Weckbecker G, et al. A novel somatostatin mimic with broad somatotropin release inhibitory factor receptor binding and superior therapeutic potential. J Med Chem. 2003;46:2334–44.
34. Ma P, Wang Y, Hoek JVD, Nedelman J, Schran H, Tran LL, et al. Pharmacokinetic-pharmacodynamic comparison of a novel multiligand somatostatin analog, SOM230, with octreotide in patients with acromegaly. Clin Pharmacol Ther. 2005;78:69–80.
35. Adnan Z. Sodium glucose co-transporter inhibitors in patients with acromegaly and diabetes. Trends Endocrinol Metab. 2019;30(2):77–9.
36. Unger N, Ueberberg B, Schulz S, Saeger W, Mann K, Petersenn S. Differential expression of somatostatin receptor subtype 1-5 proteins in numerous human normal tissues. Exp Clin Endocrinol Diabetes. 2012;120:482–9.
37. Quarella M, Walser D, Brandle M, Fournier JY, Bilz S. Rapid onset of diabetic ketoacidosis after SGLT2 inhibition in a patient with unrecognized acromegaly. J Clin Endocrinol Metab. 2017;102(5):1451–3.
38. Cozzolino A, Feola T, Simonelli I, Puliani G, Pozza C, Giannetta E, et al. Somatostatin analogs and glucose metabolism in acromegaly: a meta-analysis of prospective interventional studies. J Clin Endocrinol Metab. 2018;103:2089–99.
39. Gadelha MR, Bronstein MD, Brue T, Coculescu M, Fleseriu M, Guitelman M, et al. Pasireotide versus continued treatment with octreotide or lanreotide in patients with inadequately controlled acromegaly (PAOLA): a randomised, phase 3 trial. Lancet Diabetes Endocrinol. 2004;2:875–84.
40. Zinman B, Wanner C, Lachin JM, Fitchett D, Bluhmki E, Hantel, et al. Empagliflozin, cardiovascular outcomes, and mortality in type 2 diabetes. N Engl J Med. 2015;373:2117–28.
41. Ferrannini E, Muscelli E, Frascerra S, Baldi S, Mari A, Heise T, et al. Metabolic response to sodium glucose cotransporter 2 inhibition in type 2 diabetic patients. J Clin Invest. 2014;124:499–508.
42. van der Lely AJ, Bernabeu I, Cap J, Caron P, Colao A, Marek J, et al. Coadministration of lanreotide Autogel and pegvisomant normalizes IGF1 levels and is well tolerated in patients with acromegaly partially controlled by somatostatin analogs alone. Eur J Endocrinol. 2011;164:325–33.
43. Droste M, Domberg J, Buchfelder M, Mann K, Schwanke A, Stalla G, et al. Therapy of acromegalic patients exacerbated by concomitant type 2 diabetes requires higher pegvisomant doses to normalise IGF1 levels. Eur J Endocrinol. 2014;171:59–68.
44. Neggers SJ, Kopchick JJ, Jørgensen JOL, van der Lely AJ. Hypothesis: extra-hepatic acromegaly: a new paradigm? Eur J Endocrinol. 2011;164:11–6.
45. Yoshida N, Goto H, Suzuki H, Nagasawa K, Takeshita A, Okubo M, et al. Ketoacidosis as the initial clinical condition in nine patients with acromegaly: a review of 860 cases at a single institute. Eur J Endocrinol. 2013;169(1):127–32.

Chapter 9
Musculoskeletal Disorders of Acromegaly

Jill B. Feffer

The musculoskeletal system is affected by growth hormone (GH) excess in many ways. Downstream effects of GH excess are mediated by both endocrine and paracrine IGF-1. Patients with acromegaly are at increased risk for conditions known to increase fracture risk especially type 2 diabetes mellitus and hypogonadism. In addition, both systemic and local IGF-1 affect bone health. Systemic IGF-1 is produced by the liver and accelerates bone remodeling in two ways: (1) increasing anabolic activity via osteoblast differentiation and production of osteoprotegerin and (2) activating osteoclasts via production of RANK ligand [1]. Paracrine IGF-1 causes chondrocyte proliferation, joint space widening, and periarticular ligament laxity [1, 2]. GH also increases activity of 1-α-hydroxylase, thereby depleting its substrate 25-hydroxy vitamin D and causing hypercalciuria [3].

Multiple studies confirm associations between active acromegaly and decreased trabecular areal bone density [4, 5]. Some support increase in cortical bone density including the femur, a site classified in research settings as a hybrid with some trabecular and some cortical bone [4, 6]. Mazziotti et al. reported increasing risk of vertebral fracture among male patients, particularly those with active acromegaly and longer disease duration, while Bonadonna et al. reported fracture risk is increased among postmenopausal women commensurate with time since menopause onset [7, 8]. Mazziotti et al. also reported that acromegaly increases prevalence of vertebral facture prevalence tenfold, with patients suffering from active acromegaly having a risk more than twice as high as those achieving biochemical control [9]. Fortunately, bisphosphonates reduce incident vertebral fractures in patients with active acromegaly [10].

Patients with acromegaly commonly complain of joint pain due to accelerated development of degenerative osteoarthritis, especially in the larger joints, and hypermobility [11–13]. The sacroiliac joint is often involved, resulting in stiffness

J. B. Feffer (✉)
Division of Endocrinology, Diabetes and Metabolism, NYU Grossman School of Medicine, New York, NY, USA

L. S. Blevins Jr., M. K. Aghi (eds.), *Acromegaly*, Contemporary Endocrinology,
https://doi.org/10.1007/978-3-031-16258-9_9

and reduced range of motion that mimics the inflammatory arthritis of ankylosing spondylitis [14]. Degenerative arthritis can progress to diffuse idiopathic skeletal hypertrophy (DISH), resulting in chronic pain and motor deficits [15]. Bony overgrowth and soft tissue hypertrophy cause nerve entrapment including carpal and the more specific cubital tunnel syndromes [13, 16]. Patients with acromegaly experience temporomandibular joint dysfunction and obstructive sleep apnea and are, consequently, three times more likely than the general population to die from respiratory compromise due to upper airway obstruction [17].

Initial treatment is transsphenoidal resection of the causative pituitary adenoma. The likelihood of remission after surgery negatively correlates with tumor size [18]. In two series, 75–81.8% of patients with GH-secreting microadenomas achieved biochemical remission after surgery; this rate dropped to 45.8–48% for GH-secreting macroadenomas [19, 20]. Remission is defined as 3-month postoperative bloodwork showing age-appropriate normal IGF-1 and random GH < 1 μg/L. If disease activity is detected after surgery, external beam radiation can be utilized to target residual tumor, and systemic treatment can be initiated using one or a combination of somatostatin receptor ligands (octreotide, lanreotide, pasireotide), dopamine agonists (bromocriptine, cabergoline), or a GH receptor antagonist (pegvisomant).

These therapies can normalize biomarkers of acromegaly and hypercalciuria, but symptoms and skeletal complications may not follow suit [21]. For example, Boswell found that 70% of patients still complained of joint pain and/or had radiologic evidence of osteoarthritis 10 years after onset of acromegaly [12, 21]. Similarly, Geer et al. reported that in a cohort averaging 9 years post-surgery maintained on systemic therapy, 76% and 57% of patients still experienced soft tissue swelling and carpal tunnel syndrome, respectively, with majorities complaining that the symptoms are constant [22]. DISH has even been diagnosed after 30 years of remission [23]. Notably, the risk of vertebral fracture conferred by acromegaly does not decrease to that of age-adjusted controls even 3 years later [24]. This risk does not correlate with presence of osteopenia or osteoporosis on DEXA bone density scan [1, 8]. The presence of hypogonadism in male patients and presence of adrenal insufficiency each further increase fracture risk in patients with controlled acromegaly [10]. Additionally, residual symptoms of joint and back pain continue to adversely impact quality of life [22, 25].

Overall, musculoskeletal disorders of acromegaly are pervasive and can be insidious in onset. Healthcare providers must therefore maintain a high index of suspicion and should screen patients with acromegaly at diagnosis and repeatedly for symptoms of musculoskeletal complications including fracture, arthritis, soft tissue swelling, carpal tunnel syndrome, and obstructive sleep apnea. Unfortunately, biochemical remission may not resolve all symptoms so screening should continue indefinitely and comorbidities may need to be directly treated. The high prevalence of morphometric vertebral fractures in patients with active acromegaly supports implementation of screening x-ray of the thoracic and lumbar spine at diagnosis for all patients, regardless of presence or absence of joint or back pain. Moreover, Claessen et al. reported that 20% of patients with controlled acromegaly experienced incident vertebral fractures so a healthcare provider's threshold for imaging should remain low for at least 3 years after remission is achieved [24]. Finally, postmenopausal women and men who develop hypogonadism should have serial DEXA scans with vertebral fracture assessment because significant decline portends increased fracture risk even if T-scores remain in the osteopenic range between –1 and –1.4 [26].

References

1. Gadelha MR, Kasuki L, Lim DST, Fleseriu M. Systemic complications of acromegaly and the impact of the current treatment landscape: an update. Endocr Rev. 2019;40(1):268–332.
2. Arlien-Søborg MC, Grøndahl C, Bæk A, Dal J, Madsen M, Høgild ML, et al. Fibroblast activation protein is a GH target: a prospective study of patients with acromegaly before and after treatment. J Clin Endocrinol Metab. 2020;105(1):33.
3. Kamenický P, Blanchard A, Gauci C, Salenave S, Letierce A, Lombès M, et al. Pathophysiology of renal calcium handling in acromegaly: what lies behind hypercalciuria? J Clin Endocrinol Metab. 2012;97(6):2124–33.
4. Madeira M, Neto LV, de Paula Paranhos Neto F, Barbosa Lima IC, Carvalho de Mendonça LM, Gadelha MR, et al. Acromegaly has a negative influence on trabecular bone, but not on cortical bone, as assessed by high-resolution peripheral quantitative computed tomography. J Clin Endocrinol Metab. 2013;98(4):1734–41.
5. Silva PPB, Amlashi FG, Yu EW, Pulaski-Liebert KJ, Gerweck AV, Fazeli PK, et al. Bone microarchitecture and estimated bone strength in men with active acromegaly. Eur J Endocrinol. 2017;177(5):409–20.
6. Kotzmann H, Bernecker P, Hübsch P, Pietschmann P, Woloszczuk W, Svoboda T, et al. Bone mineral density and parameters of bone metabolism in patients with acromegaly. J Bone Miner Res. 1993;8(4):459–65.
7. Bonadonna S, Mazziotti G, Nuzzo M, Bianchi A, Fusco A, De Marinis L, et al. Increased prevalence of radiological spinal deformities in active acromegaly: a cross-sectional study in postmenopausal women. J Bone Miner Res. 2005;20(10):1837–44.
8. Mazziotti G, Bianchi A, Bonadonna S, Cimino V, Patelli I, Fusco A, et al. Prevalence of vertebral fractures in men with acromegaly. J Clin Endocrinol Metab. 2008;93(12):4649–55.
9. Mazziotti G, Bianchi A, Porcelli T, Mormando M, Maffezzoni F, Cristiano A, et al. Vertebral fractures in patients with acromegaly: a 3-year prospective study. J Clin Endocrinol Metab. 2013;98(8):3402–10.
10. Mazziotti G, Battista C, Maffezzoni F, Chiloiro S, Ferrante E, Prencipe N, et al. Treatment of acromegalic osteopathy in real-life clinical practice: the BAAC (Bone Active Drugs in Acromegaly) study. J Clin Endocrinol Metab. 2020;105(9):363.
11. Biermasz NR, Wassenaar MJ, van der Klaauw AA, Pereira AM, Smit JW, Roelfsema F, et al. Pretreatment insulin-like growth factor-I concentrations predict radiographic osteoarthritis in acromegalic patients with long-term cured disease. J Clin Endocrinol Metab. 2009;94(7):2374–9.
12. Boswell SB, Patel DB, White EA, Gottsegen CJ, Forrester DM, Masih S, et al. Musculoskeletal manifestations of endocrine disorders. Clin Imaging. 2014;38(4):384–96.
13. Podgorski M, Robinson B, Weissberger A, Stiel J, Wang S, Brooks PM. Articular manifestations of acromegaly. Aust NZ J Med. 1988;18(1):28–35.
14. Ugur K, Karatas A, Oz B, Artas H, Aydin S, Koca SS. Imaging of sacroiliac joints in patients with acromegaly. Sci Rep. 2019;9(1):11645.
15. Scarpa R, De Brasi D, Pivonello R, Marzullo P, Manguso F, Sodano A, et al. Acromegalic axial arthropathy: a clinical case-control study. J Clin Endocrinol Metab. 2004;89(2):598–603.

16. Tagliafico A, Resmini E, Ferone D, Martinoli C. Musculoskeletal complications of acromegaly: what radiologists should know about early manifestations. Radiol Med. 2011;116(5):781–92.
17. Yoshizawa T, Iwazaki M, Jitsuiki K, Ishikawa K, Ohsaka H, Yanagawa Y. Suffocation due to thoracic deformity caused by acromegaly. Intern Med. 2017;56(8):949–51.
18. Park SH, Ku CR, Moon JH, Kim EH, Kim SH, Lee EJ. Age- and sex-specific differences as predictors of surgical remission among patients with acromegaly. J Clin Endocrinol Metab. 2018;103(3):909–16.
19. Nomikos P, Buchfelder M, Fahlbusch R. The outcome of surgery in 668 patients with acromegaly using current criteria of biochemical 'cure'. Eur J Endocrinol. 2005;152(3):379–87.
20. Sun H, Brzana J, Yedinak CG, Gultekin SH, Delashaw JB, Fleseriu M. Factors associated with biochemical remission after microscopic transsphenoidal surgery for acromegaly. J Neurol Surg B Skull Base. 2014;75(1):47–52.
21. Parkinson C, Kassem M, Heickendorff L, Flyvbjerg A, Trainer PJ. Pegvisomant-induced serum insulin-like growth factor-I normalization in patients with acromegaly returns elevated markers of bone turnover to normal. J Clin Endocrinol Metab. 2003;88(12):5650–5.
22. Geer EB, Sisco J, Adelman DT, Ludlam WH, Haviv A, Liu S, et al. Patient reported outcome data from acromegaly patients treated with injectable somatostatin receptor ligands (SRLs) in routine clinical practice. BMC Endocr Disord. 2020;20(1):117.
23. Frade-Sosa B, Florez H, Isern-Kebschull J, Halperin I, Guañabens N. Fusion of sacroiliac joints in acromegaly: a challenging finding. Rheumatology. 2020;59(4):898.
24. Claessen KM, Kroon HM, Pereira AM, Appelman-Dijkstra NM, Verstegen MJ, Kloppenburg M, et al. Progression of vertebral fractures despite long-term biochemical control of acromegaly: a prospective follow-up study. J Clin Endocrinol Metab. 2013;98(12):4808–15.
25. Geer EB, Sisco J, Adelman DT, Ludlam WH, Haviv A, Gelbaum D, et al. Observed discordance between outcomes reported by acromegaly patients and their treating endocrinology medical provider. Pituitary. 2020;23(2):140–8.
26. Katznelson L, Laws ER Jr, Melmed S, Molitch ME, Murad MH, Utz A, et al. Acromegaly: an endocrine society clinical practice guideline. J Clin Endocrinol Metab. 2014;99(11):3933–51.

Chapter 10
Acromegaly and Cancer

Tamis Bright

Acromegaly and Cancer Mortality

For many years, cardiovascular disease was the leading cause of death in acromegaly. A 2004 review of the published data on mortality in acromegaly between 1970 and 2001 reported that 60% of patients died from cardiovascular disease, 25% from respiratory disease, and only 15% from malignancies. The most common cancer deaths in that review were due to lung, colorectal, and breast [1]. With advances in treatment modalities, the life expectancy in acromegaly has improved [2, 3], and cancer has surpassed cardiovascular disease in many studies as the leading cause of death. Seven recent studies published between 2009 and 2018 were reviewed by Gadelha et al. [4] with four studies showing malignancies as the leading cause of death (27–36%) and cardiovascular disease as the second most common cause [5–8]. Cardiovascular disease was still the leading cause of death in two of the studies, but malignancy was now second at 21 and 22% [9, 10]. A study by Ritvonen [11] found cardiovascular disease to be the primary cause (34%) with cancer second (27%) in the first decade after diagnosis, but then cancer became the primary cause in the next two decades at 35%. Even though cancer is a common cause of death in patients with acromegaly, overall mortality due to cancer is not elevated compared to the general population. In the four studies with cancer as the most common cause of death, the standardized mortality ratio (SMR), the ratio of the observed number of deaths in acromegaly divided by the expected deaths in the general population, was not increased [5–8]. The other three studies reported the mortality due to cancer compared to expected deaths in their control populations or calculated the SMR specifically for cancer deaths, and none showed an excess mortality from cancer [9–11], which is consistent with other reports in the literature [12–15]. Therefore, while cancer is now frequently the most common cause of death in patients with

T. Bright (✉)
Texas Tech University Health Sciences Center El Paso, El Paso, TX, USA
e-mail: tamis.bright@ttuhsc.edu

L. S. Blevins Jr., M. K. Aghi (eds.), *Acromegaly*, Contemporary Endocrinology,
https://doi.org/10.1007/978-3-031-16258-9_10

acromegaly, death due to malignancy is not increased when compared to the general population.

Disease Control and Cancer Mortality

The study mentioned above by Ritvonen [11] illustrates how improved therapies have changed the cause of mortality over time. The ability to control GH and IGF-1 levels allows patients with acromegaly to live longer, and with advancing age, they have an elevated risk for developing cancer similar to the general population. The control of GH and IGF-1 levels significantly impacts mortality. A 2008 meta-analysis showed in patients with controlled GH levels less than 2.5 ng/mL following treatment, mortality was not increased compared to the general population (SMR 1.1; 95% confidence interval (CI), 0.9–1.4), but mortality was increased if the final GH was greater than 2.5 ng/mL with a SMR 1.9 (95% CI, 1.5–2.4). Similarly, a normal serum IGF-1 for age and sex at the last follow-up after treatment was associated with an SMR of 1.1 (95% CI, 0.9–1.4), which was equivalent to the general population; however, for those with continued IGF-1 elevation, the SMR was significantly higher at 2.5 (95% CI, 1.6–4.0) [2].

Bolfi [3] compared 17 studies published before 2008 and nine studies published after 2008. The overall mortality in acromegaly in the earlier studies was greater (SMR 1.76; 95% CI, 1.52–2.4), while in those done after 2008, the mortality was not different from the general population (SMR 1.35; 95% CI, 0.99–1.85). For patients with a normal IGF-1 and a random GH <2.5 ng/mL, the overall mortality was not increased (SMR 0.88; 95% CI, 0.76–1.2). However, if GH levels were uncontrolled, the mortality was higher (SMR 2.04; 95% CI, 1.5–2.9). This relationship was true for studies published both before and after 2008. In the studies published after 2008, when life expectancy improved, a greater number of deaths due to cancer was detected, but the SMR due to malignancies was not increased over the general population. The authors concluded that as the SMR has declined in acromegaly, the causes of death related to aging shift in the same direction in acromegaly as observed in the general population.

Uncontrolled GH and IGF-1 levels impact cancer mortality as well as overall mortality. In a study of 208 cases of acromegaly, elevated GH >5 ng/mL at the last follow-up was significantly associated with an increased observed to expected mortality ratio of 2.6 (95% CI, 1.9–3.6) in comparison to a mortality rate no different than expected, 1.1 (95% CI, 0.5–2.1) for those with a controlled last follow-up GH <1 ng/ml. An uncontrolled last follow-up IGF-1 value also conveyed a higher overall mortality ratio of 3.5 (95% CI, 2.8–4.2). Although the overall cancer-related mortality was not greater than the general population in this study, those with elevated GH or IGF-1 levels at last follow-up had significantly higher mortality from cancer compared to those with normal IGF-1 values or controlled GH levels below 2 ng/mL [13].

A multicenter cohort study of 1362 patients in the United Kingdom [14] concluded similar to previous authors that the overall mortality rate due to all malignant diseases was not elevated (SMR 1.16; 95% CI, 0.92–1.44), but when analyzed based on the posttreatment GH level, there was an increased mortality from cancer associated with the highest GH levels: GH ≥10.0 ng/mL yielded a SMR 1.81 (95% CI, 1.13–2.74). When the data was examined for the individual types of cancer, only colon cancer mortality was higher than expected (SMR 2.47; 95% CI, 1.31–4.22). Worsening colon cancer mortality also correlated with elevated posttreatment GH levels. There was no increase in mortality if the GH was well controlled <2.5 ng/mL, SMR 0.51 (95% CI, 0.01–2.84), but if GH was increased, the SMR also increased: GH 2.5–9.9 ng/mL, SMR 3.08 (95% CI, 1.13–6.71), and for GH ≥10.0 ng/mL, SMR 4.59 (95% CI, 1.25–11.75). They noted no difference in mortality due to lung cancer or rectal cancer, and there was a nonsignificant increase in mortality from breast cancer in women.

In summary, although the overall mortality from cancer is no different in well-controlled acromegaly, uncontrolled GH and IGF-1 levels significantly impact overall mortality and mortality due to malignancy compared to the general population. Uncontrolled GH may also have varying effects on mortality from different tumor types with one study demonstrating elevated colon cancer mortality.

Evidence for Involvement of the GH/IGF Axis in Cancer Development

Height and Cancer

Even though the cancer mortality rates are not higher in controlled acromegaly compared to the general population, there may still be a greater incidence of cancer in acromegaly. A number of large epidemiologic studies have demonstrated an elevated risk of cancer in the general population for individuals who are taller [16–20]. In the Million Women Study, the relative risk (RR) for total cancer was 1.16 (95% CI, 1.14–1.17) for every 10 cm increase in height. A statistically significant higher risk of cancer was found for 10 of the 17 sites assessed with the RR per 10 cm increase in height ranging between 1.14 to 1.32 for colon, rectum, malignant melanoma, breast, endometrium, ovary, kidney, CNS, non-Hodgkin's lymphoma, and leukemia [16].

In a prospective cohort study investigating 24 cancer sites, 414,923 participants from the UK Biobank were recruited between 2006 and 2010 [21]. A small but statistically increased risk of cancer was found for each 5 cm change in height for all-cause cancer in both men and women; lung cancer, lymphatic cancer, non-Hodgkin's lymphoma, melanoma, and leukemia in men; and breast cancer, melanoma, lymphatic cancer, and non-Hodgkin lymphoma in women. However, even though IGF-1 levels rose linearly with increasing height, they found no strong evidence to support IGF-1 modifying the association between height and cancer [21].

The 2018 expert report by the World Cancer Research Fund/American Institute for Cancer Research reviewed 206 studies with 240,806 participants and found a significant greater risk of cancer per 5 cm increase height for pancreas, colorectal, breast, ovary, endometrium, prostate, kidney, and malignant melanoma [22].

The greater cancer risk associated with increasing height is felt to be due in part to the more numerous cells in taller individuals which augments the possible targets, which may undergo malignant transformation [23, 24]. However, GH, IGF-1, IGF-2, and IGF-binding protein 3 (IGFBP3) also play a significant role in cancer development.

GH/IGF-1 and Cancer in General Populations

In individuals *without* acromegaly, a number of studies have indicated that higher levels of IGF-1 within the normal range beget an elevated risk of cancer, including colorectal, prostate, breast, and thyroid [25–28]. The hazard ratio (HR) of colorectal cancer per 1 standard deviation increment of IGF-1 was 1.11 (95% CI, 1.05–1.17), determined from samples collected from 397,380 participants in the UK Biobank [26]. The odds ratio (OR) for prostate cancer was 1.47 (95% CI, 1.23–1.77) in a meta-analysis of men with higher than the median IGF-1 compared to those with low IGF-1 [29]. A pooled analysis from 17 studies, including 4790 cases with 9428 matched controls, showed the OR for breast cancer in women in the highest versus the lowest quintile of IGF-1 concentration was 1.28 (95% CI, 1.14–1.44) [27]. In 345 cases of differentiated thyroid cancer diagnosed in the approximate 520,000 participants in the European Prospective Investigation into Cancer and Nutrition study (EPIC), there was a positive association between IGF-1 concentrations and risk of differentiated thyroid carcinoma with the OR for a doubling in IGF-1 concentration of 1.48 (95% CI, 1.06–2.08) [28].

Conversely, lower levels of GH and IGF-1 can decrease cancer risk. A common thymine (T) to adenine (A) polymorphism in the GH gene results in lower levels of GH and IGF-1. Individuals with the A/A genotypes had lower IGF-1 levels and IGF-1/IGFBP3 ratios than the T/T or T/A genotypes and a significantly lower risk of colorectal cancer [30]. In the prospective, case-controlled Physicians Health Study, after controlling for IGF-1 and other covariates, men with the highest quintile of IGFBP3 compared to those in the lowest quintile had a lower risk of developing colorectal cancer (RR 0.28; 95% CI, 0.12–0.66) [31]. Individuals with an inactivating mutation in the GH receptor (GHR), which results in low levels of IGF-1 (Laron syndrome), have a much lower risk of developing cancer when compared to their relatives without the mutation, 1% versus 17% [32]. Studies of gene expression in cell lines derived from individuals with Laron syndrome have differences in expression of genes involved in cell cycle, metabolic control, cell signaling, apoptosis, and autophagia in addition to having enhanced levels of expression for tumor suppressor proteins and lower oncogenic proteins [33]. Knockout animal models which lack GHR also have a much lower cancer incidence when compared to the wild type [34].

GH/IGF Receptor Signaling in Cancer

Consequently, the GH/IGF axis has been implicated in the development of cancer in the general population, not just acromegaly, and it has become an important area for research in understanding and treating malignancies. Although GH is produced mainly by the pituitary and IGF-1 by the liver, they are also synthesized by a number of other tissues and have been established to have local autocrine/paracrine activity [35, 36]. GHR and IGF-1 receptors (IGF1R) are transmembrane tyrosine kinase receptors that are expressed on cells throughout the body [37, 38]. The IGF1R, composed of 2 alpha and 2 beta subunits, is activated by IGF-1 and to a lesser degree by insulin and IGF-2 [39]. IGF1R can also form hybrid receptors with insulin receptors (IR), containing an alpha and beta subunit from each [39]. IGF bioavailability is regulated by binding to the six IGF binding proteins, which have a greater affinity for IGF-1 than does the IGF1R, and the majority of IGF-1 is bound by IGFBP3 [40]. Because GH and IGF-1 regulate normal protein synthesis, cellular proliferation, angiogenesis, and cell survival, these hormones, receptors, and their signaling pathways are potential targets for triggering the development of cancers or for promoting cancer growth and metastasis. Binding of ligands to the GHR and IGF1R results in activation of receptor tyrosine kinase activity and subsequent downstream signaling cascades. The IGF2R has no intracellular signaling activity; it only acts to bind IGF-2, thereby decreasing its bioavailability. However, if IGF2R numbers are decreased, there is augmented IGF-2 binding to IGF1R [41]. GHR signal transduction is through activation of Janus kinase 2 (JAK2) and the Src family kinases, which in turn activate the signal transducer and activator of transcription (STAT), mitogen-activated protein kinase (MAPK)/extracellular signal-regulated kinases (ERK), and phosphatidylinositol-3-kinase (PI3K)/AKT pathways, resulting in gene transcription with subsequent growth and metabolism [42, 43]. The IGF1R also utilizes the PI3K/AKT and MAPK/ERK signaling pathways for cell growth, proliferation, and cell survival [39, 44] (Fig. 10.1).

There is a growing body of evidence linking the signaling transduction cascades of the GH/IGF system to cancer growth and proliferation. Growth hormone receptor mRNA was detected with variable expression in all 60 of the cancer cell lines from the National Cancer Institute's NCI60 panel except colon cancer. Cell lines positive for GHR mRNA included breast, CNS, leukemia, melanoma, non-small cell lung, ovarian, prostate, and renal cancer [45]. Numerous studies have demonstrated increased expression of GHR and IGF1R in tissue samples from patients with multiple different malignancies, including cancers of the breast, ovary, endometrium, prostate, kidney, lung, liver, stomach, thyroid, pancreas, CNS, skin, colon, and liver [26, 37, 46–54].

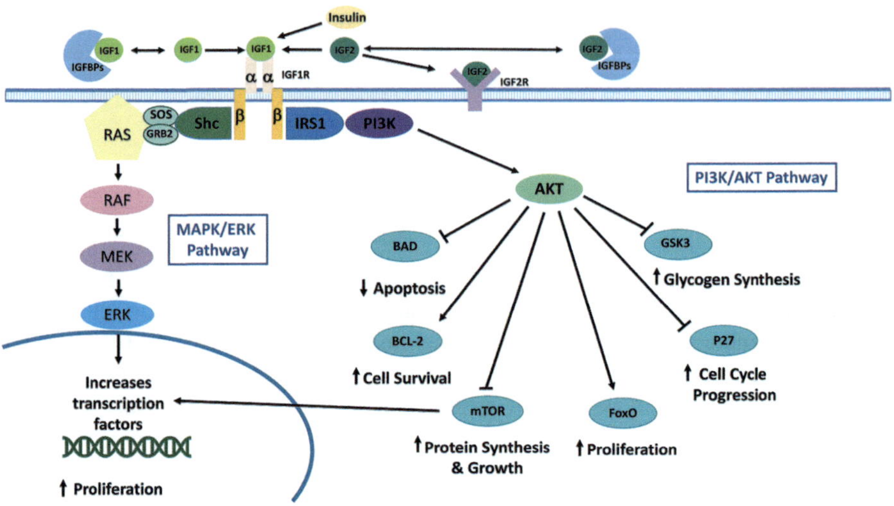

Fig. 10.1 IGF receptors. IGF1 and IGF2 circulate bound to the 6 IGFBPs. The IGF2R only binds IGF2 and has no signaling activity. The IGF1R has the highest affinity for IGF1 but can also bind IGF2 and insulin. Binding of a ligand to the IGF1 receptor leads to activation of both the PI3K/AKT and the MAPK/ERK signal transduction pathways through phosphorylation. Activated AKT phosphorylates several proteins, either upregulating or downregulating their function, leading to prolonged cell survival, cell cycle progression, growth, proliferation, protein and glycogen synthesis, and decreased apoptosis. Activation of the MAPK/ERK pathway increases transcription factors that regulate cell proliferation. *BCL-2* B-cell lymphoma 2, *BAD* BCL-2 associated agonist of cell death, *p27* cyclin-dependent kinase inhibitor 1B, *ERK* extracellular signal-regulated kinases, *FoxO* forkhead family transcription factors, *GSK3* glycogen synthase kinase 3, *GRB2* growth factor receptor-bound protein 2, *IGF* insulin-like growth factor, *IGFBP* IGF binding protein, *IGF1R* IGF1 receptor, *IGF2R* IGF2 receptor, *IRS1* insulin receptor substrate 1, *mTOR* mechanistic target of rapamycin, *MAPK* mitogen-activated protein kinases, *MEK* mitogen-activated protein kinase, *PI3K* phosphatidylinositol 3-kinase, *SOS* Son of Sevenless, *Shc* Src homology domain-containing protein

In vitro studies adding GH or IGF-1 to cancer cell lines or forced expression of the GH gene resulted in enhanced proliferation, migration, angiogenesis, invasion, and anti-apoptosis, and these actions were mitigated with receptor antagonists [48, 51, 55–57]. Many tumors have the ability to secrete IGF-1 and/or GH resulting in autocrine and/or paracrine action further enhancing proliferation, migration, and angiogenesis [46, 47, 51, 56]. However, various tissues may have different pathways for autocrine expressed GH compared to exogenous hormone. In mammary epithelial cells, autocrine GH amplified oncogenic transformation and invasion, but exogenous GH did not [57].

Animal data support the role of GH and IGF-1 in cancer. As above, the GHR knockout mouse developed fewer tumors than the wild type. The spontaneous dwarf rat, which has an inactivating mutation in the GH gene, has less mammary tumors compared to controls when exposed to carcinogens but the same occurrence if GH is replaced. Discontinuation of GH injections led to rapid regression of tumors, and subsequent resumption of GH injections resulted in a quick reappearance of tumors at the original tumor sites [58]. Transgenic animal models with overexpression of GH, IGF-1, IGF1R, or constitutively active IGF1R have more numerous mammary, epidermal, prostate, pancreatic, and salivary tumors [4, 58, 59].

Despite the increasing evidence implicating GH and IGF-1 in tumor development, neither are considered to directly induce DNA damage that would lead to mutations [60]. Large, long-term studies of the pharmacological use of GH in pediatric and adult patients without predisposing risk factors have not shown a higher risk of cancer [61–63]. It is thought, rather, that GH and IGF-1 lead to a permissive antiapoptotic environment allowing damaged cell survival and malignant transformation [64]. Tumor cells can then hijack the GH/IGF-1 signaling pathways promoting multiple factors that allow for growth, invasion, and metastasis [60].

Exposing colon epithelial cell cultures to prolonged elevated GH levels resulted in greater unrepaired DNA damage. In a mouse model, animals exposed to high circulating GH resulted in a 60% increase in unrepaired DNA damage in colon tissue [65]. The researchers demonstrated that GH blocks ataxia-telangiectasia mutated (ATM) kinase activation, which normally would be triggered in response to DNA damage. ATM kinase phosphorylates a number of proteins involved in cell-cycle checkpoint control, apoptotic responses, and DNA repair. With lower ATM kinase activity, DNA is left unrepaired, and cells do not undergo apoptosis, which can then lead to tumor transformation. Conversely, DNA repair was improved in cells with GHR suppression and in GHR knockout mice [65].

Loss of tumor suppressors decreases the cell's ability to protect against malignant transformation. Loss-of-function mutations in tumor suppressor genes (p53, breast cancer gene-1 (BRCA1), von-Hippel Lindau protein (vHL), and Wilms' tumor-1 (WT1)) have been implicated in decreased transcriptional suppression of the IGF1R promotor. Gain-of-function mutations of oncogenes can also amplify IGF1R transcription. Both types of mutations result in greater expression of IGF-1 receptors, which is felt to be necessary for malignant transformation of cells. Therefore, high levels of GH can lead to unrepaired DNA damage, which may result in mutations that amplify IGF1R quantity. Enhanced IGF1R expression coupled with autocrine secretion of IGF-1 or high levels from acromegaly then activates the augmented number of receptors, increasing proliferation and cell survival, as well as potentiating invasion, angiogenesis, and metastasis of tumor cells [60, 66].

Studies show autocrine/paracrine secretion of GH and IGF-1 is involved in oncogenic transformation through epithelial-mesenchymal transition (EMT). Epithelial cells normally exhibit a polarity with an apicobasal axis and create junctions between adjacent cells to form layers. In contrast, mesenchymal cells are loosely organized in a three-dimensional extracellular matrix [67]. EMT is a process whereby epithelial cells lose their polarity and cell-to-cell junctions to convert into mesenchymal cells with invasive and migratory properties which is an essential progression for cancer transformation [67]. IGF-1 and GH have the potential to facilitate EMT through multiple different signaling pathways. Some examples of factors involved in EMT which are upregulated by GH and IGF-1 are trefoil factor

3 (TFF3), matrix metalloprotease 2 and 9 (MMP2 and MMP9), zinc finger E-box binding homeobox 1 (ZEB1), and hypoxia-inducible factor 1 alpha (HIF1a) [68–71].

Overexpression of the secretory peptide TFF3 results in EMT through activation of the mesenchymal signaling pathway and suppression of apoptosis and E-cadherin, a glycoprotein that plays a critical role in cellular adhesion [72]. Overexpression of TFF3 promoted the proliferation, migration, and invasiveness in a colon cancer cell line, and a knockdown of TFF3 had the opposite effect [73]. TFF3 expression was greater in papillary thyroid cancer tissue when compared to adjacent noncancerous tissue and correlated with lymph node metastasis and grade [74]. Increased TFF3 expression in colorectal cancer tissue samples was associated with poor prognosis [73]. Autocrine secretion of GH augmented the expression of TTF3 and in mammary epithelial cells stimulated oncogenic transformation [68].

The enzymes MMP2 and MMP9 are type IV collagenases. They degrade basement membranes and the extracellular matrix as well as promote angiogenesis, processes necessary for tumor growth, invasion, and conversion from carcinoma in situ to metastatic disease [75, 76]. Metalloproteases have been implicated in EMT in multiple cancers, including gastric, pancreatic, colorectal, liver, lung, ovarian, mammary, and prostate [76]. MMP9 promotes angiogenesis through enhanced release of vascular endothelial growth factor (VEGF) [75] and VEGF expression correlates with tumor size and metastasis in many tumors [71, 77, 78]. In papillary thyroid cancer, concomitant elevated expression of VEGF and MMP-9 correlated with the presence of lymph node metastasis, tumor stage, and the degree of tumor infiltration [79]. Autocrine production of GH amplifies the activity of both MMP2 and MMP9, resulting in oncogenic transformation of breast cancer cells which was prevented by an MMP inhibitor [69].

Increased levels of the transcription factor ZEB1 up- or downregulates expression of a number of target genes, including decreasing E-cadherin, resulting in EMT with enhanced proliferation and dissemination of malignant cells and a worse clinical prognosis in most cancers [80]. Likewise, the transcription factor HIF1a is critical for tumor growth and survival. It regulates over 100 downstream genes, which are involved in glucose metabolism, cell proliferation, migration, and angiogenesis [81]. Paracrine/autocrine activation of the IGF1R has been shown to elevate both ZEB1 and HIF1a through PI3K and MAPK/ERK pathways, resulting in EMT [70, 71] (Fig. 10.2).

These examples show some of the multiple factors modulated by GH or IGF-1, which are involved in oncogenic transformation and demonstrate the complexity of the signaling pathways that promote malignancy. Oncogenic transformation is a multistep, multihit process of DNA damage, loss of repair and apoptosis, and hyperproliferation, resulting in an in situ lesion, which subsequently develops angiogenesis and EMT, ultimately leading to invasion and metastasis.

Because of the intricate association of the GH/IGF axis in cancer and indications that expression of autocrine GH, IGF-1, and IGF1R increases resistance to radiation and traditional chemotherapy [60, 82], novel agents are under development to target this axis. Pegvisomant, the GHR antagonist, decreased proliferation in cell-line studies and improved endometrial cancer responsiveness to radiation treatment in animal models [83, 84]. Anti-IGF1R monoclonal antibodies were effective in

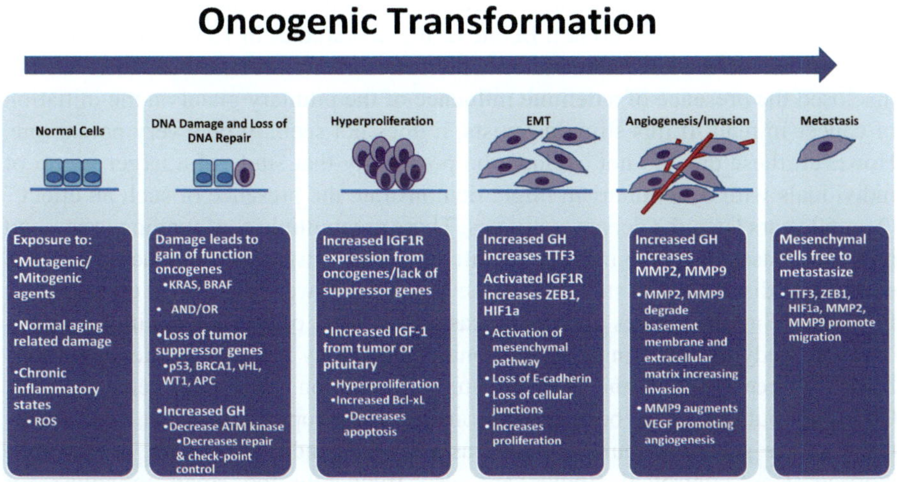

Fig. 10.2 Oncogenic transformation.
Stages in oncogenic transformation of normal epithelial cells into neoplastic cells. Examples of oncogenes, tumor suppressor genes, and signaling proteins involved in the GH/IGF axis are noted. *ROS* reactive oxygen species, *GH* growth hormone, *ATM kinase* ataxia-telangiectasia mutated kinase, *IGF1R* insulin-like growth factor 1 receptor, *IGF-1* insulin-like growth factor 1, *Bcl-xL* B-cell lymphoma-extra large, *EMT* epithelial mesenchymal transition, *TTF3* trefoil factor 3, *ZEB1* zinc finger E-box binding homeobox 1, *HIF1a* hypoxia-inducible factor 1 alpha, *MMP2 and MMP9* matrix metalloprotease 2 and 9, *VEGF* vascular endothelial growth factor

multiple cell-line studies, but thus far positive results have been seen only in patients with sarcoma [82] and in a phase 1 trial for highly proliferative breast cancer in combination with other chemotherapy [41]. Another successful treatment strategy targets the downstream signaling pathways. Multiple tyrosine kinase inhibitors are effective in different cancers [85]. Currently, an antibody, xentuzumab, that binds to both IGF-1 and IGF-2 is being studied, which blocks their activation of the IGF receptors and the IR. Xentuzumab had antiproliferative effects against a range of cancer cell lines, including colon, sarcoma, lung cancer, and multiple myeloma [86]. Phase 1 data shows antitumor activity with xentuzumab in solid tumors [87], and trials are ongoing in lung and breast cancer [41]. Growth hormone, IGF-1, and their receptors have become a promising area of cancer research, and a number of other agents, which target various steps of the GH/IGF axis, are under investigation as potential treatments.

Cancer Incidence in Acromegaly

Because higher levels of IGF-1 lead to greater cancer incidence in the general population and GH and IGF-1 are involved in multiple cancer-promoting pathways as described, it was expected that patients with acromegaly would also experience more malignancies. However, controversy has persisted for decades concerning whether acromegaly increases the incidence of cancer with some studies showing a greater risk, while others do not. In one of the first studies in 1957, Mustacchi [88] stated in his discussion, "To conclude, the material analyzed in this report has not disclosed the presence of a definite influence of the pituitary gland on the initiation of cancer in man. If this stimulus exists, it does not seem to be a very potent one. However, these data do not exclude the possibility that study of a larger group of individuals with dyspituitarism might demonstrate the presence of such an effect." Over 60 years later, the debate continues. There are multiple confounding issues and potential biases that have made a definitive answer elusive. Because acromegaly is such a rare disease, most studies lack the statistical power to detect an elevated risk for cancer. Smaller studies are usually case-controlled, often with significant differences in study design. Single-institutional studies may have more intense surveillance or screening for cancers in the study population, increasing detection bias. Control populations have been drawn from various groups that may not be representative of the general population, such as a single gender, inpatients, or the well-worried. Case-controlled studies are also frequently too small to adjust for confounding factors, such as age, smoking, and gender. These differences have led in general to higher estimates of cancer in the single-center, case-controlled studies of acromegaly as compared to population-based studies [89]. Population-based studies eliminate some of the potential biases and may give a better estimate of the cancer risk [90]. Population-based studies with large numbers improve statistical power and decrease selection and detection biases, but they can also be difficult to compare since different geographic regions have varying rates of cancer [91]. Another limitation to acromegaly cancer studies is that in order to obtain a reasonable sample size, the majority of studies have included patients diagnosed years ago when treatment methods were not as efficacious. Therefore, there is potential for exposure to elevated levels or GH and IGF-1 for longer periods in patients diagnosed many years ago compared to more recently diagnosed patients who are more likely to have controlled levels [3]. The risk of cancer may be high in the lag time prior to diagnosing acromegaly, which can frequently be unrecognized for 5–10 years [5, 92, 93], so some studies include cancers identified prior to the diagnosis of acromegaly and others do not. As treatment modalities have improved and life expectancy has lengthened, cancer incidence has increased as the population ages [11]. These factors have led to very mixed study groups with significant variations in treatments, life expectancies, cancer screening, and control populations making comparisons challenging.

Three, large reviews have collectively examined 23 studies for cancer incidence, including both case controlled and population studies [89, 94, 95]. Boguszewski and Ayuk found in their 2016 review of 17 series between 1957 and 2015 that the overall prevalence of cancer in acromegaly was 10.8% (4.8–21.3%) [94]. The results were mixed, with some studies with no increased risk, some with an increased risk, two with an increase in women only, and one with an increase in men only. Because of the small patient number in many of the reports, they separately reviewed the largest five population-based studies with patients numbering between 331 and 1634 that also reported the standardized incidence ratio (SIR). The SIR is the ratio of the observed number of cancer cases in the study population divided by the expected cases in the general population. They concluded that even in the largest five population studies, there were conflicting results with a higher SIR in three studies, SIR 1.5–1.6 [15, 96, 97], and either lower or no difference than the general population studied in two, SIR 0.75–0.76 [14, 98].

Terzolo et al. [95] revisited the question in 2017 with a review of nine studies that had both SIR data and at least 200 patients, and their own nationwide cohort study in Italy. The nine studies with greater than 200 patients included 609 cancers in 6248 patients, resulting in a 9.7% prevalence of cancer (6.4–14.4%). Five of the nine studies [15, 96, 97, 99, 100] had increased risk (SIR 1.5–3.39), while four [8, 14, 89, 98] did not show a greater risk compared to the general population. In their national cohort, they studied 1512 patients, finding 124 patients diagnosed with cancer (8.2%) between 1980 and 2002. The SIR for all cancers was 1.41; 95% CI, 1.18–1.68. When they excluded cancers diagnosed prior to the acromegaly diagnosis, the SIR was still increased (SIR 1.28; 95% CI, 1.07–1.55).

Dal et al. [89] performed a meta-analysis of 14 studies with SIR data between 1957 and 2018 with a total of 8555 patients. Their analysis showed the pooled SIR for cancer in acromegaly was 1.5; 95% CI, 1.2–1.8.

In addition, in a recent national cohort study which was published since the three reviews above, Wu et al. reported on 87 cancers (7.3%) in 1195 acromegaly cases diagnosed between 1997 and 2013 in Taiwan and found an elevated SIR of 1.91; 95% CI, 1.55–2.35 [101].

Interestingly, although two studies [7, 102] noted development of malignancy correlated with an increased fasting GH at diagnosis, the majority of studies that included the hormone levels did not find an association of either GH or IGF-1 levels at baseline or posttreatment with the development of cancer [8, 14, 15, 89, 95, 98–100].

Table 10.1 shows the 11 studies with 200 or more cases, which also reported SIR data and Dal's meta-analysis for comparison. Seven of the 11 studies and the meta-analysis show a higher risk of cancer in acromegaly. Therefore, the current data suggests that Mustacchi's 1957 conclusion was on target with the necessity of exceptionally large studies to see the trend toward a small increase incidence of cancer in acromegaly over the general population.

Table 10.1 Studies of cancer incidence in acromegaly with >200 cases reporting SIR data and the meta-analysis by Dal

Study pub year (reference)	Study period	*n*	Observed cancer	Expected cancer	SIR	95% CI
Ron 1991 [96]	1969–1985	1041	116	72.3	1.6	1.3–1.9 (men)
Orme 1998 [14]	1958–1995	1239	79	104	0.76	0.6–0.95
Popovic 1998 [99]	1991–1997	220	23	6.49	3.39	2.12–5.12
Baris 2002 [97]	1965–1993	1643	177	117	1.5	1.3–1.8
Kauppinen-Makelin 2010 [15]	1980–2006	331	48	33.1	1.5	1.1–1.9
Petroff 2015 [98]	NA	446	46	61.3	0.75	0.55–1.0
Terzolo 2017 [95]	1980–2012	1512	124	87.8	1.41	1.18–1.68
Maione 2017 [8]	1999–2012	999	102	NA	1.34	0.94–1.87 (men)
					1.24	0.77–1.73 (women)
Wolinski 2017 [155]	2005–2016	200	27	8.3	3.3	2.2–4.7
Dal 2018 [89]	1978–2013	529	81	72.7	1.1	0.9–1.4
Wu 2020 [101]	1997–2013	1195	87	45.6	1.91	1.55–2.35
Dal meta-analysis [89]	1957–2016	8555			1.5	1.2–1.8

Specific Cancer Incidence

Identifying specific cancers that potentially have an elevated risk in acromegaly again suffers from the need for exceptionally large sample sizes to reach significance, because the expected number of occurrences of a specific cancer even in large population-based studies is frequently less than ten cases for common cancers, like colon or breast, and less than one case for cancers with lower frequency, like thyroid. Therefore, due to the small numbers, many studies report only the overall incidence of cancer not data for the individual cancer types. There are five large studies with greater than 1000 acromegaly cases each that report SIR data for specific types of cancers and four of the five [95–97, 101] did show a greater incidence of a number of cancers with only one showing no additional risk of any type of cancer [14]. For the four studies reporting an elevated risk, the results were variable for which cancers were higher, except three found an increased risk of colon cancer.

Orme did not find a greater risk of cancer overall or of any individual cancers in a study of 1239 individuals in the United Kingdom [14]. Ron's VA study of 1041 men reported an increase in cancers of the colon, esophagus, and CNS [96]. The studies by Baris [97] with 1643 cases and Terzolo [95] with 1512 cases both noted an elevated risk for cancers of the colon, thyroid, and kidney. In addition, Baris found a greater risk of small intestine, rectal, CNS, and bone cancers, but the authors note that the higher risk of CNS and bone cancers in their study was likely due to pituitary radiation treatment, not the acromegaly. Wu noted an increase in cancers of the stomach, CNS, endocrine glands, and lymphoma [101]. They unfortunately did not report which endocrine glands developed cancer.

Additionally, Dal's meta-analysis included pooled data for individual cancers from 14 studies (which included the studies above except Wu [101]) with 8554 individuals and reported elevated risk for colorectal, thyroid, gastric, breast, and urinary tract cancer [89]. However, the urinary tract cancer confidence intervals included one.

Consequently, even in these large studies, there is inconsistency in the specific cancers that were increased, which also may be influenced by other risk factors in the populations in which the studies were done, the control of the patients, and the treatments available at the time. The risks for colon, thyroid, and breast cancer in acromegaly have been studied the most extensively.

Colon Cancer and Acromegaly

Colon cancer has the most robust and compelling data for a greater risk in acromegaly. Normal colonic epithelium is organized in crypts with actively dividing cells at the base, which then move to the luminal surface and undergo apoptosis and shedding [103]. Increased epithelial cell proliferation leads to polyp formation. Histologically, colon polyps are divided into hyperplastic and adenomatous polyps. Adenomatous polyps have the potential to dedifferentiate into colon cancer. All hyperplastic polyps were initially thought to be benign; however, larger, particularly proximal, and serrated hyperplastic polyps have been noted to have premalignant features [104].

It has been well-documented that there is a greater risk of both hyperplastic and adenomatous colon polyps and more proximal polyps in acromegaly. Biopsies of the colonic mucosa in acromegaly showed amplified epithelial cell proliferation which correlated with GH and IGF-1 levels [105]. In a meta-analysis by Rokkas of nine studies published between 1994 and 2006, hyperplastic polyps were found in 22% of 573 acromegaly cases versus 7% of controls and adenomatous polyps in 23% of 641 cases versus 12% of controls. The pooled odds ratios by both the fixed and random effects models for adenomatous polyps were OR 2.486 (95% CI, 1.908–3.238) and OR 2.537 (95% CI, 1.914–3.364), respectively [106]. In patients with acromegaly who had all visible polyps removed, 14% had newly developed adenomas on repeat colonoscopy, done approximately 2.5 years later, which was significantly related to GH and IGF-1 levels [107]. In another study with colonoscopies done approximately 4 years apart, the incidence of polyps was 38%, 36%, and 37% at the initial, second, and third surveillance, respectively. Patients with an initial adenoma had a 4.4-fold increased risk of an adenoma on the second colonoscopy and an 8.8-fold increased risk on the third colonoscopy. Even with a normal initial colonoscopy, a persistently elevated IGF-1 level led to a 7.5-fold risk of a subsequent adenoma, compared to those with a normal colonoscopy at the initial screening and controlled IGF-1 levels [108].

Acromegaly cases also have a greater risk of multiple polyps [109–111], ascending or transverse colon polyps [94], and a higher prevalence of polyps occurring at a younger age as compared to controls: below 40 years old (19.3% versus 4.4% of controls), below 50 years old (25% versus 9.6%), and below 55 years old (20% versus 3%) [110, 112]. Therefore, a full colonoscopy is necessary in acromegaly to reach all potential polyps, and it should be done even in younger patients. However, a full colonoscopy may not always be obtained because the colon is on average 20% longer and is more likely to have complex looping, and transit time in acromegaly is prolonged, so bowel preparation may be inadequate [113]. Thus, a full colonoscopy is technically more difficult and can have a higher risk of procedure-related complications, such as pain, perforation, and bleeding [90]. Since the procedure is technically challenging, this adds bias when determining cancer risk, because more experienced physicians are most likely to be requested to do the procedure, and they then may find more lesions to biopsy. Because the studies are not blinded, the perception that patients with acromegaly have more colon cancer leads to more biopsies taken and more cancer detected [90]. The incidence of colon cancer in the general population also varies greatly by region due to environmental and dietary exposure as well as by age, gender, and genetic risks [114], so studies from different regions may not be comparable. Consequently, there are a number of potential biases that may confound the data for colon cancer incidence.

Even taking these biases into consideration, patients with acromegaly have more polyps, which expands the number of targets at risk for cancer. Premalignant polyps undergo a slow, stepwise malignant transformation into colon cancer, which is felt to occur over at least 10 years [115]. In Rokkas' meta-analysis, colon cancer was more likely in acromegaly patients compared to controls, 4.6% versus 1.2%, with the pooled odds ratio of OR 4.351 (95% CI, 1.533–12.354) [106]. As mentioned above, three of the five large studies showed a greater risk of colon cancer with SIR 1.67–3.1 [95–97]. Although the study by Orme [14] had a nonsignificant increase in colon cancer incidence (SIR, 1.68; 95% CI, 0.87–2.93; $P = 0.06$), they did observe increased colon cancer mortality (SMR 2.47; 95% CI, 1.31–4.22), which correlated with uncontrolled GH levels. Dal's meta-analysis of 14 studies showed an elevated risk for colorectal cancer (pooled SIR 2.6; 95% CI, 1.7–4.0). They observed that a higher colorectal cancer incidence was reported in 13 out of 14 studies they reviewed [89].

There is in vitro and in vivo evidence that supports an elevated colon cancer risk in acromegaly. Both normal colon and colon cancer cells express GHR [116]. As previously discussed, exposure of colon epithelial cells to prolonged excessive GH levels resulted in greater amounts of unrepaired DNA damage [65]. The mutations in unrepaired DNA may initiate the stepwise transformation of adenomas into carcinomas. Allelic loss or mutations may decrease expression of tumor suppressor genes, particularly adenomatous polyposis coli (APC) and p53, or activate oncogenes, KRAS or BRAF [77, 117], which can trigger malignant transformation. Growth hormone, via its receptor activated signaling pathway, increases STAT5, and when STAT5 was elevated in tumor samples, it correlated with worsening invasion, stage, and survival in colon cancer [118, 119]. Amplified IGF-1 receptor expression in colon cancer cell lines enhanced growth, decreased apoptosis, and promoted migration [120], and blockade of IGF1R inhibited these effects [121]. In addition to inducing the previously discussed factors which lead to EMT, overexpression of IGF1R in colon cancer cells activated AKT in the PI3K pathway, which in turn augmented expression of B-cell lymphoma-extra large, (Bcl-xL), which is an antiapoptotic protein [120]. Colon cancer cells from patient biopsy samples also overexpressed IGF-1 and IGF1R compared to normal or adenomatous mucosa [120, 122], and the level of IGF1R expression correlated with higher tumor stage [122]. Colon cancer patients without acromegaly given octreotide for 2 weeks prior to surgery had a significant reduction in proliferation of tumor cells and IGF-1 levels compared to untreated patients [123]. In patients with acromegaly, there is decreased apoptosis [124] and increased proliferation [105, 125] in colonic epithelial cells correlating with higher IGF-1 and GH levels.

In summary, elevated levels of IGF-1 are associated with increased polyps in patients with acromegaly and in the general population [26, 107, 108]. Growth hormone and IGF-1 can promote the development of polyps through stimulating epithelial cell proliferation and subsequently may be permissive in allowing cells with DNA damage to propagate by decreasing DNA repair and enhancing antiapoptotic effects. Elevated circulating IGF-1 in acromegaly may then have an additive role to the autocrine/paracrine action from tumor produced IGF-1 activating the amplified number of IGF-1 receptors, thereby augmenting tumor proliferation, invasion, and metastasis. Nearly all studies have noted a greater risk of colon cancer in acromegaly [89], and increased GH levels were associated with higher colon cancer mortality [14].

Based on the evidence of the greater risk of polyps and the above studies with an increased risk of colon cancer, the current Endocrine Society [126], Pituitary Society [127], and Acromegaly Consensus Group [128] guidelines recommend a colonoscopy at diagnosis for all patients, since even younger patients are at a higher risk for polyps. The Pituitary Society and the Acromegaly Consensus Group recommend repeat colonoscopy as per standard population guidelines. The Endocrine Society recommendations are based on the findings of the initial colonoscopy and the level of control of the acromegaly. A repeat colonoscopy is suggested every 5 years in patients with a polyp on initial screening or for those with persistently elevated IGF-1. In patients without polyps and normal IGF-1 levels, then repeat screening every 10 years is appropriate [126].

Thyroid Cancer and Acromegaly

Thyroid cancer, like colon cancer, has been scrutinized in acromegaly more than other types of cancers. Thyroid cells have IGF1R and secrete IGF-1 [129]. In vitro studies show IGF-1 promotes thyroid cell growth [130, 131] and also potentiates TSH-mediated thyroid growth [130]. An elevated IGF-1 level above the upper tertile in a population study showed a greater OR for goiter relative to an IGF-1 level below the lower tertile [132].

Therefore, it is not surprising that cases with acromegaly have a greater number of goiters compared to controls [1, 131, 133–136]. Goiters have been noted in 25–92% of cases [1] with a correlation between GH and IGF-1 levels with the size of the gland in some studies [131, 137–140], but not all [141, 142]. The majority of the goiters are nodular, 40–78%, but only rarely toxic [1, 133, 142]. Goiters are associated with the years of disease duration (1, 131, 138,) and with advancing age [1, 131, 143]. Control of GH and IGF-1 levels have been shown to decrease the volume of the gland, but not the nodules [131, 138]. Biopsies of thyroid nodules have demonstrated higher levels of IGF-1 and IGF1R compared to normal tissue [52, 144, 145].

The elevated incidence of thyroid nodules has led to concern for a greater risk of thyroid cancer in acromegaly, and there is epidemiologic evidence to support the risk. Higher serum levels of IGF-1 in the general population have been associated with differentiated thyroid cancer (DTC) [28]. Patients with DTC had elevated levels of serum IGF-1 and IGF1R compared to controls or cases with multinodular goiters [146]. IGF-1 levels were also higher in biopsies of DTC than in benign nodular disease or adjacent normal tissue [144], and in papillary thyroid cancer, the expression of IGF-1 was related to tumor size [147]. The IGF-1 staining in tissue samples was greater in papillary tumors in patients with acromegaly compared to papillary cancers in control patients [134]. However, there was no difference in the last reported IGF-1 level in patients with acromegaly and thyroid cancer compared to those without thyroid cancer [102, 134].

From the five large population-based studies that reported SIR data for individual cancers, two studies showed no increased thyroid cancer risk [14, 96], and Wu [101] reported on a composite of endocrine gland cancers without specific thyroid numbers. Two studies showed a greater risk of thyroid cancer (Baris [97] with SIR 3.7; 95% CI, 1.8–10.9 and Terzolo [95] SIR 3.99; 95% CI, 2.32–6.87). However, the number of thyroid cancer cases was quite small in all of these studies, even though each included over 1000 cases of acromegaly, and CI were also very wide; two studies had only one case [14, 96], one had three cases [97], and one had eight cases [95]. Dal's meta-analysis had a much higher SIR, but the CI again was very wide: pooled SIR for thyroid cancer 9.2; 95% CI, 4.2–19.9 [89].

In a 2016 review of nine studies with a total of 50 thyroid cancers in 1579 acromegaly cases, the rate of thyroid cancer reported was 3.2% (range 1.2–10.6%) versus 0.3% in controls, and the vast majority (91%) were papillary [136]. The predominance of papillary cancer over the other types of thyroid cancer has been noted in the majority of studies [133–136]. In a meta-analysis of seven studies, the pooled prevalence for thyroid cancer was 5.4%, the pooled OR was 4.1 (95% CI, 2.0–8.3), and RR was 3.9 (95% CI, 1.9–7.8) [133]. Some studies are now reporting thyroid as the most common cancer in acromegaly [102, 135, 148]. However, there is a wide range of thyroid cancer rates reported, which can in part be explained by different methodology. More recent studies [133, 134, 149] have elevated rates of thyroid cancer compared to the older studies [14, 96, 97, 99]. Screening methods have changed over the years, which makes comparisons of the studies difficult. The oldest studies would not have had ultrasound surveillance, some studies have done ultrasounds only on patients with palpable nodules, and many recent studies screen all patients with ultrasounds, which amplifies the numbers of nodules detected and subsequently biopsied. Some centers follow the 2015 American Thyroid Association guidelines [150] and biopsy only lesions ≥1 cm, but others biopsy all suspicious lesions no matter the size [139, 143, 148], which leads to much higher rates of cancer, since microcarcinomas are included. For example, the thyroid cancer rate was 1.4% in a 1998 study [99], which would not have done routine thyroid ultrasounds. In a study with ultrasounds performed on all patients, but biopsies of only nodules ≥1 cm, the cancer rate was 7.2% versus 0.7% for the general population [149], compared to a study with biopsies done on all suspicious nodules, no matter the size, resulting in a rate of 11% [143]. This has led to significant variation in the reported incidence of thyroid cancer in acromegaly and the uncertainty of whether there is a greater risk, or it is due to surveillance bias.

In studies that report the number of nodules undergoing fine-needle aspiration, the rate of thyroid cancer in nodules ≥1 cm in acromegaly was 8.5–25% [102, 139, 149, 151] with only one study [149] reporting a higher rate (25%) than the rate of cancer in nodules of the general population, which is 7–15% [151]. In a study comparing patients with papillary thyroid cancer and acromegaly with matched papillary thyroid cancer patients without acromegaly, there was no difference in mean age of diagnosis of thyroid cancer, histology, tumor size, risk of recurrence, or response to treatment in the acromegaly group, concluding that there was no worse evolution or prognosis of disease [152].

Based off a comparable rate of cancer in nodules, similar outcomes to other DTC cases, and no increase in thyroid cancer mortality, current guidelines from the Endocrine Society [126] and the Acromegaly Consensus Group [128] recommend careful examination and surveillance of patients with acromegaly for thyroid disease and thyroid ultrasounds only in those with palpable thyroid nodules. The recommendation is to manage thyroid nodules the same as in patients without acromegaly [126].

Breast Cancer and Acromegaly

Due to the very large numbers necessary to show a statistically significant increased incidence of cancer in acromegaly, both the gender specific cancers, prostate and breast, suffer from halving the population numbers. However, much of the extensive research discussed thus far, demonstrating the considerable role that GH, IGF-1, and their receptors play in oncogenic transformation and proliferation of tumors, has been done in breast cancer. The autocrine/paracrine action of the hormones and the upregulation of receptors has been shown both in vitro and in vivo to promote proliferation, angiogenesis, and invasion of breast cancer [47, 56–58]. The pooled analysis of studies on IGF-1 and breast cancer in individuals without acromegaly showed a greater risk with higher IGF-1 levels [27, 153]. An older study by Nabarro [154] did have a larger number of acromegaly cases with breast cancer, 11 versus the expected 2.6. Wolinski [155] also noted an increased risk with seven women with breast cancer out of 200 cases of acromegaly (5.4%) and none in the controls but did not report the SIR. However, the individual studies that reported SIR information for acromegaly [14, 15, 89, 95, 97, 98, 101] did not find a greater risk for breast cancer. Yet Dal's meta-analysis did show an increased risk for the pooled SIR 1.6; 95% CI, 1.1–2.3 [89]. Since a consistently elevated risk has not been reported, current guidelines are to screen women with acromegaly the same as the general population [126, 128]. Given the extensive data on the GH/IGF-1 axis in promoting and potentiating breast cancer, it seems prudent to stress compliance with appropriate breast cancer screening guidelines in women with acromegaly.

Prostate Cancer and Acromegaly

Normal prostate cells express GH, GHR, and IGF1R [156, 157]. Prostate cancer cell lines overexpress IGF1R and increase proliferation with the addition of IGF-1 [158]. Enhanced expression of IGF1R correlated with the progression of androgen-sensitive prostate cancer becoming androgen-independent cancer in animal models [159]. Transfecting prostate cancer cells with an IGF1R antisense construct dramatically reduced endogenous IGF1R mRNA. Injecting cancer cells with the construct into animals resulted in a 90% reduction in tumor growth, compared to controls injected with cancer cells without the construct [160]. Prostate cancer biopsies also show IGF1R expression is greater, compared to prostate hypertrophy or normal tissue, and expression increases with advanced states of prostate cancer [157].

A number of studies have noted a link between higher IGF-1 levels in the population and prostate cancer [29, 153, 161]. In one study of 3700 men with prostate cancer who had an IGF-1 serum level done approximately 5 years prior to their cancer diagnosis, the higher the IGF-1, the greater the risk for subsequently developing prostate cancer: OR of the highest versus lowest quintile (1.38; 95% CI, 1.19–1.60) [161]. These studies show there is epidemiologic, in vitro, and in vivo evidence for a potential greater risk for prostate cancer in acromegaly.

Prostate volume was significantly enlarged in uncontrolled acromegaly compared to controls and correlated with disease duration and age. Acromegaly cases had a significantly greater prevalence of structural abnormalities, including calcifications, nodules, cysts, and vesicle inflammation, compared to controls (78.2 versus

23.3%) [162]. Prostate hypertrophy also occurred in untreated patients less than 40 years old, despite having secondary hypogonadism, and the hypertrophy improved with treatment of the IGF-1 and GH levels [163].

Previously, none of the large acromegaly trials [14, 15, 89, 95, 97, 98, 101] showed an elevated risk of prostate cancer over the general population. Since prostate cancer usually develops in older men, a higher occurrence in acromegaly may not have been noted when life expectancy was shorter. However, a recent, large cohort study by Watts [164] is the first to show a greater risk of prostate cancer in acromegaly. Using the English national Hospital Episode Statistics and mortality data from 1999 to 2017, men ≥35 years old diagnosed with acromegaly (n = 2495) were compared to a reference cohort of 4.3 million men admitted for minor surgeries or conditions. They excluded men diagnosed with prostate cancer prior to the diagnosis of acromegaly or within 6 months of entry into the cohorts. During the median follow-up time of 7.7 years, the control cohort developed 127,299 cases of prostate cancer and had 29,022 prostate cancer deaths. For men diagnosed with acromegaly, they found 96 prostate cancer cases, resulting in a HR for prostate cancer of 1.33 (95% CI, 1.09–1.63). When divided by age group, those 35–64 years old had a HR 1.25 (95% CI, 1.02–1.78) and 65 and older showed a HR 1.29 (95% CI, 0.97–1.72). There were also 19 prostate cancer deaths with a HR of 1.44 (95% CI, 0.92–2.26), but it did not reach statistical significance. The authors note that they may not have investigated all cases of acromegaly or prostate cancer incidences, because data was obtained from hospitalization records and not all cases would be hospitalized.

The recent guidelines [126, 128] were written prior to the latest study showing the elevated risk of prostate cancer, so the current recommendations do not have any additional screening for the general population. With the study by Watts showing the increase in prostate cancer, particularly in younger men, it may be reasonable to begin screening men with acromegaly for prostate cancer at a younger age, especially for patients who are uncontrolled. Unfortunately, the available screening tests, the prostate specific antigen (PSA) and digital rectal exam (DRE), have a number of limitations. Many other conditions can elevate PSA, leading to potential false positives, and prostate cancer can have a normal DRE and PSA, producing false negatives. Wider screening can also lead to more frequent biopsies, and overtreatment of cancers that otherwise would not have impacted the patient's health [165]. Further studies will need to determine the benefit-risk analysis of potential recommendations for any additional prostate cancer screening in men with acromegaly.

Other Cancers and Acromegaly

There is conflicting data for urinary tract cancer in both general population studies and those in acromegaly. A greater risk of kidney cancer was identified in the general population in a meta-analysis of 18,766 cases, RR 1.23 (95% CI, 1.18–1.28) for each 10 cm increase in height [17]. However, there was no association of prediagnostic IGF-1 levels and subsequent overall risk of bladder and urothelial cell cancer in the population study of the EPIC cohort including 843 cases matched with controls [166]. There is minimal information on urinary tract cancer in acromegaly, and most studies did not include SIR data for this cancer. For the large series that did report SIR, no greater risk in urinary tract cancer was found in three studies [14, 89, 96], but two did note an increased risk (Baris SIR 3.2; 95% CI, 1.6–5.5 and Terzolo 2.87; 95% CI, 1.55–5.34). In addition, although the SIR was not elevated in the complete 24-year observation time of their study, Kauppinen-Mäkelin found a greater incidence of bladder and kidney cancer during the first 5 years after acromegaly diagnosis (SIR 7.77; 95% CI, 2.12–19.9), but again confidence intervals were very wide [15]. With the limited data, there are no recommendations for additional surveillance for urinary tract cancer in acromegaly.

Similar to the other cancers, IGF-1 and IGF1R are expressed in gastric cancer cell lines as well as gastric cancer biopsies, and the addition of IGF-1 augmented proliferation of the cell lines [167]. In acromegaly studies, two reported an increase in stomach cancer, Wu [101] (SIR 3.95; 95% CI, 1.97–7.89) and Dal's meta-analysis [89] (pooled SIR 2.0; 95% CI, 1.4–2.9), although the majority of the individual studies [14, 89, 95–97] did not show a higher risk of gastric cancer.

Various studies have noted elevated risks for other cancers in acromegaly, such as CNS, esophagus, small intestine, and hematologic [96, 97, 101], but numbers are small, confidence intervals are broad, and these cancers have not been shown to consistently occur more frequently in acromegaly compared to the general population.

Summary of Cancer Incidence

In summary, only colon cancer, thyroid cancer, and now prostate cancer have enough data to suggest a greater risk in acromegaly. Although studies have not shown a higher risk for breast cancer, there is still significant concern due to the extensive epidemiologic data plus the in vitro and in vivo studies with compelling evidence for the involvement of the GH/IGF axis in breast cancer development and metastasis. Similar to the prior studies on prostate cancer, numbers may just be too small to determine the risk, because the gender specific cancer halves the population studied. Other cancers do not have enough data to determine risk, but uncontrolled levels of IGF-1 have the potential to worsen any malignancy, since the majority of cancer cells studied harbor elevated numbers of IGF1R. Due to the improved treatment modalities for acromegaly and subsequent lengthened life expectancy, cancer incidence will also increase as a function of normal aging. Recognizing the significant role that the GH/IGF-1 axis plays in malignancy development and progression, it is essential to maintain excellent control of acromegaly as well as emphasize cancer prevention and order appropriate screening tests.

Diabetes and Cancer Incidence in Acromegaly

In addition to GH and IGF-1, insulin resistance plays a role in acromegaly and cancer. Acromegaly causes insulin resistance, and type 2 diabetes (DM2) occurred in 11–53% of patients in a review of studies between 2007 and 2017 [4]. Diabetes is associated with a greater risk of a number of cancers in the general population, including liver, pancreas, colorectal, kidney, bladder, endometrial, breast, and non-Hodgkin's lymphoma with the RR ranging from 1.18 to 2.51 [168]. However, diabetes decreases the risk of prostate cancer [168–170]. Overall, diabetes is associated with a 10% increase in the RR of developing cancer with strongest evidence for intrahepatic cholangiocarcinoma, breast, endometrial, and colorectal carcinoma [169]. The risk of cancer is even higher in Asians with diabetes, RR 1.23 (95% CI, 1.09–1.39) [171]. Overall cancer mortality is also greater in diabetes, RR 1.16 (95% CI, 1.04–1.30) [169] with studies indicating an increase in breast, colorectal, endometrial, and prostate cancer death [168]; even though prostate cancer incidence is decreased by diabetes, mortality is elevated [172]. Mortality from any cancer was also higher in Asians with diabetes (HR 1.26;95% CI, 1.21–1.31), with positive associations for lymphoma, colorectal, liver, bile duct, gallbladder, pancreas, breast, endometrial, ovary, prostate, kidney, and thyroid cancers. Diabetes was not statistically significantly associated with mortality from leukemia or cancers of the bladder, cervix, esophagus, stomach, or lung [173].

In a study comparing patients with acromegaly and diabetes to acromegaly without diabetes, 26% of the cases had diabetes, and 22.6% of those with diabetes developed malignant tumors versus 9.2% without diabetes, OR 2.873 (95% CI, 1.572–5.250). In cases with diabetes, IGF-1 was significantly higher compared to those without diabetes, but IGF-1 was not different in those with malignancy verses those without [100]. Not surprisingly, patients older than 50 were more likely to develop cancer than the younger patients, but those older than 50 with diabetes had a greater risk of malignancy, 26.58%, compared to older patients without diabetes, 11.68%. The authors noted that the OR for developing cancer was greater in their patients with acromegaly and diabetes compared to studies of cancer risk with diabetes alone, suggesting that the acromegaly potentiates the risk of cancer. Prior to treatment, Hba1c was higher in patients with diabetes and malignancy, 8.24%, versus 7.1% in those with diabetes without malignancy, but it did not reach significance. Following acromegaly treatment, Hba1c was 6.3% in patients with malignancy verses 6.5% in those without [100].

Insulin resistance and diabetes may result in an elevated cancer risk through a number of processes. Hyperglycemia leads to oxidative stress and production of reactive oxidative species (ROS), which can cause DNA damage through oxidation of nucleobases [174]. Errors during repair of the damaged bases can also result in mutations [175]. Oxidative stress leads to worsening insulin resistance, with resultant increases in hyperglycemia and hyperinsulinemia. Glycation of proteins from hyperglycemia creates advanced glycation end products (AGEs), and accumulation of AGEs promotes more oxidative stress and chronic inflammation, creating a microenvironment conducive to tumorigenesis [174]. AGEs attach to the receptor for advanced glycation end products (RAGE), which are present on normal cells, and have been reported on a number of cancers including gastric, prostate, lung, pancreas, and liver [176]. Activation of the RAGE results in a heightened inflammatory environment with upregulation of VEGF and metalloproteinase-2, and decreased E-cadherin [176], many of the same pathways activated by IGF-1 which result in EMT.

Hyperinsulinemia decreases IGFBP1 and IGFBP2, which increases bioavailable IGF-1 [168], and insulin can also bind to the IGF1R, although with a lower affinity than IGF-1 [39]. Consequently, insulin resistance with hyperinsulinemia can potentiate IGF1R signaling through both elevated insulin and IGF-1. Insulin receptors and IGF1R share common signaling cascades through P3IK for metabolism and growth, and MAPK/ERK for mitogenesis and proliferation, but activation of the IR usually results in preferentially metabolic effects and less mitogenic effects compared to the IGF1R [177]. Insulin receptors, however, exist in alpha and beta isoforms, IRA and IRB. The IRA isoform activates the mitogenic pathway more than the metabolic pathway and IRB the converse [168, 177]. Tumors overexpress IR, particularly the IRA isoform, which is significantly elevated in cancers of the breast, prostate, colorectum, liver, endometrium, and in multiple myeloma [177]. In breast cancer, a high IRA/IRB ratio and hyperinsulinemia correlated with more aggressive and hormone-resistant tumors with worse prognosis [177]. The IRA isoform also has a high affinity for IGF-2 as well as proinsulin and can bind IGF-1, but with lower affinity, whereas the IRB isoform has low affinity for IGF-2, proinsulin, and IGF-1. In addition, tumors can express hybrid insulin/IGF-1 receptors, which are activated mainly by IGF-1, but also IGF-2 and insulin [177]. Many tumors have upregulated IGF-2 expression, including glioblastomas, Wilms' tumors, sarcomas, breast, esophageal, colorectal, endometrial, ovarian, hepatocellular, lung, and prostate cancers [178–180].

Hyperglycemia and hyperinsulinemia decrease sex hormone-binding globulin synthesis, increasing free estrogen and testosterone. Elevated levels of free estrogen and testosterone are associated with greater risks of breast, endometrial, and prostate cancers [181].

Diabetes leads to dysregulation in a number of noncoding RNAs (ncRNAs), which control gene expression through posttranscriptional regulation. These ncRNAs can inhibit or augment protein translation or induce mRNA degradation, thereby modifying cell signaling. Many of these ncRNAs are involved in IGF1R and IR expression, so dysregulation from uncontrolled diabetes can lead to overexpression of IGF1R and IRA [182].

Therefore, the combination of hyperglycemia and hyperinsulinemia may lead to DNA damage by ROS, potentiate tumors by increasing sex hormones, facilitate EMT through RAGE, and augment IGF1R and IR expression via ncRNAs. Activation of the overexpressed receptors by elevated bioavailable IGF-1 and hyperinsulinemia leads to tumor proliferation with excess glucose providing the energy substrate. In uncontrolled diabetes with uncontrolled acromegaly, the high levels of insulin and IGF-1 enhance activation of IGF1R, IR, and hybrid IR/IGF1R in normal and tumor cells in addition to paracrine/autocrine stimulation by secretion of IGF-1 and/or IGF-2 by cancers. Consequently, cancer risk in acromegaly is potentiated by the insulin resistance that it induces.

Conclusion

Well-controlled acromegaly has the same cancer mortality rate as the general population. However, if acromegaly is uncontrolled, cancer mortality is higher, with a potentially greater mortality from colorectal cancer in particular. There is a large body of evidence implicating the GH/IGF axis in promotion and proliferation of malignancy. The associated insulin resistance with hyperinsulinemia and hyperglycemia induced by acromegaly also compounds the cancer risk. Although it has been debated for years if acromegaly leads to higher overall rates of cancer, recent, large population studies and meta-analyses show a greater incidence of cancer. Colon polyps are increased, and colon cancer incidence is higher in nearly all studies of patients with acromegaly. Accordingly, current screening guidelines recommend a colonoscopy at diagnosis and a repeat colonoscopy in 5 years in patients with a polyp on initial screening or for those with persistently elevated IGF-1. For patients without polyps and normal IGF-1 levels, every 10-year repeat colonoscopies are appropriate.

There is also a greater incidence of thyroid nodules and nodular goiter in acromegaly. There may be an increased risk of papillary thyroid cancer, but it is most likely due to expanded ultrasound surveillance and inclusion of microcarcinomas. The differentiated thyroid cancers diagnosed in acromegaly behave similarly to those in patients without acromegaly, with no worse morbidity or mortality. Hence, current acromegaly guidelines recommend careful thyroid examination in all patients and thyroid ultrasound only for those with palpable nodules. Recommendations for fine-needle aspiration of thyroid nodules in acromegaly are the same as in the general population.

In the most recent study, prostate cancer risk appears to be greater in acromegaly, but whether this should change screening guidelines will need to be studied. The data for other cancers is still inadequate to conclude if the risk is elevated in acromegaly, so standard screening guidelines should be followed. However, there is substantial evidence that cancers of nearly every type develop IGF1R as part of their malignant transformation, allowing for proliferation, invasion, and metastasis. Therefore, it is essential to achieve and maintain control of GH and IGF-1 as well as glucose levels to avoid creating an environment conducive to carcinogenesis. In patients with acromegaly, it is important to emphasize cancer prevention and promote performance of appropriate screening tests to mitigate the cancer risk.

References

1. Colao A, Ferone D, Marzullo P, Lombardi G. Systemic complications of acromegaly: epidemiology, pathogenesis, and management. Endocr Rev. 2004;25(1):102–52. https://doi.org/10.1210/er.2002-0022.
2. Holdaway IM, Bolland MJ, Gamble GD. A meta-analysis of the effect of lowering serum levels of GH and IGF-1 on mortality in acromegaly. Eur J Endocrinol. 2008;159(2):89–95. https://doi.org/10.1530/EJE-08-0267.
3. Bolfi F, Neves AF, Boguszewski CL, Nunes-Nogueira VS. Mortality in acromegaly decreased in the last decade: a systematic review and meta-analysis. Eur J Endocrinol. 2018;179(1):59–71. https://doi.org/10.1530/EJE-18-0255.
4. Gadelha MR, Kasuki L, Lim DST, Fleseriu M. Systemic complications of acromegaly and the impact of the current treatment landscape: an update. Endocr Rev. 2019;40(1):268–332. https://doi.org/10.1210/er.2018-00115.
5. Arosio M, Reimondo G, Malchiodi E, et al. Predictors of morbidity and mortality in acromegaly: an Italian survey. Eur J Endocrinol. 2012;167(2):189–98. https://doi.org/10.1530/EJE-12-0084.
6. Bogazzi F, Colao A, Rossi G, et al. Comparison of the effects of primary somatostatin analogue therapy and pituitary adenomectomy on survival in patients with acromegaly: a retrospective cohort study. Eur J Endocrinol. 2013;169(3):367–76. https://doi.org/10.1530/EJE-13-0166.
7. Mercado M, Gonzalez B, Vargas G, et al. Successful mortality reduction and control of comorbidities in patients with acromegaly followed at a highly specialized multidisciplinary clinic. J Clin Endocrinol Metab. 2014;99(12):4438–46. https://doi.org/10.1210/jc.2014-2670.
8. Maione L, Brue T, Beckers A, et al. Changes in the management and comorbidities of acromegaly over three decades: the French acromegaly registry. Eur J Endocrinol. 2017;176(5):645–55. https://doi.org/10.1530/EJE-16-1064.
9. Esposito D, Ragnarsson O, Granfeldt D, Marlow T, Johannsson G, Olsson DS. Decreasing mortality and changes in treatment patterns in patients with acromegaly from a nationwide study. Eur J Endocrinol. 2018;178(5):459–69. https://doi.org/10.1530/EJE-18-0015. Errata: https://doi.org/10.1530/EJE-18-0015e.
10. Sherlock M, Ayuk J, Tomlinson JW, et al. Mortality in patients with pituitary disease. Endocr Rev. 2010;31(3):301–42. https://doi.org/10.1210/er.2009-0033.
11. Ritvonen E, Löyttyniemi E, Jaatinen P, Ebeling T, Moilanen L, Nuutila P, Kauppinen-Mäkelin R, Schalin-Jäntti C. Mortality in acromegaly: a 20-year follow-up study. Endocr Relat Cancer. 2016;23(6):469–80. https://doi.org/10.1530/ERC-16-0106.
12. Ayuk J, Clayton RN, Holder G, Sheppard MC, Stewart PM, Bates AS. Growth hormone and pituitary radiotherapy, but not serum insulin-like growth factor-I concentrations, predict excess mortality in patients with acromegaly. J Clin Endocrinol Metab. 2004;89(4):1613–7. https://doi.org/10.1210/jc.2003-031584.
13. Holdaway IM, Rajasoorya RC, Gamble GD. Factors influencing mortality in acromegaly. J Clin Endocrinol Metab. 2004;89(2):667–74. https://doi.org/10.1210/jc.2003-031199.
14. Orme SM, McNally RJ, Cartwright RA, Belchetz PE. Mortality and cancer incidence in acromegaly: a retrospective cohort study. United Kingdom Acromegaly Study Group. J Clin Endocrinol Metab. 1998;83(8):2730–4. https://doi.org/10.1210/jcem.83.8.5007.
15. Kauppinen-Mäkelin R, Sane T, Välimäki MJ, Markkanen H, Niskanen L, Ebeling T, Jaatinen P, Juonala M, Finnish Acromegaly Study Group, Pukkala E. Increased cancer incidence in acromegaly--a nationwide survey. Clin Endocrinol. 2010;72(2):278–9. https://doi.org/10.1111/j.1365-2265.2009.03619.x.
16. Green J, Cairns BJ, Casabonne D, et al. Height and cancer incidence in the Million Women Study: prospective cohort, and meta-analysis of prospective studies of height and total cancer risk. Lancet Oncol. 2011;12(8):785–94. https://doi.org/10.1016/S1470-2045(11)70154-1.

17. Liang S, Lv G, Chen W, Jiang J, Wang J. Height and kidney cancer risk: a meta-analysis of prospective studies. J Cancer Res Clin Oncol. 2015;141(10):1799–807. https://doi.org/10.1007/s00432-014-1870-5.
18. Schouten LJ, Rivera C, Hunter DJ, et al. Height, body mass index, and ovarian cancer: a pooled analysis of 12 cohort studies. Cancer Epidemiol Biomark Prev. 2008;17(4):902–12. https://doi.org/10.1158/1055-9965.EPI-07-2524.
19. Song X, Gong X, Zhang T, Jiang W. Height and risk of colorectal cancer: a meta-analysis. Eur J Cancer Prev. 2018;27(6):521–9. https://doi.org/10.1097/CEJ.0000000000000390.
20. Aarestrup J, Bjerregaard LG, Meyle KD, et al. Birthweight, childhood overweight, height and growth and adult cancer risks: a review of studies using the Copenhagen School Health Records Register. Int J Obes. 2020;44(7):1546–60. https://doi.org/10.1038/s41366-020-0523-9.
21. Parra-Soto S, Ho FK, Pell JP, Celis-Morales C. Does insulin-like growth factor moderate the association between height and risk of cancer at 24 sites? Br J Cancer. 2020;123(11):1697–704. https://doi.org/10.1038/s41416-020-01059-1.
22. World Cancer Research Fund/American Institute for Cancer Research. Continuous Update Project Expert Report 2018. Height and birthweight and the risk of cancer. Available at Diet, Nutrition, Physical Activity and Cancer: a Global Perspective (wcrf.org).
23. Nunney L. Size matters: height, cell number and a person's risk of cancer. Proc Biol Sci. 1889;2018(285):20181743. https://doi.org/10.1098/rspb.2018.1743.
24. Stefan N, Häring HU, Hu FB, Schulze MB. Divergent associations of height with cardiometabolic disease and cancer: epidemiology, pathophysiology, and global implications. Lancet Diabetes Endocrinol. 2016;4(5):457–67. https://doi.org/10.1016/S2213-8587(15)00474-X.
25. Gunnell D, Okasha M, Smith GD, Oliver SE, Sandhu J, Holly JM. Height, leg length, and cancer risk: a systematic review. Epidemiol Rev. 2001;23(2):313–42. https://doi.org/10.1093/oxfordjournals.epirev.a000809.
26. Murphy N, Carreras-Torres R, Song M, et al. Circulating levels of insulin-like growth factor 1 and insulin-like growth factor binding protein 3 associate with risk of colorectal cancer based on serologic and mendelian randomization analyses. Gastroenterology. 2020;158(5):1300–1312.e20. https://doi.org/10.1053/j.gastro.2019.12.020.
27. Endogenous Hormones and Breast Cancer Collaborative Group, Key TJ, Appleby PN, Reeves GK, Roddam AW. Insulin-like growth factor 1 (IGF1), IGF binding protein 3 (IGFBP3), and breast cancer risk: pooled individual data analysis of 17 prospective studies. Lancet Oncol. 2010;11(6):530–42. https://doi.org/10.1016/S1470-2045(10)70095-4.
28. Schmidt JA, Allen NE, Almquist M, et al. Insulin-like growth factor-I and risk of differentiated thyroid carcinoma in the European prospective investigation into cancer and nutrition. Cancer Epidemiol Biomark Prev. 2014;23(6):976–85. https://doi.org/10.1158/1055-9965.EPI-13-1210-T.
29. Shi R, Berkel HJ, Yu H. Insulin-like growth factor-I and prostate cancer: a meta-analysis. Br J Cancer. 2001;85(7):991–6. https://doi.org/10.1054/bjoc.2001.1961.
30. Le Marchand L, Donlon T, Seifried A, Kaaks R, Rinaldi S, Wilkens LR. Association of a common polymorphism in the human GH1 gene with colorectal neoplasia. J Natl Cancer Inst. 2002;94(6):454–60. https://doi.org/10.1093/jnci/94.6.454.
31. Ma J, Pollak MN, Giovannucci E, et al. Prospective study of colorectal cancer risk in men and plasma levels of insulin-like growth factor (IGF)-I and IGF-binding protein-3. J Natl Cancer Inst. 1999;91(7):620–5. https://doi.org/10.1093/jnci/91.7.620.
32. Guevara-Aguirre J, Balasubramanian P, Guevara-Aguirre M, et al. Growth hormone receptor deficiency is associated with a major reduction in pro-aging signaling, cancer, and diabetes in humans. Sci Transl Med. 2011;3(70):70ra13. https://doi.org/10.1126/scitranslmed.3001845.
33. Laron Z, Kauli R, Lapkina L, Werner H. IGF-1 deficiency, longevity and cancer protection of patients with Laron syndrome. Mutat Res Rev Mutat Res. 2017;772:123–33. https://doi.org/10.1016/j.mrrev.2016.08.002.
34. Ikeno Y, Hubbard GB, Lee S, et al. Reduced incidence and delayed occurrence of fatal neoplastic diseases in growth hormone receptor/binding protein knockout mice. J Gerontol A Biol Sci Med Sci. 2009;64(5):522–9. https://doi.org/10.1093/gerona/glp017.

35. Harvey S. Extrapituitary growth hormone. Endocrine. 2010;38(3):335–59. https://doi.org/10.1007/s12020-010-9403-8.
36. Kasprzak A, Szaflarski W. Role of alternatively spliced messenger RNA (mRNA) isoforms of the insulin-like growth factor 1 (IGF1) in selected human tumors. Int J Mol Sci. 2020;21(19):6995. https://doi.org/10.3390/ijms21196995.
37. Lincoln DT, Sinowatz F, Temmim-Baker L, Baker HI, Kölle S, Waters MJ. Growth hormone receptor expression in the nucleus and cytoplasm of normal and neoplastic cells. Histochem Cell Biol. 1998;109(2):141–59. https://doi.org/10.1007/s004180050212.
38. Forbes BE, Blyth AJ, Wit JM. Disorders of IGFs and IGF-1R signaling pathways. Mol Cell Endocrinol. 2020;518:111035. https://doi.org/10.1016/j.mce.2020.111035.
39. Hakuno F, Takahashi SI. 40 years of IGF1: IGF1 receptor signaling pathways. J Mol Endocrinol. 2018;61(1):T69–86. https://doi.org/10.1530/JME-17-0311.
40. Bach LA. IGF-binding proteins. J Mol Endocrinol. 2018;61(1):T11–28. https://doi.org/10.1530/JME-17-0254.
41. Iams WT, Lovly CM. Molecular pathways: clinical applications and future direction of insulin-like growth factor-1 receptor pathway blockade. Clin Cancer Res. 2015;21(19):4270–7. https://doi.org/10.1158/1078-0432.CCR-14-2518.
42. Frank SJ. Classical and novel GH receptor signaling pathways. Mol Cell Endocrinol. 2020;518:110999. https://doi.org/10.1016/j.mce.2020.110999.
43. Lu M, Flanagan JU, Langley RJ, Hay MP, Perry JK. Targeting growth hormone function: strategies and therapeutic applications. Signal Transduct Target Ther. 2019;4:3. https://doi.org/10.1038/s41392-019-0036-y.
44. Li H, Batth IS, Qu X, et al. IGF-IR signaling in epithelial to mesenchymal transition and targeting IGF-IR therapy: overview and new insights. Mol Cancer. 2017;16(1):6. https://doi.org/10.1186/s12943-016-0576-5.
45. Sustarsic EG, Junnila RK, Kopchick JJ. Human metastatic melanoma cell lines express high levels of growth hormone receptor and respond to GH treatment. Biochem Biophys Res Commun. 2013;441(1):144–50. https://doi.org/10.1016/j.bbrc.2013.10.023.
46. Gebre-Medhin M, Kindblom LG, Wennbo H, Törnell J, Meis-Kindblom JM. Growth hormone receptor is expressed in human breast cancer. Am J Pathol. 2001;158(4):1217–22. https://doi.org/10.1016/S0002-9440(10)64071-0.
47. Wu ZS, Yang K, Wan Y, Qian PX, Perry JK, Chiesa J, Mertani HC, Zhu T, Lobie PE. Tumor expression of human growth hormone and human prolactin predict a worse survival outcome in patients with mammary or endometrial carcinoma. J Clin Endocrinol Metab. 2011;96(10):E1619–29. https://doi.org/10.1210/jc.2011-1245.
48. Buckels A, Zhang Y, Jiang J, Athar M, Afaq F, Shevde-Samant L, Frank SJ. Autocrine/paracrine actions of growth hormone in human melanoma cell lines. Biochem Biophys Rep. 2019;21:100716. https://doi.org/10.1016/j.bbrep.2019.100716.
49. Wu X, Liu F, Yao X, Li W, Chen C. Growth hormone receptor expression is up-regulated during tumorigenesis of human colorectal cancer. J Surg Res. 2007;143(2):294–9. https://doi.org/10.1016/j.jss.2007.03.056.
50. García-Caballero T, Mertani HM, Lambert A, Gallego R, Fraga M, Pintos E, Forteza J, Chevallier M, Lobie PE, Vonderhaar BK, Beiras A, Morel G. Increased expression of growth hormone and prolactin receptors in hepatocellular carcinomas. Endocrine. 2000;12(3):265–71. https://doi.org/10.1385/ENDO:12:3:265.
51. Samani AA, Yakar S, LeRoith D, Brodt P. The role of the IGF system in cancer growth and metastasis: overview and recent insights. Endocr Rev. 2007;28(1):20–47. https://doi.org/10.1210/er.2006-0001.
52. Karagiannis A, Kassi E, Chatzigeorgiou A, Koutsilieris M. IGF bioregulation system in benign and malignant thyroid nodular disease: a systematic review. In Vivo. 2020;34(6):3069–91. https://doi.org/10.21873/invivo.12141.
53. Quinn KA, Treston AM, Unsworth EJ, et al. Insulin-like growth factor expression in human cancer cell lines. J Biol Chem. 1996;271(19):11477–83. https://doi.org/10.1074/jbc.271.19.11477.

54. Hellawell GO, Turner GD, Davies DR, Poulsom R, Brewster SF, Macaulay VM. Expression of the type 1 insulin-like growth factor receptor is up-regulated in primary prostate cancer and commonly persists in metastatic disease. Cancer Res. 2002;62(10):2942–50. PMID: 12019176.
55. Messias de Lima CF, Dos Santos Reis MD, da Silva Ramos FW, Ayres-Martins S, Smaniotto S. Growth hormone modulates in vitro endothelial cell migration and formation of capillary-like structures. Cell Biol Int. 2017;41(5):577–84. https://doi.org/10.1002/cbin.10747.
56. Brunet-Dunand SE, Vouyovitch C, Araneda S, et al. Autocrine human growth hormone promotes tumor angiogenesis in mammary carcinoma. Endocrinology. 2009;150(3):1341–52. https://doi.org/10.1210/en.2008-0608.
57. Zhu T, Starling-Emerald B, Zhang X, et al. Oncogenic transformation of human mammary epithelial cells by autocrine human growth hormone. Cancer Res. 2005;65(1):317–24. PMID: 15665309.
58. Kopchick JJ, List EO, Kelder B, Gosney ES, Berryman DE. Evaluation of growth hormone (GH) action in mice: discovery of GH receptor antagonists and clinical indications. Mol Cell Endocrinol. 2014;386(1–2):34–45. https://doi.org/10.1016/j.mce.2013.09.004.
59. Clayton PE, Banerjee I, Murray PG, Renehan AG. Growth hormone, the insulin-like growth factor axis, insulin and cancer risk. Nat Rev Endocrinol. 2011;7(1):11–24. https://doi.org/10.1038/nrendo.2010.171.
60. Werner H, Laron Z. Role of the GH-IGF1 system in progression of cancer. Mol Cell Endocrinol. 2020;518:111003. https://doi.org/10.1016/j.mce.2020.111003.
61. Stochholm K, Johannsson G. Reviewing the safety of GH replacement therapy in adults. Growth Hormon IGF Res. 2015;25(4):149–57. https://doi.org/10.1016/j.ghir.2015.06.006.
62. Stochholm K, Kiess W. Long-term safety of growth hormone-a combined registry analysis. Clin Endocrinol. 2018;88(4):515–28. https://doi.org/10.1111/cen.13502.
63. Raman S, Grimberg A, Waguespack SG, et al. Risk of neoplasia in pediatric patients receiving growth hormone therapy--a report from the pediatric endocrine society drug and therapeutics committee. J Clin Endocrinol Metab. 2015;100(6):2192–203. https://doi.org/10.1210/jc.2015-1002.
64. Jenkins PJ, Mukherjee A, Shalet SM. Does growth hormone cause cancer? Clin Endocrinol. 2006;64(2):115–21. https://doi.org/10.1111/j.1365-2265.2005.02404.x.
65. Chesnokova V, Zonis S, Barrett R, et al. Excess growth hormone suppresses DNA damage repair in epithelial cells. JCI Insight. 2019;4(3):e125762. https://doi.org/10.1172/jci.insight.125762.
66. Werner H. Tumor suppressors govern insulin-like growth factor signaling pathways: implications in metabolism and cancer. Oncogene. 2012;31(22):2703–14. https://doi.org/10.1038/onc.2011.447.
67. Thiery JP, Acloque H, Huang RY, Nieto MA. Epithelial-mesenchymal transitions in development and disease. Cell. 2009;139(5):871–90. https://doi.org/10.1016/j.cell.2009.11.007.
68. Xu XQ, Emerald BS, Goh EL, et al. Gene expression profiling to identify oncogenic determinants of autocrine human growth hormone in human mammary carcinoma. J Biol Chem. 2005;280(25):23987–4003. https://doi.org/10.1074/jbc.M503869200.
69. Mukhina S, Mertani HC, Guo K, Lee KO, Gluckman PD, Lobie PE. Phenotypic conversion of human mammary carcinoma cells by autocrine human growth hormone. Proc Natl Acad Sci U S A. 2004;101(42):15166–71. https://doi.org/10.1073/pnas.0405881101.
70. Graham TR, Zhau HE, Odero-Marah VA, et al. Insulin-like growth factor-I-dependent up-regulation of ZEB1 drives epithelial-to-mesenchymal transition in human prostate cancer cells [published correction appears in cancer res. 2008;68(10):4012]. Cancer Res. 2008;68(7):2479–88. https://doi.org/10.1158/0008-5472.CAN-07-2559.
71. Beppu K, Nakamura K, Linehan WM, Rapisarda A, Thiele CJ. Topotecan blocks hypoxia-inducible factor-1alpha and vascular endothelial growth factor expression induced by insulin-like growth factor-I in neuroblastoma cells. Cancer Res. 2005;65(11):4775–81. https://doi.org/10.1158/0008-5472.CAN-04-3332.

72. Zhang Y, Liu Y, Wang L, Song H. The expression and role of trefoil factors in human tumors. Transl Cancer Res. 2019;8(4):1609–17. https://doi.org/10.21037/tcr.2019.07.48.
73. Yusufu A, Shayimu P, Tuerdi R, Fang C, Wang F, Wang H. TFF3 and TFF1 expression levels are elevated in colorectal cancer and promote the malignant behavior of colon cancer by activating the EMT process. Int J Oncol. 2019;55(4):789–804. https://doi.org/10.3892/ijo.2019.4854.
74. Lin X, Zhang H, Dai J, et al. TFF3 contributes to epithelial-mesenchymal transition (EMT) in papillary thyroid carcinoma cells via the MAPK/ERK signaling pathway. J Cancer. 2018;9(23):4430–9. https://doi.org/10.7150/jca.24361.
75. Bergers G, Brekken R, McMahon G, et al. Matrix metalloproteinase-9 triggers the angiogenic switch during carcinogenesis. Nat Cell Biol. 2000;2(10):737–44. https://doi.org/10.1038/35036374.
76. Scheau C, Badarau IA, Costache R, et al. The role of matrix metalloproteinases in the epithelial-mesenchymal transition of hepatocellular carcinoma. Anal Cell Pathol (Amst). 2019;2019:9423907. https://doi.org/10.1155/2019/9423907.
77. Malki A, ElRuz RA, Gupta I, Allouch A, Vranic S, Al Moustafa AE. Molecular mechanisms of colon cancer progression and metastasis: recent insights and advancements. Int J Mol Sci. 2020;22(1):130. https://doi.org/10.3390/ijms22010130.
78. Kong D, Zhou H, Neelakantan D, et al. VEGF-C mediates tumor growth and metastasis through promoting EMT-epithelial breast cancer cell crosstalk. Oncogene. 2020;40(5):964–79. https://doi.org/10.1038/s41388-020-01539-x.
79. Šelemetjev S, Đoric I, Paunovic I, Tatic S, Cvejic D. Coexpressed high levels of VEGF-C and active MMP-9 are associated with lymphatic spreading and local invasiveness of papillary thyroid carcinoma. Am J Clin Pathol. 2016;146(5):594–602. https://doi.org/10.1093/ajcp/aqw184.
80. Drápela S, Bouchal J, Jolly MK, Culig Z, Souček K. ZEB1: a critical regulator of cell plasticity, DNA damage response, and therapy resistance. Front Mol Biosci. 2020;7:36. https://doi.org/10.3389/fmolb.2020.00036.
81. Masoud GN, Li W. HIF-1α pathway: role, regulation and intervention for cancer therapy. Acta Pharm Sin B. 2015;5(5):378–89. https://doi.org/10.1016/j.apsb.2015.05.007.
82. Osher E, Macaulay VM. Therapeutic targeting of the IGF axis. Cell. 2019;8(8):895. https://doi.org/10.3390/cells8080895.
83. Evans A, Jamieson SM, Liu DX, Wilson WR, Perry JK. Growth hormone receptor antagonism suppresses tumour regrowth after radiotherapy in an endometrial cancer xenograft model. Cancer Lett. 2016;379(1):117–23. https://doi.org/10.1016/j.canlet.2016.05.031.
84. Minoia M, Gentilin E, Molè D, et al. Growth hormone receptor blockade inhibits growth hormone-induced chemoresistance by restoring cytotoxic-induced apoptosis in breast cancer cells independently of estrogen receptor expression. J Clin Endocrinol Metab. 2012;97(6):E907–16. https://doi.org/10.1210/jc.2011-3340.
85. Wu P, Nielsen TE, Clausen MH. Small-molecule kinase inhibitors: an analysis of FDA-approved drugs. Drug Discov Today. 2016;21(1):5–10. https://doi.org/10.1016/j.drudis.2015.07.008.
86. Friedbichler K, Hofmann MH, Kroez M, et al. Pharmacodynamic and antineoplastic activity of BI 836845, a fully human IGF ligand-neutralizing antibody, and mechanistic rationale for combination with rapamycin. Mol Cancer Ther. 2014;13(2):399–409. https://doi.org/10.1158/1535-7163.MCT-13-0598.
87. de Bono J, Lin CC, Chen LT, et al. Two first-in-human studies of xentuzumab, a humanised insulin-like growth factor (IGF)-neutralising antibody, in patients with advanced solid tumours. Br J Cancer. 2020;122(9):1324–32. https://doi.org/10.1038/s41416-020-0774-1.
88. Mustacchi P, Shimkin M. Occurrence of cancer in acromegaly and in hypopituitarism. Cancer. 1957;10(1):100–4. https://doi.org/10.1002/1097-0142(195701/02)10:1<100::aid-cncr2820100113>3.0.co;2-v.

89. Dal J, Leisner MZ, Hermansen K, Farkas DK, Bengtsen M, Kistorp C, Nielsen EH, Andersen M, Feldt-Rasmussen U, Dekkers OM, Sørensen HT, Jørgensen JOL. Cancer incidence in patients with acromegaly: a cohort study and meta-analysis of the literature. J Clin Endocrinol Metab. 2018;103(6):2182–8. https://doi.org/10.1210/jc.2017-02457.
90. Renehan AG, Brennan BM. Acromegaly, growth hormone and cancer risk. Best Pract Res Clin Endocrinol Metab. 2008;22(4):639–57. https://doi.org/10.1016/j.beem.2008.08.011.
91. Bray F, Ferlay J, Soerjomataram I, Siegel RL, Torre LA, Jemal A. Global cancer statistics 2018: GLOBOCAN estimates of incidence and mortality worldwide for 36 cancers in 185 countries [published correction appears in CA Cancer J Clin. 2020;70(4):313]. CA Cancer J Clin. 2018;68(6):394–424. https://doi.org/10.3322/caac.21492.
92. Holdaway IM, Rajasoorya C. Epidemiology of acromegaly. Pituitary. 1999;2(1):29–41. https://doi.org/10.1023/a:1009965803750.
93. Reid TJ, Post KD, Bruce JN, Nabi Kanibir M, Reyes-Vidal CM, Freda PU. Features at diagnosis of 324 patients with acromegaly did not change from 1981 to 2006: acromegaly remains under-recognized and under-diagnosed. Clin Endocrinol. 2010;72(2):203–8. https://doi.org/10.1111/j.1365-2265.2009.03626.x.
94. Boguszewski CL, Ayuk J. MANAGEMENT OF ENDOCRINE DISEASE: acromegaly and cancer: an old debate revisited. Eur J Endocrinol. 2016;175(4):R147–56. https://doi.org/10.1530/EJE-16-0178.
95. Terzolo M, Reimondo G, Berchialla P, et al. Acromegaly is associated with increased cancer risk: a survey in Italy. Endocr Relat Cancer. 2017;24(9):495–504. https://doi.org/10.1530/ERC-16-0553.
96. Ron E, Gridley G, Hrubec Z, Page W, Arora S, Fraumeni JF Jr. Acromegaly and gastrointestinal cancer [published correction appears in cancer 1992;69(2):549]. Cancer. 1991;68(8):1673–7. https://doi.org/10.1002/1097-0142(19911015)68:8<1673::aid-cncr2820680802>3.0.co;2-0.
97. Baris D, Gridley G, Ron E, et al. Acromegaly and cancer risk: a cohort study in Sweden and Denmark. Cancer Causes Control. 2002;13(5):395–400. https://doi.org/10.1023/a:1015713732717.
98. Petroff D, Tönjes A, Grussendorf M, et al. The incidence of cancer among acromegaly patients: results from the German acromegaly registry. J Clin Endocrinol Metab. 2015;100(10):3894–902. https://doi.org/10.1210/jc.2015-2372.
99. Popovic V, Damjanovic S, Micic D, et al. Increased incidence of neoplasia in patients with pituitary adenomas. Pituitary Study Group. Clin Endocrinol (Oxf). 1998;49(4):441–5. https://doi.org/10.1046/j.1365-2265.1998.00536.x.
100. Cheng S, Gomez K, Serri O, Chik C, Ezzat S. The role of diabetes in acromegaly associated neoplasia. PLoS One. 2015;10(5):e0127276. https://doi.org/10.1371/journal.pone.0127276.
101. Wu JC, Huang WC, Chang HK, Ko CC, Lirng JF, Chen YC. Natural history of acromegaly: incidences, re-operations, cancers, and mortality rates in a national cohort. Neuroendocrinology. 2020;110(11–12):977–87. https://doi.org/10.1159/000505332.
102. Gullu BE, Celik O, Gazioglu N, Kadioglu P. Thyroid cancer is the most common cancer associated with acromegaly. Pituitary. 2010;13(3):242–8. https://doi.org/10.1007/s11102-010-0224-9.
103. Jenkins PJ. Acromegaly and cancer. Horm Res. 2004;62(Suppl 1):108–15. https://doi.org/10.1159/000080768.
104. Jass JR. Hyperplastic polyps and colorectal cancer: is there a link? Clin Gastroenterol Hepatol. 2004;2(1):1–8. https://doi.org/10.1016/s1542-3565(03)00284-2.
105. Cats A, Dullaart RP, Kleibeuker JH, et al. Increased epithelial cell proliferation in the colon of patients with acromegaly. Cancer Res. 1996;56(3):523–6. PMID: 8564965.
106. Rokkas T, Pistiolas D, Sechopoulos P, Margantinis G, Koukoulis G. Risk of colorectal neoplasm in patients with acromegaly: a meta-analysis. World J Gastroenterol. 2008;14(22):3484–9. https://doi.org/10.3748/wjg.14.3484.

107. Jenkins PJ, Frajese V, Jones AM, et al. Insulin-like growth factor I and the development of colorectal neoplasia in acromegaly. J Clin Endocrinol Metab. 2000;85(9):3218–21. https://doi.org/10.1210/jcem.85.9.6806.
108. Dworakowska D, Gueorguiev M, Kelly P, et al. Repeated colonoscopic screening of patients with acromegaly: 15-year experience identifies those at risk of new colonic neoplasia and allows for effective screening guidelines. Eur J Endocrinol. 2010;163(1):21–8. https://doi.org/10.1530/EJE-09-1080.
109. Terzolo M, Tappero G, Borretta G, et al. High prevalence of colonic polyps in patients with acromegaly. Influence of sex and age. Arch Intern Med. 1994;154(11):1272–6. PMID: 8203994.
110. Delhougne B, Deneux C, Abs R, Chanson P, Fierens H, Laurent-Puig P, Duysburgh I, Stevenaert A, Tabarin A, Delwaide J, Schaison G, Belaïche J, Beckers A. The prevalence of colonic polyps in acromegaly: a colonoscopic and pathological study in 103 patients. J Clin Endocrinol Metab. 1995;80(11):3223–6. https://doi.org/10.1210/jcem.80.11.7593429.
111. Colao A, Balzano A, Ferone D, et al. Increased prevalence of colonic polyps and altered lymphocyte subset pattern in the colonic lamina propria in acromegaly. Clin Endocrinol. 1997;47(1):23–8. https://doi.org/10.1046/j.1365-2265.1997.00253.x.
112. Terzolo M, Reimondo G, Gasperi M, et al. Colonoscopic screening and follow-up in patients with acromegaly: a multicenter study in Italy. J Clin Endocrinol Metab. 2005;90(1):84–90. https://doi.org/10.1210/jc.2004-0240.
113. Renehan AG, Painter JE, Bell GD, Rowland RS, O'Dwyer ST, Shalet SM. Determination of large bowel length and loop complexity in patients with acromegaly undergoing screening colonoscopy. Clin Endocrinol. 2005;62(3):323–30. https://doi.org/10.1111/j.1365-2265.2005.02217.x.
114. Center MM, Jemal A, Ward E. International trends in colorectal cancer incidence rates. Cancer Epidemiol Biomark Prev. 2009;18(6):1688–94. https://doi.org/10.1158/1055-9965.EPI-09-0090.
115. Selby JV, Friedman GD, Quesenberry CP Jr, Weiss NS. A case-control study of screening sigmoidoscopy and mortality from colorectal cancer. N Engl J Med. 1992;326(10):653–7. https://doi.org/10.1056/NEJM199203053261001.
116. Lincoln DT, Kaiser HE, Raju GP, Waters MJ. Growth hormone and colorectal carcinoma: localization of receptors. In Vivo. 2000;14(1):41–9. PMID: 10757060.
117. Chesnokova V, Zonis S, Zhou C, et al. Growth hormone is permissive for neoplastic colon growth [published correction appears in proc Natl Acad sci U S a. 2016 Aug 30;113(35):E5251]. Proc Natl Acad Sci U S A. 2016;113(23):E3250–9. https://doi.org/10.1073/pnas.1600561113.
118. Dworakowska D, Grossman AB. Colonic cancer and acromegaly. Front Endocrinol (Lausanne). 2019;10:390. https://doi.org/10.3389/fendo.2019.00390.
119. Mao YL, Li ZW, Lou CJ, Pang D, Zhang YQ. Phospho-STAT5 expression is associated with poor prognosis of human colonic adenocarcinoma. Pathol Oncol Res. 2011;17(2):333–9. https://doi.org/10.1007/s12253-010-9321-3.
120. Sekharam M, Zhao H, Sun M, et al. Insulin-like growth factor 1 receptor enhances invasion and induces resistance to apoptosis of colon cancer cells through the Akt/Bcl-x(L) pathway. Cancer Res. 2003;63(22):7708–16. PMID: 14633695.
121. Lahm H, Amstad P, Wyniger J, et al. Blockade of the insulin-like growth-factor-I receptor inhibits growth of human colorectal cancer cells: evidence of a functional IGF-II-mediated autocrine loop. Int J Cancer. 1994;58(3):452–9. https://doi.org/10.1002/ijc.2910580325.
122. Hakam A, Yeatman TJ, Lu L, et al. Expression of insulin-like growth factor-1 receptor in human colorectal cancer. Hum Pathol. 1999;30(10):1128–33. https://doi.org/10.1016/s0046-8177(99)90027-8.
123. Cascinu S, Del Ferro E, Grianti C, et al. Inhibition of tumor cell kinetics and serum insulin growth factor I levels by octreotide in colorectal cancer patients. Gastroenterology. 1997;113(3):767–72. https://doi.org/10.1016/s0016-5085(97)70170-7.

124. Bogazzi F, Russo D, Locci MT, et al. Apoptosis is reduced in the colonic mucosa of patients with acromegaly. Clin Endocrinol. 2005;63(6):683–8. https://doi.org/10.1111/j.1365-2265.2005.02405.x.
125. Dutta P, Bhansali A, Vaiphei K, et al. Colonic neoplasia in acromegaly: increased proliferation or deceased apoptosis? Pituitary. 2012;15:166–73. https://doi.org/10.1007/s11102-011-0300-9.
126. Katznelson L, Laws ER Jr, Melmed S, et al. Acromegaly: an endocrine society clinical practice guideline. J Clin Endocrinol Metab. 2014;99(11):3933–51. https://doi.org/10.1210/jc.2014-2700.
127. Fleseriu M, Biller BMK, Freda PU, et al. A pituitary society update to acromegaly management guidelines. Pituitary. 2020;24(1):1–13. https://doi.org/10.1007/s11102-020-01091-7.
128. Giustina A, Barkan A, Beckers A, et al. A consensus on the diagnosis and treatment of acromegaly comorbidities: an update. J Clin Endocrinol Metab. 2020;105(4):dgz096. https://doi.org/10.1210/clinem/dgz096.
129. Tode B, Serio M, Rotella CM, et al. Insulin-like growth factor-I: autocrine secretion by human thyroid follicular cells in primary culture. J Clin Endocrinol Metab. 1989;69(3):639–47. https://doi.org/10.1210/jcem-69-3-639.
130. Tramontano D, Cushing GW, Moses AC, Ingbar SH. Insulin-like growth factor-I stimulates the growth of rat thyroid cells in culture and synergizes the stimulation of DNA synthesis induced by TSH and Graves'-IgG. Endocrinology. 1986;119(2):940–2. https://doi.org/10.1210/endo-119-2-940.
131. Chen Z, Jiang X, Feng Y, et al. Decrease in acromegaly-associated thyroid enlargement after normalization of IGF-1 levels: a prospective observation and in vitro study. Endocr Pract. 2020;26(4):369–77. https://doi.org/10.4158/EP-2019-0353.
132. Völzke H, Friedrich N, Schipf S, et al. Association between serum insulin-like growth factor-I levels and thyroid disorders in a population-based study. J Clin Endocrinol Metab. 2007;92(10):4039–45. https://doi.org/10.1210/jc.2007-0816.
133. Woliński K, Stangierski A, Gurgul E, et al. Thyroid lesions in patients with acromegaly - case-control study and update to the meta-analysis. Endokrynol Pol. 2017;68(1):2–6. https://doi.org/10.5603/EP.2017.0001.
134. Tita P, Ambrosio MR, Scollo C, et al. High prevalence of differentiated thyroid carcinoma in acromegaly. Clin Endocrinol. 2005;63(2):161–7. https://doi.org/10.1111/j.1365-2265.2005.02316.x.
135. Kaldrymidis D, Papadakis G, Tsakonas G, et al. High incidence of thyroid cancer among patients with acromegaly. J BUON. 2016;21(4):989–93. PMID: 27685924.
136. Tirosh A, Shimon I. Complications of acromegaly: thyroid and colon. Pituitary. 2017;20(1):70–5. https://doi.org/10.1007/s11102-016-0744-z.
137. Miyakawa M, Saji M, Tsushima T, Wakai K, Shizume K. Thyroid volume and serum thyroglobulin levels in patients with acromegaly: correlation with plasma insulin-like growth factor I levels. J Clin Endocrinol Metab. 1988;67(5):973–8. https://doi.org/10.1210/jcem-67-5-973.
138. Cheung NW, Boyages SC. The thyroid gland in acromegaly: an ultrasonographic study. Clin Endocrinol. 1997;46(5):545–9. https://doi.org/10.1046/j.1365-2265.1997.1680985.x.
139. Uchoa HB, Lima GA, Corrêa LL, et al. Prevalence of thyroid diseases in patients with acromegaly: experience of a Brazilian center. Arq Bras Endocrinol Metabol. 2013;57(9):685–90. https://doi.org/10.1590/s0004-27302013000900003.
140. Wu X, Gao L, Guo X, et al. GH, IGF-1, and age are important contributors to thyroid abnormalities in patients with acromegaly. Int J Endocrinol. 2018;2018:6546832. https://doi.org/10.1155/2018/6546832.
141. Cannavò S, Squadrito S, Finocchiaro MD, et al. Goiter and impairment of thyroid function in acromegalic patients: basal evaluation and follow-up. Horm Metab Res. 2000;32(5):190–5. https://doi.org/10.1055/s-2007-978620.

142. Gasperi M, Martino E, Manetti L, et al. Prevalence of thyroid diseases in patients with acromegaly: results of an Italian multi-center study. J Endocrinol Investig. 2002;25(3):240–5. https://doi.org/10.1007/BF03343997.
143. Mian C, Ceccato F, Barollo S, et al. AHR over-expression in papillary thyroid carcinoma: clinical and molecular assessments in a series of Italian acromegalic patients with a long-term follow-up. PLoS One. 2014;9(7):e101560. https://doi.org/10.1371/journal.pone.0101560.
144. Baştürk E, Kement M, Yavuzer D, et al. The role of insulin-like growth factor 1 in the development of benign and malignant thyroid nodules. Balkan Med J. 2012;29(2):133–8. https://doi.org/10.5152/balkanmedj.2011.034.
145. Liu YJ, Qiang W, Shi J, Lv SQ, Ji MJ, Shi BY. Expression and significance of IGF-1 and IGF-1R in thyroid nodules. Endocrine. 2013;44(1):158–64. https://doi.org/10.1007/s12020-012-9864-z.
146. Lawnicka H, Motylewska E, Borkowska M, et al. Elevated serum concentrations of IGF-1 and IGF-1R in patients with thyroid cancers. Biomed Pap Med Fac Univ Palacky Olomouc Czech Repub. 2020;164(1):77–83. https://doi.org/10.5507/bp.2019.018.
147. Maiorano E, Ciampolillo A, Viale G, et al. Insulin-like growth factor 1 expression in thyroid tumors. Appl Immunohistochem Mol Morphol. 2000;8(2):110–9. https://doi.org/10.1097/00129039-200006000-00005.
148. Dagdelen S, Cinar N, Erbas T. Increased thyroid cancer risk in acromegaly. Pituitary. 2014;17(4):299–306. https://doi.org/10.1007/s11102-013-0501-5.
149. dos Santos MC, Nascimento GC, Nascimento AG, et al. Thyroid cancer in patients with acromegaly: a case-control study. Pituitary. 2013;16(1):109–14. https://doi.org/10.1007/s11102-012-0383-y.
150. Haugen BR, Alexander EK, Bible KC, et al. 2015 American Thyroid Association management guidelines for adult patients with thyroid nodules and differentiated thyroid cancer: the American Thyroid Association guidelines task force on thyroid nodules and differentiated thyroid cancer. Thyroid. 2016;26(1):1–133. https://doi.org/10.1089/thy.2015.0020.
151. Lai NB, Garg D, Heaney AP, Bergsneider M, Leung AM. No benefit of dedicated thyroid nodule screening in patients with acromegaly. Endocr Pract. 2020;26(1):16–21. https://doi.org/10.4158/EP-2019-0254.
152. Danilowicz K, Sosa S, Gonzalez Pernas MS, et al. Acromegaly and thyroid cancer: analysis of evolution in a series of patients. Clin Diabetes Endocrinol. 2020;6(1):24. https://doi.org/10.1186/s40842-020-00113-4.
153. Renehan AG, Zwahlen M, Minder C, O'Dwyer ST, Shalet SM, Egger M. Insulin-like growth factor (IGF)-I, IGF binding protein-3, and cancer risk: systematic review and meta-regression analysis. Lancet. 2004;363(9418):1346–53. https://doi.org/10.1016/S0140-6736(04)16044-3.
154. Nabarro JD. Acromegaly. Clin Endocrinol. 1987;26(4):481–512. https://doi.org/10.1111/j.1365-2265.1987.tb00805.x.
155. Wolinski K, Stangierski A, Dyrda K, et al. Risk of malignant neoplasms in acromegaly: a case-control study. J Endocrinol Investig. 2017;40(3):319–22. https://doi.org/10.1007/s40618-016-0565-y.
156. Bidosee M, Karry R, Weiss-Messer E, Barkey RJ. Growth hormone affects gene expression and proliferation in human prostate cancer cells. Int J Androl. 2011;34(2):124–37. https://doi.org/10.1111/j.1365-2605.2010.01064.x.
157. Wu J, Yu E. Insulin-like growth factor receptor-1 (IGF-IR) as a target for prostate cancer therapy. Cancer Metastasis Rev. 2014;33(2–3):607–17. https://doi.org/10.1007/s10555-013-9482-0.
158. Iwamura M, Sluss PM, Casamento JB, Cockett AT. Insulin-like growth factor I: action and receptor characterization in human prostate cancer cell lines. Prostate. 1993;22(3):243–52. https://doi.org/10.1002/pros.2990220307.
159. Nickerson T, Chang F, Lorimer D, Smeekens SP, Sawyers CL, Pollak M. In vivo progression of LAPC-9 and LNCaP prostate cancer models to androgen independence is associated with

increased expression of insulin-like growth factor I (IGF-I) and IGF-1 receptor (IGF-IR). Cancer Res. 2001;61(16):6276–80. PMID: 11507082.
160. Burfeind P, Chernicky CL, Rininsland F, Ilan J, Ilan J. Antisense RNA to the type I insulin-like growth factor receptor suppresses tumor growth and prevents invasion by rat prostate cancer cells in vivo. Proc Natl Acad Sci U S A. 1996;93(14):7263–8. https://doi.org/10.1073/pnas.93.14.7263.
161. Roddam AW, Allen NE, Appleby P, et al. Insulin-like growth factors, their binding proteins, and prostate cancer risk: analysis of individual patient data from 12 prospective studies. Ann Intern Med. 2008;149(7):461–W88. https://doi.org/10.7326/0003-4819-149-7-200810070-00006.
162. Colao A, Marzullo P, Spiezia S, et al. Effect of growth hormone (GH) and insulin-like growth factor I on prostate diseases: an ultrasonographic and endocrine study in acromegaly, GH deficiency, and healthy subjects. J Clin Endocrinol Metab. 1999;84(6):1986–91. https://doi.org/10.1210/jcem.84.6.5776.
163. Colao A, Marzullo P, Ferone D, et al. Prostatic hyperplasia: an unknown feature of acromegaly. J Clin Endocrinol Metab. 1998;83(3):775–9. https://doi.org/10.1210/jcem.83.3.4645.
164. Watts EL, Goldacre R, Key TJ, Allen NE, Travis RC, Perez-Cornago A. Hormone-related diseases and prostate cancer: an English national record linkage study. Int J Cancer. 2020;147(3):803–10. https://doi.org/10.1002/ijc.32808.
165. Kim JH, Hong SK. Clinical utility of current biomarkers for prostate cancer detection. Investig Clin Urol. 2021;62(1):1–13. https://doi.org/10.4111/icu.20200395.
166. Lin C, Travis RC, Appleby PN, et al. Pre-diagnostic circulating insulin-like growth factor-I and bladder cancer risk in the European Prospective Investigation into Cancer and Nutrition. Int J Cancer. 2018;143(10):2351–8. https://doi.org/10.1002/ijc.31650.
167. Khandwala HM, McCutcheon IE, Flyvbjerg A, Friend KE. The effects of insulin-like growth factors on tumorigenesis and neoplastic growth. Endocr Rev. 2000;21(3):215–44. https://doi.org/10.1210/edrv.21.3.0399.
168. Vigneri P, Frasca F, Sciacca L, Pandini G, Vigneri R. Diabetes and cancer. Endocr Relat Cancer. 2009;16(4):1103–23. https://doi.org/10.1677/ERC-09-0087.
169. Tsilidis KK, Kasimis JC, Lopez DS, Ntzani EE, Ioannidis JP. Type 2 diabetes and cancer: umbrella review of meta-analyses of observational studies. BMJ. 2015;350:g7607. https://doi.org/10.1136/bmj.g7607.
170. Bansal D, Bhansali A, Kapil G, Undela K, Tiwari P. Type 2 diabetes and risk of prostate cancer: a meta-analysis of observational studies. Prostate Cancer Prostatic Dis. 2013;16(2):151–S1. https://doi.org/10.1038/pcan.2012.40.
171. Noto H, Tsujimoto T, Noda M. Significantly increased risk of cancer in diabetes mellitus patients: a meta-analysis of epidemiological evidence in Asians and non-Asians. J Diabetes Investig. 2012;3(1):24–33. https://doi.org/10.1111/j.2040-1124.2011.00183.x.
172. Lee J, Giovannucci E, Jeon JY. Diabetes and mortality in patients with prostate cancer: a meta-analysis. Springerplus. 2016;5(1):1548. https://doi.org/10.1186/s40064-016-3233-y.
173. Chen Y, Wu F, Saito E, et al. Association between type 2 diabetes and risk of cancer mortality: a pooled analysis of over 771,000 individuals in the Asia cohort consortium. Diabetologia. 2017;60(6):1022–32. https://doi.org/10.1007/s00125-017-4229-z.
174. Sruthi CR, Raghu KG. Advanced glycation end products and their adverse effects: the role of autophagy. J Biochem Mol Toxicol. 2021;35:e22710. https://doi.org/10.1002/jbt.22710.
175. Harris IS, DeNicola GM. The complex interplay between antioxidants and ROS in cancer. Trends Cell Biol. 2020;30(6):440–51. https://doi.org/10.1016/j.tcb.2020.03.002.
176. Rojas A, González I, Morales E, Pérez-Castro R, Romero J, Figueroa H. Diabetes and cancer: looking at the multiligand/RAGE axis. World J Diabetes. 2011;2(7):108–13. https://doi.org/10.4239/wjd.v2.i7.108.
177. Belfiore A, Malaguarnera R, Vella V, et al. Insulin receptor isoforms in physiology and disease: an updated view. Endocr Rev. 2017;38(5):379–431. https://doi.org/10.1210/er.2017-00073.

178. Simpson A, Petnga W, Macaulay VM, Weyer-Czernilofsky U, Bogenrieder T. Insulin-like growth factor (IGF) pathway targeting in cancer: role of the IGF axis and opportunities for future combination studies. Target Oncol. 2017;12(5):571–97. https://doi.org/10.1007/s11523-017-0514-5.
179. Livingstone C. IGF2 and cancer. Endocr Relat Cancer. 2013;20(6):R321–39. https://doi.org/10.1530/ERC-13-0231.
180. Brouwer-Visser J, Huang GS. IGF2 signaling and regulation in cancer. Cytokine Growth Factor Rev. 2015;26(3):371–7. https://doi.org/10.1016/j.cytogfr.2015.01.002.
181. Wang M, Yang Y, Liao Z. Diabetes and cancer: epidemiological and biological links. World J Diabetes. 2020;11(6):227–38. https://doi.org/10.4239/wjd.v11.i6.227.
182. Chen B, Li J, Chi D, et al. Non-coding RNAs in IGF-1R signaling regulation: the underlying pathophysiological link between diabetes and cancer. Cell. 2019;8(12):1638. https://doi.org/10.3390/cells8121638.

Chapter 11
Mortality in Acromegaly

Basma Abdulhadi, Charles Couch Farmer, and T. Brooks Vaughan

Introduction

Known in formal academic terms since at least 1886 when described by Pierre Marie, acromegaly has occupied our interest ever since in the medical literature and in fiction and the arts. Likely references to acromegaly and gigantism exist throughout history, including Dickens' memorable observation of a male with gigantism while on a trip to Kentucky: "He had a weakness in the knees and trustfulness in his long face. He was only 25 years old… He went bobbing down the cabin, among men of six feet high and upward, like a lighthouse walking among lampposts" [1]. In 1892 Massalongo first suggested that the cause of acromegaly was due to pituitary hyperfunction, and in 1909 Cushing first reported that the clinical symptoms of acromegaly remitted after partial hypophysectomy. Evans and Long later confirmed the pituitary source of growth hormone in 1921 by intraperitoneal injection of anterior pituitary extracts in rats. Growth hormone was later isolated in 1957, and the first radioimmunoassay became available in 1963, which is when GH levels were shown to be elevated in patients with acromegaly [2].

Arriving at a clear understanding of the mortality risks associated with acromegaly is obviously of great interest and has been attempted since the 1970s [3]. Known causes of mortality associated with acromegaly are predominantly macrovascular, respiratory, and potentially malignant in nature. Defining this risk clearly has proven to be a difficult task as our ability to measure excess growth hormone

B. Abdulhadi · C. C. Farmer · T. B. Vaughan (✉)
Division of Endocrinology, Diabetes and Metabolism,
University of Alabama at Birmingham School of Medicine,
Birmingham, AL, USA
e-mail: babdulhadi@uabmc.edu; cfarmer@uabmc.edu; tbvaughan@uabmc.edu

L. S. Blevins Jr., M. K. Aghi (eds.), *Acromegaly*, Contemporary Endocrinology,
https://doi.org/10.1007/978-3-031-16258-9_11

levels in the laboratory has become more sensitive over time and treatment options for these patients have happily become more effective. A move toward multimodal therapy in the modern era has allowed us to become more selective in choosing invasive options. The adverse sequela of the disease must be teased out from other confounding factors including mortality risks associated with specific treatment modalities (medications, surgery, and radiotherapy), accompanying pituitary dysfunction, and common comorbidities such as diabetes and sleep apnea. This chapter will review the current state of the literature regarding acromegaly, associated therapies and conditions, and mortality.

GH and IGF-1 Levels as Predictors of Mortality

Serum GH and IGF-1 levels are used by clinicians as biomarkers of acromegalic disease activity. The Endocrine Society Clinical Practice Guidelines for Acromegaly defines the goals of management as achieving an age-normalized serum IGF-1 value and a random GH level of less than 1.0 μg/L (or less than 1.0 μg/L on a growth hormone suppression test if random levels are not in this range) [4]. Older estimates of mortality have indicated that despite the use of pituitary surgery and radiotherapy, mortality in patients with acromegaly was significantly increased compared to the general population [5]. More recent studies, however, have found that mortality from acromegaly approaches that of the general population if treatment is successful in controlling the biochemical activity of the disease [5]. This improved mortality estimate in more recent studies likely reflects the wider range of therapeutics that have become available as well as the use of tighter cutoffs to indicate control of disease.

Serum GH levels have been identified by multiple studies as the single most important and consistent predictor of mortality in patients with acromegaly. A meta-analysis by Holdaway et al. included 18 studies with a total of 4806 patients with acromegaly and used the last available GH level to predict the standardized mortality ratio (SMR) [5]. Overall mortality was increased in patients with acromegaly compared to that of the general population despite almost all patients receiving treatment in this cohort (SMR 1.7, 95% CI 1.5–2.0) [5]. Stratification of patients into groups according to last available GH levels revealed that those with final GH values <2.5 μg/L had mortality risk similar to that of the general population with SMR 1.1, (CI 0.9–1.4). For patients with a final GH levels above 2.5 μg/L, the standardized mortality ratio was 1.9 (CI 1.5–2.4), significantly higher than the general population [5].

The association between levels of IGF-1 and mortality in patients with acromegaly is less clear than has been established with GH levels. Holdaway et al. found that patients with normal last visit IGF-1 levels had a similar mortality to that of the general population (SMR 1.1 with CI 0.9–1.4), whereas those with elevated IGF-1 levels had an increased standardized mortality ratio (SMR 2.5 with CI 1.6–4.0) [5]. However, multiple other studies have failed to show a clear relationship between posttreatment IGF-1 levels and mortality [6, 7]. For example, using the West Midlands database, Ayuk and others found a relative mortality risk of 1.2 (CI .71–2.03) for those patients with elevated IGF-1 levels vs those with normal levels. Data from a Finnish database of 334 patients failed to show any relationship between IGF-1 levels and mortality [6, 7]. Both of these studies confirmed an association with GH levels and mortality like that described above.

It is important to note that the studies assessing IGF-1 and GH levels as determinants of mortality typically use the last available GH and IGF-1 levels in their analysis. This is a potentially limiting methodology, not accounting for the duration or severity of disease and thus overall exposure to higher levels of GH. It is plausible that a patient who had a longer and more severe exposure to the disease would have a greater mortality risk than a patient who was diagnosed earlier, received therapy, and achieved control or remission sooner. This is a well-understood concept from other disorders, such as diabetes where we know longer exposure and more severe elevations of blood sugar raise the risk of complications.

Sherlock et al. investigated this question and compared the use of the last available GH/IGF-1 analysis to a cumulative, time-dependent method to assess mortality risk [8]. They argued that the use of the last available IGF-1 and GH levels was an incomplete representation of the disease course. To calculate a "time-dependent" or cumulative GH effect on mortality, they used multiple data points for each patient and quantified cumulative GH exposure using "GH units-year: GHU" [8]. They considered GH levels to be constant between two consecutive GH measurements and extrapolated back in time from the most recent level. They then calculated the cumulative GHU for each patient and used multivariable Poisson regression model to calculate relative risks of mortality based on patient's last GH level and cumulative GH levels. Their results showed an overall increased all-cause mortality in patients with acromegaly as compared to the general population (SMR 1.7 (1.4–2.0), $P < 0.001$) [8]. Comparing the mortality relative risk of the last available GH level to the "time-dependent method," mortality relative risk was generally lower in the time-dependent method, and only GH values above than or equal to 5 μg/L were suggestive of an increased risk of mortality (RR 1.5, CI 0.9–2.4) [8]. When they analyzed their data using only the last available GH level, there was a statistically increased mortality risk in patients with GH levels above 1 μg/L (RR 1.8, *P* value 0.03) [8]. They concluded that using the last available GH level to estimate mortality risk led to potential overestimates. Thus, the GHU, while less convenient to calculate, may be a more accurate measure of mortality risk, accounting for the cumulative effects of GH over the years. As seen in other studies, this newer methodology also failed to show statistical significance in terms of IGF-1 levels and mortality [8].

Encouragingly, mortality rates associated with acromegaly appear to be improving over time. A meta-analysis in 2018 suggested that studies done before 2008 (1970–2007) showed elevated overall mortality rates in acromegaly, but in studies published since 2009–2018, the overall mortality was not increased (SMR 1.35, CI 0.99–1.85) [9]. However, there were clear increases in mortality in uncontrolled patients vs patients with biochemical control throughout the entire timeframe

(1970–present). The availability of somatostatin analogues vs studies in which surgery and radiotherapy were the only treatment modalities was associated with significant improvements in the SMR [9]. The benefits of specific medical therapies (somatostatin analogues, dopamine agonists, pegvisomant) are further discussed elsewhere in this volume.

Hypopituitarism and Mortality

Growth hormone-secreting pituitary tumors are most commonly macroadenomas, and stalk compression may lead to hypopituitarism which has been shown to increase mortality, predominantly due to cardiovascular disease [10]. Hypopituitarism in patients with acromegaly may also be secondary to surgery or to treatment with radiotherapy [9, 11]. A recent comparison of national acromegalic registries found that in France, approximately 31% of patients treated for acromegaly developed some degree hypopituitarism, which is substantial but improved in contrast to older studies showing rates as high as 68%. Surgery and radiotherapy were the sole treatment modalities many older studies [11].

While the benefits of biochemical normalization of GH are clear (and IGF-1 less clear), it is important to note that patients with hypopituitarism (particularly in patients with ACTH deficiency) and those who have undergone radiation therapy as part of their treatment regimen have been shown to have an increased mortality risk in multiple studies [9, 12]. ACTH deficiency and increasing doses of hydrocortisone have been shown to be associated with an increased SMR with the principle cause of death being cardiovascular disease [12]. The increase in cardiovascular death was associated with increasing hydrocortisone doses [HC dose >0 and ≤20 mg/day, 10% cardiovascular mortality; HC dose >20 and ≤25 mg/day, 33.3% cardiovascular mortality; HC dose >25 and ≤30 mg/day, 38.5% cardiovascular mortality; and HC >30 mg/day, 44.4% cardiovascular mortality] [12].

This suggests a need for caution in aiming for lower GH levels to lower mortality rates. Achieving this goal may require the use of radiotherapy and or repeated surgeries which may ultimately create new mortality risks in these patients, thus the need for individualized treatment goals in every patient.

Although there is a large body of literature investigating thyroid abnormalities and overall mortality, there is, to date, no data independently associating central hypothyroidism with mortality [13]. Hypogonadism associated with acromegaly is potentially due to mass effect, surgery, radiotherapy, or co-secretion of prolactin by a GH-producing pituitary adenoma. In a 2001 study of patients with hypopituitarism of any cause, only untreated gonadotropin deficiency was associated with increased mortality [14].

Growth hormone deficiency plays a potential role in the excess cardiovascular mortality seen in hypopituitarism, but treatment of GH deficiency has not been definitively shown to reduce mortality [10, 15, 16]. Since patients with acromegaly commonly develop growth hormone deficiency due to treatment, the question of growth hormone replacement in these patients has been of particular concern as the concept may seem counterintuitive. Available data suggests these patients may benefit from growth hormone replacement in terms of quality of life, body composition, muscle mass, bone density, and lipid profiles, all of which are typically seen in patients with treated GH deficiency [17–19]. Norrman et al. noted an increase in cerebrovascular events in the treatment arm of small cohort but noted that the patients with events had prior radiotherapy [19]. Most data show benefits outweighing risks, but longer-term follow-up is needed [17].

Radiotherapy and Mortality

Conventional radiation therapy was first described in patients with acromegaly in 1909 and remained first-line treatment for decades due to its apparent low morbidity and efficacy in relieving most of the outward signs of acromegaly. Since immunoassays were not yet available, outcomes were described in terms of reversal of visual field deficits. Once immunoassays became available in 1963, it was found that conventional radiation therapy was rarely effective in reducing GH levels to normal. Therapy went on to involve megavoltage radiation and proton beam therapy which were more efficacious in reducing GH levels, but concerns were raised regarding damage to adjacent brain. Panhypopituitarism and visual deficits began to become apparent around 1976. Due to this, neurosurgical measures including transsphenoidal surgery came into favor and showed a more rapid reduction in GH levels [2].

Assessing the independent effects of radiotherapy on mortality in acromegaly has been extremely challenging. There are no randomized trials comparing various forms of radiotherapy (fractionated vs radiosurgery) [20]. There are several relevant issues that may be confounders. Radiotherapy itself is not rapidly effective, and the data we have suggests regarding conventional radiotherapy and acromegaly suggests a mean time to remission among patients that can range from 5 to 15 years [21]. Radiosurgery, a newer and more precise modality with multiple techniques may be associated a more rapid time to remission [21, 22]. Radiosurgery should pose less risk for collateral injury to adjacent tissue. A significant confounder is likely that tumors in which radiotherapy and radiosurgery are employed tend to be larger and associated with higher GH and IGF-1 levels. Radiotherapy frequently leads to associated hypopituitarism, discussed above, which may affect mortality rates. To date, there is not clear evidence of a risk of second malignancy after pituitary radiotherapy [23, 24].

Data in acromegaly specifically indicates an increase in all-cause mortality after conventional radiotherapy with an SMR of 1.58 (CI 1.22–2.04) [25]. As might be expected due to radiation effects on the cerebral vasculature, the strongest risk is in cerebrovascular mortality (SMR 4.42, CI 2.71–7.22), and this is persistent even when controlled for GH and IGF-1 levels, suggesting the effect was independent of underlying disease activity [25]. Hypopituitarism associated with radiotherapy continues to be a significant confounder, with one study showing no association with mortality and specific radiation doses or regimens but an association with the duration of radiation-induced hypopituitarism [26].

Cancer Incidence, Mortality, and Acromegaly

Mentioned here but covered in detail elsewhere in this text, opinions regarding acromegaly and the associated incidence of cancer and risk of cancer mortality have varied over the years [27]. Of concern is the clear role that GH and IGF-1 can play in cell proliferation [28]. Despite this, data related to incident cancers do not show a consistent pattern [28, 29]. Neoplasms of the thyroid and colon have received the most attention in acromegaly.

Colon polyps have classically been associated with acromegaly, and this has been described in multiple studies, although whether the true incidence of these polyps differs from the general population is unclear [27]. Some relatively large retrospective reports have shown no increased incidence in cancers, but there are concerns that cancer-associated mortality may be increased in acromegaly [30].

Patients with acromegaly have a high prevalence of a variety of thyroid abnormalities, and each patient deserves evaluation. Although both goiters and multinodular goiters are quite common in acromegalic patients, thyroid cancer is rare, and the Endocrine Society Guidelines currently recommend thyroid ultrasound only in the case of a palpable nodule or nodularity although some experts would recommend a more aggressive approach [4, 29, 31]. Uncontrolled acromegaly may increase the risk of thyroid cancer, but not the mortality, and patients with acromegaly may be subject to overdiagnosis from increased surveillance [29]. There is a lack of consensus at this point regarding the general need increased cancer surveillance in acromegaly, particularly with thyroid ultrasound and colonoscopy [27, 32, 33].

Other Causes of Mortality

Covered in more detail elsewhere in this volume, excess growth hormone production leads to metabolic changes and comorbidities including hypertension, cardiovascular disease, diabetes mellitus, respiratory system dysfunction, and, more controversially, malignant neoplasms. Working to prevent, identify, and adequately treat these comorbidities remains a cornerstone in the treatment of patients with acromegaly [9]. Conclusive data related to sex, race, and economic disparities are lacking in acromegaly. There is limited information regarding sexual differences in acromegaly, with some data suggesting that women have increased mortality in the first 20 years after diagnosis compared to men, possibly due to being diagnosed at a later age [32].

Recent data suggests that adequate treatment significantly reduces mortality in these patients as evidenced by a shift in leading cause of death from cardiovascular disease to malignancy [34]. A meta-analysis published in 2018 looked at 17 studies published before 2008 and 9 studies published after 2008, and it showed that mortality has gone from being increased [SMR 1.76 (95% CI 1.52–2.40)] to being equal to the average population [SMR 1.35 (95% CI 0.99–1.85)] [9]. Hypertension, diabetes, hypopituitarism, and sleep apnea were some of the most frequently reported comorbidities in the Spanish Acromegaly Registry. Compared to those never exposed to somatostatin analogues, patients treated with these drugs had a higher incidence of diabetes (42% compared with 33.5%; 95% CI 2.7–14.3; $P = 0.005$) and sleep apnea (16.3% compared with 10.5%; 95% CI 1.3–10.4; $P = 0\ 0.013$). Hypertension prevalence in acromegalic patients varies widely between 18% and 62% likely given lack of standardized defining criteria and evolving guidelines.

Cardiovascular Disease

GH and IGF-1 levels may also affect mortality by altering cardiovascular mortality in patients with acromegaly. It was noted that even patients with acromegaly who lacked the traditional cardiac risk factors had increased cardiovascular mortality, and this correlated with increased levels of GH and IGF-1 [35]. Controlling GH and IGF-1 levels during the early stages of disease may improve and reverse the cardiomyopathy that results during the course of the disease thus improving overall mortality risk in those patients [12].

Approximately 50% of acromegaly patients develop hypertriglyceridemia and reduced HDL levels. LDL levels are more variable and tend to be normal or increased. These derangements contribute to cardiovascular disease which is one of the most prevalent comorbidities in patients with acromegaly with arterial hypertension being the most common disorder. Hypertension is present in at least one third of acromegaly patients. The main driver of hypertension in these patients is sodium and water retention leading to increased plasma volume. Aldosterone and renin tend to be suppressed and total body sodium is increased, possibly due to a direct effect from GH on sodium transport [35]. Hypertension was found to be more prevalent in those acromegalic patients with high IGF-I concentrations than in the total acromegalic or normal populations. It has been shown to be an independent predictor of mortality in some studies of patients with acromegaly [36].

Prolonged excess GH exposure leads to cardiac remodeling and changes in the vasculature further contributing to cardiovascular disease. GH excess leads to concentric myocardial hypertrophy, interstitial fibrosis via increased collagen deposition, and increased left ventricular mass coined as acromegaly cardiomyopathy. Progressive ventricular dilation eventually leads to biventricular failure, although acromegalic cardiomyopathy can be improved by lowering GH concentration [35].

Valvular heart disease, secondary to collagen and mucopolysaccharide deposition, is present in up to 75% of patients at diagnosis with the mitral and aortic valve being most affected. LVH prevalence ranges from 11% to 78% in these patients, although systolic dysfunction appears to be uncommon. Coronary artery disease does not appear to be increased in patients with acromegaly, and GH excess does not seem to directly contribute to atherosclerosis [35]. Atherosclerosis prevalence is controversial due to its multifactorial nature and concomitant cardiovascular risk factors in acromegaly.

Treating acromegaly patients with first-generation somatostatin analogs has been shown to improve cardiomyopathy, reduce LVH, and possibly improve diastolic dysfunction [37]. A study in 2004 showed that increased mortality in acromegaly was due to cardiovascular disease (60%), respiratory disease (25%), and malignancy (15%), but more recent studies published over the past 10 years have shown a shift in mortality with malignancy now surpassing cardiovascular disease [9, 35]. In a 20-year follow-up study of Finnish acromegaly patients from January 1980 to December 1999, cause of death moved from 44% cardiovascular and 28% cancer related in the first decade to 23% cardiovascular and 35% cancer related over the next decade with males being more adversely affected than females [32].

Sleep Apnea

GH excess causes a variety of changes in the human body including upper respiratory tract changes. Tongue swelling, changes in the cartilage and mucosa along the respiratory tract, lung volume changes (including reduced elasticity and increased distensibility), and anatomical changes to the craniofacial region (including macroglossia, deformities in the jaw, goiter, thickening of the vocal cords, and epiglottis hypertrophy) all contribute to respiratory diseases being a common comorbidity in acromegaly patients. Obstructive sleep apnea has been found to be present in a vast majority of patients and severity has been found to correspond with higher GH and IGF-1 levels with males more affected than females. Central sleep apnea is found in approximately one third of patients. Treatment appears to aid the central component but not necessarily the obstructive component [38].

Sleep apnea reportedly affects between 67% and 75% of acromegalic patients when investigated prospectively, but the Spanish Registry only documented a prevalence of roughly 13% [39]. This possibly reflects a low awareness of the problem by many physicians leading to not specifically asking about snoring and sleep apnea in their acromegalic patients. Sleep apnea is also more frequent in those treated with somatostatin analogues, probably reflecting both a more active disease and lower postoperative cure rate than in those who had not required medical treatment, and increased awareness of the problem in the past decade when these analogues became available. Sleep apnea is well-known to cause an increase in mortality, and concerningly it is not clear that appropriate treatment with positive airway pressure improves that mortality rate. A large meta-analysis in 2013 showed an increased RR for CVD of 1.79, CI 1.47–2.18; fatal and nonfatal stroke of 2.15, CI 1.42–3.24; and death from all causes of 1.92, CI 1.38–2 [40, 41]. A recent study showed no improvement in risk using PAP. Although some of the mortality studies looking at IGF-1 and GH attempt to control for sleep apnea, it is likely to be a confounding factor in this data.

Diabetes

Diabetes mellitus is more prevalent in acromegaly than in the general population, greater in the Spanish acromegalic population (especially in those exposed to somatostatin analogues) than in New Zealand (20%) but lower than in Canada (40% plus 22% glucose intolerance) [7, 11, 36, 39]. Type 2 diabetes has been shown independently to have a relative risk of mortality of 1.26, CI 1.2–1.32 [42]. Growth hormone excess leads to metabolic derangements affecting both glycemic and lipid metabolism. Examples include insulin resistance, impaired insulin sensitivity/impaired glucose tolerance, and increased gluconeogenesis. GH is an anabolic hormone that, in excess, leads to sustained lipolysis and lipid oxidation in addition to inhibiting lipoprotein lipase in adipose tissue. These changes lead to increased synthesis of triglycerides, reduced HDL, and reduced body fat. GH also reduces glucose uptake via lower expression of GLUT-1 and 4 transporters. IGF-1 typically promotes free fatty acid uptake into liver and adipose tissues, but its effect is counteracted by GH in acromegaly leading to higher prevalence of glucose and lipid abnormalities [35].

Approximately 50% of patients with acromegaly will go on to develop impaired glucose tolerance, and approximately 30–56% will develop diabetes. Family history, BMI, age, GH levels, and IGF-1 levels all contribute to the risk. Treatment improves these comorbidities and surgery completely cures diabetes in approximately two thirds of patients [2, 35].

Conclusions

In summary, a variety of factors influence mortality in acromegaly (see Table 11.1). The most well established is growth hormone, although debate continues regarding how to measure this (last available GH vs a time-dependent method). IGF-1 has proven to be a far less reliable predictor of mortality. Radiotherapy appears to be a mortality risk factor, but we do not have mortality data for judiciously applied stereotactic radiosurgery. A variety of comorbidities likely affect mortality rates, with sleep apnea being very common and serious. It is unproven that treating sleep apnea with positive airway pressure lowers mortality and there is inadequate data in patients with acromegaly to draw conclusions. Cardiovascular disease and diabetes are risk factors that are likely more modifiable. To date, we have no data directly comparing the relative mortality benefits of various pharmaceutical therapies for acromegaly. Thankfully, there is a consensus that mortality risks have diminished over time and causes of mortality have shifted toward those seen in the general

Table 11.1 Influences on mortality in acromegaly

Marker of mortality	Pooled SMR (selected studies)	CI	Comment
GH >2.5 μg (last available)	1.9 [5]	1.5–2.4	Wide agreement across studies
IGF-1 above normal (last available)	2.5 [5]	1.6–4.0	Increased SMR with IGF-1 not seen in all studies
GH >2.5 μg (time-dependent)	1.2 [8]	0.8–1.9	
GH >5 μg (time-dependent)	1.7 [8]	1.1–2.8	
IGF-1 (time-dependent)	No increase at any level [8]		
OSA	1.92 [40]	1.38–2.69	Patients without acromegaly
ACTH deficiency	1.7 [12]	1.2–2.5	SMR higher at higher replacement doses
DM (general population)	1.26 [42]	1.2–1.32	Patients without acromegaly
Conventional radiotherapy, all-cause	2.1 [12] 1.58 [25]	1.7–2.6 1.22–2.04	
Cerebrovascular mortality after conventional radiotherapy	4.42 [25]	2.71–7.22	

population. This is probably due to more selective use of radiotherapy and surgery and a broader armamentarium of effective medical therapies. How to best balance aggressive lowering of GH levels without introducing now mortality risks continues to be a fundamental question that must be individualized for each patient. We have limited data regarding race, sex, and healthcare disparities in acromegaly [43]. The ongoing use of national acromegaly registries is necessary to understand the disease and to improve outcomes [44].

References

1. Beckers A, Aaltonen LA, Daly AF, Karhu A. Familial isolated pituitary adenomas (FIPA) and the pituitary adenoma predisposition due to mutations in the aryl hydrocarbon receptor interacting protein (AIP) gene. Endocr Rev. 2013;34(2):239–77.
2. Wass JA. Acromegaly: treatment after 100 years. BMJ. 1993;307(6918):1505–6.
3. Wright AD, Hill DM, Lowy C, Fraser TR. Mortality in acromegaly. Q J Med. 1970;39(153):1–16.
4. Katznelson L, Laws ER Jr, Melmed S, Molitch ME, Murad MH, Utz A, et al. Acromegaly: an endocrine society clinical practice guideline. J Clin Endocrinol Metab. 2014;99(11):3933–51.
5. Holdaway IM, Bolland MJ, Gamble GD. A meta-analysis of the effect of lowering serum levels of GH and IGF-I on mortality in acromegaly. Eur J Endocrinol. 2008;159(2):89–95.
6. Ayuk J, Clayton RN, Holder G, Sheppard MC, Stewart PM, Bates AS. Growth hormone and pituitary radiotherapy, but not serum insulin-like growth factor-I concentrations, predict excess mortality in patients with acromegaly. J Clin Endocrinol Metab. 2004;89(4):1613–7.

7. Kauppinen-Makelin R, Sane T, Reunanen A, Valimaki MJ, Niskanen L, Markkanen H, et al. A nationwide survey of mortality in acromegaly. J Clin Endocrinol Metab. 2005;90(7):4081–6.
8. Sherlock M, Reulen RC, Aragon-Alonso A, Ayuk J, Clayton RN, Sheppard MC, et al. A paradigm shift in the monitoring of patients with acromegaly: last available growth hormone may overestimate risk. J Clin Endocrinol Metab. 2014;99(2):478–85.
9. Bolfi F, Neves AF, Boguszewski CL, Nunes-Nogueira VS. Mortality in acromegaly decreased in the last decade: a systematic review and meta-analysis. Eur J Endocrinol. 2018;179(1):59–71.
10. Rosen T, Bengtsson BA. Premature mortality due to cardiovascular disease in hypopituitarism. Lancet. 1990;336(8710):285–8.
11. Maione L, Brue T, Beckers A, Delemer B, Petrossians P, Borson-Chazot F, et al. Changes in the management and comorbidities of acromegaly over three decades: the French Acromegaly Registry. Eur J Endocrinol. 2017;176(5):645–55.
12. Sherlock M, Reulen RC, Alonso AA, Ayuk J, Clayton RN, Sheppard MC, et al. ACTH deficiency, higher doses of hydrocortisone replacement, and radiotherapy are independent predictors of mortality in patients with acromegaly. J Clin Endocrinol Metab. 2009;94(11):4216–23.
13. Rodondi N, den Elzen WP, Bauer DC, Cappola AR, Razvi S, Walsh JP, et al. Subclinical hypothyroidism and the risk of coronary heart disease and mortality. JAMA. 2010;304(12):1365–74.
14. Tomlinson JW, Holden N, Hills RK, Wheatley K, Clayton RN, Bates AS, et al. Association between premature mortality and hypopituitarism. West Midlands Prospective Hypopituitary Study Group. Lancet. 2001;357(9254):425–31.
15. van Bunderen CC, van Nieuwpoort IC, Arwert LI, Heymans MW, Franken AA, Koppeschaar HP, et al. Does growth hormone replacement therapy reduce mortality in adults with growth hormone deficiency? Data from the Dutch National Registry of Growth Hormone Treatment in adults. J Clin Endocrinol Metab. 2011;96(10):3151–9.
16. Diez JJ, Sangiao-Alvarellos S, Cordido F. Treatment with growth hormone for adults with growth hormone deficiency syndrome: benefits and risks. Int J Mol Sci. 2018;19(3):893.
17. Giavoli C, Profka E, Verrua E, Ronchi CL, Ferrante E, Bergamaschi S, et al. GH replacement improves quality of life and metabolic parameters in cured acromegalic patients with growth hormone deficiency. J Clin Endocrinol Metab. 2012;97(11):3983–8.
18. Ronchi CL, Giavoli C, Ferrante E, Verrua E, Bergamaschi S, Ferrari DI, et al. Prevalence of GH deficiency in cured acromegalic patients: impact of different previous treatments. Eur J Endocrinol. 2009;161(1):37–42.
19. Norrman LL, Johannsson G, Sunnerhagen KS, Svensson J. Baseline characteristics and the effects of two years of growth hormone (GH) replacement therapy in adults with GH deficiency previously treated for acromegaly. J Clin Endocrinol Metab. 2008;93(7):2531–8.
20. Chanson P, Dormoy A, Dekkers OM. Use of radiotherapy after pituitary surgery for nonfunctioning pituitary adenomas. Eur J Endocrinol. 2019;181(1):D1–d13.
21. Castinetti F, Morange I, Dufour H, Regis J, Brue T. Radiotherapy and radiosurgery in acromegaly. Pituitary. 2009;12(1):3–10.
22. Landolt AM, Haller D, Lomax N, Scheib S, Schubiger O, Siegfried J, et al. Stereotactic radiosurgery for recurrent surgically treated acromegaly: comparison with fractionated radiotherapy. J Neurosurg. 1998;88(6):1002–8.
23. van Varsseveld NC, van Bunderen CC, Ubachs DH, Franken AA, Koppeschaar HP, van der Lely AJ, et al. Cerebrovascular events, secondary intracranial tumors, and mortality after radiotherapy for nonfunctioning pituitary adenomas: a subanalysis from the Dutch National Registry of Growth Hormone Treatment in Adults. J Clin Endocrinol Metab. 2015;100(3):1104–12.
24. Sattler MG, van Beek AP, Wolffenbuttel BH, van den Berg G, Sluiter WJ, Langendijk JA, et al. The incidence of second tumours and mortality in pituitary adenoma patients treated with postoperative radiotherapy versus surgery alone. Radiother Oncol. 2012;104(1):125–30.
25. Ayuk J, Stewart PM. Mortality following pituitary radiotherapy. Pituitary. 2009;12(1):35–9.
26. Erfurth EM, Bulow B, Svahn-Tapper G, Norrving B, Odh K, Mikoczy Z, et al. Risk factors for cerebrovascular deaths in patients operated and irradiated for pituitary tumors. J Clin Endocrinol Metab. 2002;87(11):4892–9.

27. Melmed S. Acromegaly and cancer: not a problem? J Clin Endocrinol Metab. 2001;86(7):2929–34.
28. Cohen P, Clemmons DR, Rosenfeld RG. Does the GH-IGF axis play a role in cancer pathogenesis? Growth Horm IGF Res. 2000;10(6):297–305.
29. Tirosh A, Shimon I. Complications of acromegaly: thyroid and colon. Pituitary. 2017;20(1):70–5.
30. Orme SM, McNally RJ, Cartwright RA, Belchetz PE. Mortality and cancer incidence in acromegaly: a retrospective cohort study. United Kingdom Acromegaly Study Group. J Clin Endocrinol Metab. 1998;83(8):2730–4.
31. Siegel G, Tomer Y. Is there an association between acromegaly and thyroid carcinoma? A critical review of the literature. Endocr Res. 2005;31(1):51–8.
32. Ritvonen E, Loyttyniemi E, Jaatinen P, Ebeling T, Moilanen L, Nuutila P, et al. Mortality in acromegaly: a 20-year follow-up study. Endocr Relat Cancer. 2016;23(6):469–80.
33. Dekkers OM, Biermasz NR, Pereira AM, Romijn JA, Vandenbroucke JP. Mortality in acromegaly: a metaanalysis. J Clin Endocrinol Metab. 2008;93(1):61–7.
34. Kasuki L, Rocha PDS, Lamback EB, Gadelha MR. Determinants of morbidities and mortality in acromegaly. Arch Endocrinol Metab. 2019;63(6):630–7.
35. Colao A, Ferone D, Marzullo P, Lombardi G. Systemic complications of acromegaly: epidemiology, pathogenesis, and management. Endocr Rev. 2004;25(1):102–52.
36. Holdaway IM, Rajasoorya RC, Gamble GD. Factors influencing mortality in acromegaly. J Clin Endocrinol Metab. 2004;89(2):667–74.
37. Gadelha MR, Kasuki L, Lim DST, Fleseriu M. Systemic complications of acromegaly and the impact of the current treatment landscape: an update. Endocr Rev. 2019;40(1):268–332.
38. van Haute FR, Taboada GF, Correa LL, Lima GA, Fontes R, Riello AP, et al. Prevalence of sleep apnea and metabolic abnormalities in patients with acromegaly and analysis of cephalometric parameters by magnetic resonance imaging. Eur J Endocrinol. 2008;158(4):459–65.
39. Sesmilo G. [Epidemiology of acromegaly in Spain]. Endocrinol Nutr. 2013;60(8):470–4.
40. Wang X, Ouyang Y, Wang Z, Zhao G, Liu L, Bi Y. Obstructive sleep apnea and risk of cardiovascular disease and all-cause mortality: a meta-analysis of prospective cohort studies. Int J Cardiol. 2013;169(3):207–14.
41. Yu J, Zhou Z, McEvoy RD, Anderson CS, Rodgers A, Perkovic V, et al. Association of positive airway pressure with cardiovascular events and death in adults with sleep apnea: a systematic review and meta-analysis. JAMA. 2017;318(2):156–66.
42. Zghebi SS, Steinke DT, Carr MJ, Rutter MK, Emsley RA, Ashcroft DM. Examining trends in type 2 diabetes incidence, prevalence and mortality in the UK between 2004 and 2014. Diabetes Obes Metab. 2017;19(11):1537–45.
43. Lavrentaki A, Paluzzi A, Wass JA, Karavitaki N. Epidemiology of acromegaly: review of population studies. Pituitary. 2017;20(1):4–9.
44. Maione L, Chanson P. National acromegaly registries. Best Pract Res Clin Endocrinol Metab. 2019;33(2):101264.

Chapter 12
An Overview of the Approach to the Management of Acromegaly

Lewis S. Blevins Jr., Denise Feng, and AnneMarie Destruel

At the time of this writing, in early 2022, 34 years has passed since I evaluated and managed my first patient with acromegaly. Things have changed since then. Surgeons are better. Treatment goals are more well-defined. Radioimmunoassay techniques have improved greatly. There have been significant advances in radiotherapeutic techniques. Multiple classes of drugs are now available to treat patients with residual and recurrent disease. In this era, uncontrolled treated acromegaly is the exception rather than the rule. I have learned a lot managing literally hundreds of patients with this disease process as a neuroendocrinologist over the past three decades. My recommendations for treatment are evidenced-based yet highly influenced by a multitude of things learned from my patients through observations over the course of their diseases and treatments. Thus, the medical decision-making that I employ is a balance between the art of medicine and documented scientific facts based on accumulated evidence [1].

Over the past couple of decades, various organizations and working groups have published guidelines for the management of patients with acromegaly [2–4]. While these are, mostly, evidence-based, I suspect that treatment bias has been introduced in regard to the recommended choices of medications used to treat residual and recurrent disease. Still, most of these guidelines are reasonably similar, and they serve as a roadmap of sorts for practitioners with little to no experience in managing this complex disease. With experience, however, one recognizes that no two patients are alike even in the setting of anatomic and biochemical similarities. For example, if you had 100 patients with 1 cm growth hormone-producing pituitary adenomas

L. S. Blevins Jr. (✉)
Department of Neurological Surgery, University of California, San Francisco, CA, USA
e-mail: lewis.blevins@ucsf.edu

D. Feng · A. Destruel
Department of Neurosurgery, University of California—San Francisco, San Francisco, CA, USA
e-mail: denise.feng@ucsf.edu; Annemarie.destruel@ucsf.edu

L. S. Blevins Jr., M. K. Aghi (eds.), *Acromegaly*, Contemporary Endocrinology,
https://doi.org/10.1007/978-3-031-16258-9_12

and IGF-I levels at 3.5 standard deviation above mean for age and sex, you would have 100 very different patients. Organ and tissue responses to IGF-I among affected persons are very different. Some patients have a genetic risk for hypertension or metabolic syndrome and are more likely to have cardiovascular and metabolic complications of the disease. Others may be prone to sleep apnea, arthritis, or in some way predisposed to develop one or more of the other manifestations of acromegaly, including malignancies. Further, psychosocial, other social, and economic factors also play a role in modulating the disease state leading to what I like to consider as the illness. In effect, not only would those 100 patients have different manifestations of their disease, but they would have 100 different illnesses. They should be treated individually, according to need, based on innumerable factors to be considered, and not according to some general schematic that is meant to apply to a group of patients as if they all had the same disease and illness. For these reasons, I tend to recommend against the strict use of guidelines in the practice of medicine. Unfortunately, one of the unintended consequences of the presence of guidelines is that third-party payers often utilize them as the definitive guide to decision-making in the management of patients with acromegaly. In my opinion, carefully considered individualized therapy is often wrestled away from the doctors and patients. These decisions often lead to consternation among our patients and to a great deal of frustration for experienced highly specialized clinicians who have deliberately selected most appropriate treatments for their patients.

Most patients with newly diagnosed and previously untreated acromegaly undergo surgery as first-line therapy [2, 4]. Surgery is often the treatment of choice even for those patients in whom resection would not be curative due to invasive disease or other circumstances. In these patients, incomplete resection often leads to biochemical and clinical improvement. Furthermore, these patients often respond better to medical therapy, and their tumor remnants are frequently amenable to and respond better to stereotactic radiosurgery rather than conventional radiotherapy that would be required without debulking surgery [5, 6]. In some patients who harbor smaller tumors with invasive disease, and without mass effects or compromise of pituitary functions, it might be reasonable to treat with medical therapy rather than surgery as these patients would probably end up on medical therapy long-term [7]. I am inclined to first treat these patients with dopamine agonist drugs. Nonresponders are treated with somatostatin receptor ligands. Radiotherapy could also be considered although this is not my usual practice because of the risks of radiation-induced apoplexy and hypopituitarism. There have been several studies investigating the use of somatostatin receptor ligands prior to surgery in attempt to reduce tumor size in hopes of achieving a greater likelihood of gross total removal of noninvasive tumors [8–10]. There are approximately an equal number of studies suggesting better outcomes with this approach as there are studies showing no difference in outcomes between patients treated with somatostatin receptor ligands prior to surgery and those who were untreated. I have treated two patients prior to surgery, both of whom enjoyed 50% reduction in tumor size, and they were rendered disease-free as a result of surgery. It is not clear whether they would have entered remission following surgery without treatment. Importantly, growth hormone and IGF-I levels were controlled in both patients, and they experienced marked improvements in sleep apnea, cardiac dysfunction, and overall sense of well-being prior to surgery. At the present time, I only employ pre-treatment with somatostatin receptor ligands prior to surgery for those patients who have cardiomyopathy, severe obstructive sleep apnea, or other factors that significantly increase their risks of surgery at the time of diagnosis.

Treatment of patients with residual or recurrent disease requires careful consideration of several factors to determine whether to proceed with repeat surgery, radiotherapy, medical therapy, or a combination of these modalities. I firmly believe that treatment of these patients is best undertaken in a tertiary medical center or "pituitary center of excellence" by experienced providers who understand the nuances and caveats of the disease and can design and deliver an appropriate individualized therapeutic program and follow-up [11].

All patients with residual and recurrent disease should be considered for repeat surgery when tumor is present on magnetic resonance imaging studies of the sella. This is especially true if the tumor appears to be amenable to resection or if debulking of a significant amount of tumor would be possible and likely to improve clinical and biochemical features of the disease process or improve responses to medical therapy [12]. Repeat surgery is also worthwhile if removal of a sufficient amount of tumor would allow for stereotactic radiotherapy instead of conventional radiotherapy. Surgical outcomes, including control of disease and morbidity as well as mortality, are demonstrably better when these patients are operated on by experienced surgeons [13].

Radiotherapy for acromegaly is a controversial topic. Some use it regularly and others not at all given there are medications that can control disease activity. Thirty years ago, nearly all patients were treated with conventional postoperative radiotherapy [14]. While treatment would almost always prevent further tumor progression, only about two-thirds to three-quarters of patients would achieve biochemical control over the ensuing 15–20 years. Further, most patients later developed one or more partial or complete deficiencies of anterior pituitary hormones. Some suffered from profound memory loss, and others had cognitive deficits as a result of radiation-induced brain damage, while others had second neoplasm such as sarcomas and meningiomas. I have seen two patients who developed postradiation vascular anomalies with associated cerebral hemorrhage that required treatment several decades after conventional radiotherapy. Stereotactic radiosurgery has certainly proved to result in a lower likelihood of hypopituitarism and other complications, and it is also quite effective. In general, three- fourths of patients enter remission in response to stereotactic radiosurgery. While the time course of responses seems to be sooner than in patients who received conventional radiotherapy, direct comparisons cannot be made due to the selection biases of modality based on tumor burden, location, and other factors. My approach is to use radiotherapy sparingly. If a patient has progressive tumor that cannot be controlled with medical therapy nor surgery, then I will choose to recommend radiotherapy. I prefer to employ stereotactic radiosurgery, if able, rather than conventional radiotherapy but use both modalities as required. I tend to favor not irradiating younger people, and I'm more comfortable recommending radiotherapy to those in and beyond their Middle Ages. However, a young person with a tumor that is progressing and otherwise uncontrollable would receive a recommendation for treatment. Regardless, it is important to educate patients so that they can also contribute to the decision-making process. For example, I have seen plenty of patients who do not want a lifetime of medical therapy and would choose stereotactic radiosurgery, if candidates for such an approach to treatment, in hope to 1 day discontinue medical therapy.

A common approach is to debulk the tumor and then administer stereotactic radiotherapy. Medical therapy is then employed to control the biochemical and clinical features of the disease until efficacy of radiotherapy has been demonstrated and medical therapy can be discontinued. Based on analysis of factors that influence outcomes, most experts choose to withhold treatment with dopamine agonist drugs and somatostatin receptor ligands for a period of anywhere from 2 weeks to 6 months after radiotherapy as medication-induced tumor suppression might interfere with radiation-induced cell damage and apoptosis and lead to diminished efficacy of treatment [15]. Patients with uncontrolled disease who may require therapy during this waiting period are often treated with a growth hormone receptor antagonist.

Medical therapy is reviewed in detail elsewhere in this book. I do, however, wish to convey some of my thoughts regarding the caveats of the disease process and treatments that guide my decision-making and to convey my general approaches to treatment.

Patients with biochemical evidence for disease but without obvious residual tumor on imaging of the sella are best treated with medical therapy while they undergo surveillance for radiographic evidence of recurrence that would permit additional surgery and possibly radiotherapy.

I tend to employ dopamine agonist drugs in patients who have plurihormonal tumors that co-secrete growth hormone and prolactin. I find these drugs to be particularly useful in the elderly and in patients who have little to no tumor burden [16].

I also treat patients who have biochemical evidence of persistent disease and little to no tumor burden with a growth hormone receptor antagonist [17]. Appearance of or progression of residual tumor prompts consideration of surgery, radiotherapy, or transition to a somatostatin receptor ligand.

I tend to favor use of a growth hormone receptor antagonist over a somatostatin receptor ligand in patients who have hyperglycemia and diabetes mellitus [18]. The former class of drugs tends to improve glycemic control, while there is potential for the latter to worsen such.

I tend to use somatostatin receptor ligands in patients who have a significant amount of residual tumor when it is important to either reduce the size of their tumors or inhibit tumor progression [19].

Patients who develop side effects during somatostatin receptor ligand therapy are given the opportunity to transition to one of the other classes of drugs.

If there is no response whatsoever to a somatostatin receptor ligand, then I discontinue therapy and employ a different class of drug. Rarely, I will try one of the other somatostatin receptor ligands. If there is partial but significant response to treatment, then I will continue therapy and add either a dopamine agonist drug or a growth hormone receptor antagonist administered 2 to 3 times weekly [20]. Occasionally, the growth hormone receptor antagonist must be administered daily.

Regardless of drug used, my aim is to lower the IGF-I levels into the normal range [3]. I prefer to adjust treatment in my patients to achieve IGF-I levels less than 1.0 standard deviation above the mean IGF-1 for their age and sex. In patients treated with dopamine agonist drugs and somatostatin receptor ligands, a second goal is to achieve a growth hormone level of less than 1.0 ng/mL.

Most patients on chronic stable medical therapy achieve IGF-1 levels that vary within a range of 30–50 ng/mL on either side of what seems to be an estimated treatment average result. Consecutive rises in the IGF-I level over time in treated patients often suggest progression of residual disease and a need to reevaluate for tumor growth and alter therapy. Conversely, an insidious progressive decline in IGF-I levels suggests that a patient might be responding to radiotherapy, and they may be able to lower the dose of or even discontinue medical therapy. In this setting, I usually work to find the least effective dose of the medication necessary to achieve my treatment goals. Whenever circumstances permit a discontinuation of therapy, I follow IGF-I levels at 3-month intervals for a couple of years and respond accordingly.

As mentioned, this overview highlights my approach to the management of patients with acromegaly. Detailed information is presented in other chapters throughout this book. I will conclude by stating that it is imperative that patients be included in treatment decisions, setting of treatment goals, and that they partner in establishment of follow-up plans. Development and facilitation of a good doctor–patient relationship is essential to the successful management of patients with acromegaly.

References

1. Blevins LS. The art of medicine. Oper Neurosurg. 2015;11:1–2.
2. Katznelson L, Laws ER, Melmed S, Molitch ME, Murad MH, Utz A, Wass JAH. Acromegaly: an Endocrine Society clinical practice guideline. J Clin Endocrinol Metab. 2014;99:3933–51.
3. Melmed S, Bronstein MD, Chanson P, Klibanski AK, Casanueva FF, Wass JAH, Strasburger CJ, Clemmons DR, Giustina A. A consensus statement on acromegaly therapeutic outcomes. Nat Rev Endocrinol. 2018;14:552–61.
4. Fleseriu M, Biller BMK, Freda PU, Gadelha MR, Giustina A, Katznelson L, Molitch ME, Samson SL, Strasburger CJ, van der Lely AJ, Melmed S. A Pituitary Society update to acromegaly management guidelines. Pituitary. 2021;24:1–13.
5. Fahlbusch R, Kleinberg D, Biller B, Bpnert V, Buchfelder M, Cappabianca P, Carmichael J, Chandler W, Colao A, George A, Klibanski A, Knopp E, Kreutzer J, Kundurti N, Lesser M, Mamelak A, Pivonello R, Post K, Swearingen B, Vance ML, Barkan A. Surgical debulking of pituitary adenomas improves responsiveness to octreotide lar in the treatment of acromegaly. Pituitary. 2017;20:668–75.
6. Franzin A, Spatola G, Losa M, Picozzi P, Mortini P. Results of gamma knife radiosurgery in acromegaly. Int J Endocrinol. 2012;2012:342034, 6 pages. https://doi.org/10.1155/2012/342034.
7. Moyes VJ, Metcalfe KA, Drake WM. Clinical use of cabergoline as primary and adjunctive treatment for acromegaly. Eur J Endocrinol. 2008;159:541–5.

8. Jacob JJ, Bevan JS. Should all patients with acromegaly receive somatostatin analogue therapy before surgery and, if so, for how long? Clin Endocrinol. 2014;81:812–7.
9. Nunes VS, Correa JMS, Puga MES, Silva EMK, Boguszewski CL. Preoperative somatostatin analogues versus direct transsphenoidal surgery for newly-diagnosed acromegaly patients: a systematic review and meta-analysis using the GRADE system. Pituitary. 2015;18:500–8.
10. Losa M, Mortini P, Urbaz L, Ribotto P, Castrignano T, Giovanilli M. Presurgical treatment with somatostatin analogues in patients with acromegaly: effects on the remission and complication rates. J Neurosurg. 2006;104:899–906.
11. Casanueva FF, Barkan AL, Buchfelder M, Klibanski A, Laws ER, Loeffler JS, Melmed S, Mortini P, Wass J, Giustina A. Criteria for the definition of Pituitary Tumor Centers of Excellence: a Pituitary Society statement. Pituitary. 2017;20:489–98.
12. Petrossians P, Borges-Martins L, Espinoza C, Daly A, Betea D, Valdes-Socin H, Stevenaert A, Chanson P, Beckers A. Gross total resection or debulking of pituitary adenomas improves hormonal control of acromegaly by somatostatin analogs. Eur J Endocrinol. 2005;152:61–6.
13. Lissett CA, Peacey SR, Laing I, Tetlow L, Davis JR, Shalet SM. The outcome of surgery for acromegaly: the need for a specialist pituitary surgeon for all types of growth hormone (GH) secreting pituitary adenoma. Clin Endocrinol. 1998;49:653–7.
14. Hannon MJ, Barkan AL, Drake WM. The role of radiotherapy in acromegaly. Neuroendocrinology. 2016;103:42–9.
15. Sheehan JP, Pouratian N, Steiner L, Laws ER, Vance ML. Gamma knife surgery for pituitary adenomas: factors related to radiological and endocrine outcomes. J Neurosurg. 2011;114:303–9.
16. Kuhn E, Chanson P. Cabergoline in acromegaly. Pituitary. 2017;20:121–8.
17. Giustina A, Arnaldi G, Bogazzi F, Cannavo S, Colao A, De Marinis L, Degli Uberti E, Giorgino F, Grottoli S, Lania AG, Maffei P, Pivonello R, Ghigo E. Pegvisomant in acromegaly: an update. J Endocrinol Invest. 2017;40:577–89.
18. Brue T, Lindberg A, van der Lely AJ, Akerblad AC, Koltowska-Haggstrom M, Gomez R, Droste M, Hey-Hadavi J, Strasburger CJ, Camacho-Hubner C. Diabetes in patients with acromegaly treated with pegvisomant: observations from acrostudy. Endocrine. 2019;63:563–72.
19. Ben-Shlomo A, Melmed S. Somatostatin agonists for treatment of acromegaly. Mol Cell Endocrinol. 2008;286:192–8.
20. Ma L, Luo D, Ying T, Wu S, Li M, Chen C, Zhou S, Ma L, Wu Y, Zhou Y, Cui Y. Combined therapy of somatostatin analogues with pegvisomant for the treatment of acromegaly: a meta-analysis of prospective studies. BMC Endocr Disord. 2020;20:126. https://doi.org/10.1186/s12902-020-0545-2.

Chapter 13
Transsphenoidal Surgery for Acromegaly

Ryan R. L. Phelps, Jacob S. Young, José Gurrola II, and Manish K. Aghi

Introduction

Pituitary adenomas are quite common, with some reports showing that over 15% of asymptomatic, healthy individuals have incidental adenomas [1]. Tumors are categorized by their size, malignant potential, extent of local invasion, and, perhaps most importantly, their hormonal secretion. Tumors which oversecrete growth hormone (GH) can produce gigantism in younger individuals whose growth plates have not fully closed or, more commonly, lead to acromegaly in older individuals whose growth plates have closed [2]. There are rare instances of GHRH-secreting hypothalamic tumors or peripheral secretion of excess GH, but over 95% of acromegaly cases are attributable to benign GH-secreting pituitary adenomas [3].

Acromegaly can cause substantial morbidity and mortality. The signs and symptoms range from facial soft tissue overgrowth to systemic disorders like metabolic dysfunction and hypertension to respiratory obstruction and severe cardiovascular disease [4, 5]. Unfortunately, given the insidious nature of this condition, there is often a substantial delay in diagnosis after symptom onset. In fact, there is a substantial delay in diagnosis even after patients undergo surgical operations for acromegaly-induced sequelae, with 35% of patients undergoing these procedures prior to diagnosis [6]. For example, acromegaly-induced adenoid hyperplasia (Fig. 13.1a) may be surgically treated without recognition of the underlying pituitary adenoma and GH hypersecretion. This is the case for several other surgically treatable conditions of the head, throat, nose, thyroid, and musculoskeletal system as well [6].

R. R. L. Phelps · J. S. Young · J. GurrolaII
University of California, San Francisco (UCSF), San Francisco, CA, USA
e-mail: Ryan.Phelps@ucsf.edu; Jacob.Young@ucsf.edu; Jose.Gurrola@ucsf.edu

M. K. Aghi (✉)
Department of Neurological Surgery, University of California, San Francisco, CA, USA
e-mail: manish.aghi@ucsf.edu

L. S. Blevins Jr., M. K. Aghi (eds.), *Acromegaly*, Contemporary Endocrinology,
https://doi.org/10.1007/978-3-031-16258-9_13

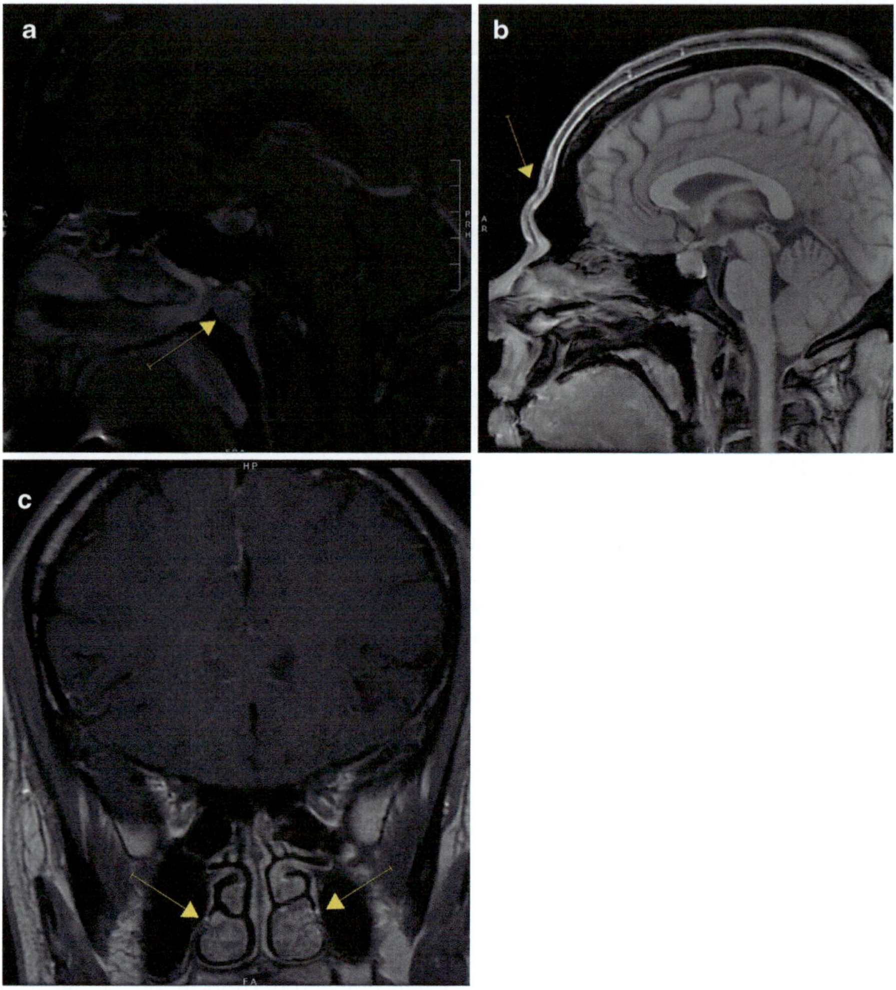

Fig. 13.1 Examples of sinonasal anatomic findings in acromegalic patients. (**a**) 36-year-old man with acromegaly-induced nasopharyngeal adenoid enlargement due to lymphoid adenomatous hyperplasia, evident on sagittal, gadolinium-enhanced T1 MRI, and intraoperatively found to have 5–8 mm cystic deposits within the adenoids. (**b**) 31-year-old man with obvious acromegalic features on exam including frontal bossing (seen here on sagittal MRI), high zygomatic arches, thickened lips and nose, enlarged hands, mild thenar wasting, deepening of the voice, and substantial muscularity. (**c**) 23-year-old woman with significant acromegaly-induced turbinate hypertrophy evident on coronal, gadolinium-enhanced T1 MRI, and evident intraoperatively during approach to the sella

Pituitary adenomas causing acromegaly are typically addressed with surgery upfront, although surgery can also be combined with medical therapy. Successful treatment largely normalizes lifespan and significantly improves quality of life as well [7, 8]. Given the severity of acromegaly sequelae, early surgical management is often indicated. The importance of surgical intervention for this condition was first acknowledged in the late nineteenth century. In 1893, an attempt to resect a somatotroph adenoma was pursued via a transcranial approach, but unfortunately it was unsuccessful [9]. The first successful resection occurred in 1907 in Vienna, which ushered in the embrace of transsphenoidal approaches that were subsequently championed by Harvey Cushing and the rest of the neurosurgical community and are still preferred today [10].

Given the systemic nature of this condition, the frequently changing subtleties regarding diagnostics and workup, and the nuances involved in surgical intervention, it is important to understand neurosurgical aspects of acromegaly management, especially as they relate to communication and coordination with a multidisciplinary team working in conjunction to provide optimal care for these patients.

Diagnosis and Referral

Most acromegaly cases are initially identified by primary care physicians, internists, or endocrinologists [11]. The physical exam is often key in initiating diagnostic workup; both patients and providers may notice classic acromegalic features such as frontal bossing (Fig. 13.1b), high zygomatic arches, thickened lips and nose, enlarged hands, voice deepening, and increased muscularity. Much of the diagnostic workup is often complete by the time neurosurgical team members become involved. However, understanding diagnostic nuances with respect to preoperative GH and insulin-like growth factor 1 (IGF-1) measurement is crucial for contextualizing postoperative and sometimes even intraoperative hormone levels. This can have implications for surgical decision-making in terms of extent of resection as well as reoperation.

The typical acromegaly workup consists of an initial IGF-1 level measurement, followed by a confirmatory GH suppression test [12]. GH and IGF-1 have a log-linear relationship, at least up until a GH level of 7 μg/L. GH secretion is pulsatile, while IGF-1 levels are more stable given the longer half-life [13]. GH regulation is complex, but secretion is largely stimulated by GHRH and ghrelin and largely inhibited by somatotropin release-inhibiting factor (SRIF) and IGF-1. The relationship between acute hyperglycemia (e.g., the oral glucose tolerance test (OGTT)) and GH suppression is incompletely understood but likely involves glucose-mediated somatostatin release from the hypothalamus, as well as some level of ghrelin involvement [14].

However, patient-specific and assay-specific factors can contribute to variations in test results and make test interpretation nuanced. For example, pregnancy and late-stage adolescence can both cause false positives due to excess IGF-1-binding proteins extending the IGF-1 half-life. Medical conditions like hepatic failure, renal failure, hypothyroidism, malnutrition, infection, and diabetes mellitus can also lead to aberrant IGF-1 levels, as can oral estrogen medication [12, 15, 16]. Given that optimal biochemical control (i.e., normalizing GH and IGF-1 levels) is the cornerstone of acromegaly treatment, the success of surgical resection can most accurately be determined if all relevant comorbidities, demographic variables, and medications are accounted for.

Similarly, the specific assays used are important to understand; some are more sensitive and/or specific than others and have different cutoffs for diagnosis. For example, the initial screening test for acromegaly—serum IGF-1 levels—can vary wildly among different laboratories, with some assays failing to diagnose up to 30% of true positives [17]. Similarly, GH measurement is laboratory-specific, with some oral glucose tolerance tests being considered positive with a GH nadir of <1 μg/L, some ultrasensitive tests requiring a nadir of <0.4 μg/L, and some having nonstandard cutoffs [18]. Regardless of the particular assays used, their specific parameters must be noted for reliable comparison with postoperative biochemical evaluation.

Once the diagnosis is established, the next steps in preoperative workup can proceed, including neurosurgical referral, pituitary imaging, and possible premedication.

Given that resection is typically the first-line treatment for acromegaly, neurosurgical referral and evaluation is almost always necessary. The decision of where to refer these patients may warrant more consideration than is necessary for other conditions. There is a large body of literature demonstrating substantial outcome variation of pituitary surgery; in particular, sites with very experienced surgeons, high volume, and high-quality multidisciplinary teams familiar with endocrine disease have improved patient outcome [19]. These variables should be considered when referring patients for pituitary tumor resection.

Preoperative Management

Preoperative Imaging

After biochemical diagnosis of acromegaly, imaging is indicated to confirm pituitary disease and to assist in preoperative planning with respect to bony, vascular, and tumor anatomy. Pituitary MRI is the imaging modality of choice. In particular, these adenomas should be evaluated with contrast-enhanced high-resolution MRI to investigate the sellar region [20]. This high-resolution imaging is necessary to understand the three-dimensional nature of the particular tumor as well as intraoperative landmarks, some of which can be used to navigate and some of which must be carefully avoided. If MRI is contraindicated or unavailable, head CT is recommended. In fact, thin-slice CT can be valuable as an adjunct regardless of MRI availability, as it can help outline bony anatomy of the sella and septations within the sphenoid sinus. In the rare case in which standard imaging fails to demonstrate a pituitary tumor in spite of biochemically confirmed diagnosis, somatostatin receptor scintigraphy and thoracic/abdominal imaging can be performed to search for ectopic GH secretion [21].

There are several acromegaly-specific anatomic variations that should be looked for on these images. For example, acromegalic patients may have particularly tortuous or ectatic internal carotid arteries (ICA) [22, 23]. This is crucial information for operative planning, as pituitary adenomas can abut or even encase the ICAs, and they must be protected and sometimes mobilized. Not only can the ICAs be tortuous or ectatic, but the intercarotid distance is often reduced in acromegalic patients as well, narrowing the operative corridor. The average distance between the ICAs in acromegalic patients relative to controls at the level of C5 is 1.64 cm versus 1.90 cm [24], and they can even nearly make contact with each other in the coronal plane [25]. CT angiography may be of significant value in these cases. Bony anatomy can also be altered by excess GH and IGF-1. Not only can bone be generally thicker in these patients, but bone window CT can also uncover common acromegaly-specific variants such as increased anterior-posterior diameter of the sphenoid sinus [26], or upward and lateral displacement of the sphenoid ostium [27]. These variations are important for the surgeon's ability to anticipate the dimensions of the operative window, prepare for intraoperative landmark navigation, and even properly select surgical tools. Imaging can also be helpful for determining whether the adenoma abuts the optic chiasm (which would be an indication for formal preoperative visual field testing [25]) or even whether there is substantial mucosal hypertrophy or polyposis [26], which could be important findings for a transnasal approach.

Premedication

Although surgical resection is a critical component of acromegaly management in the vast majority of patients, it is worth discussing the rare cases in which medications can either be used as first-line standalone treatment or simply as preparation for surgical intervention. Somatostatin receptor ligand (SRL) therapy is considered the cornerstone of medical management for acromegaly [28]. However, there is some controversy regarding the validity of consensus statements recommending SRLs over other medications, such as pegvisomant or cabergoline, and medication decisions should always be made on an individualized basis. SRLs may work through a variety of cellular mechanisms depending on the particular receptors involved, but their main effects in inhibiting hormone secretion are likely through inhibiting Ca^{2+} and activating K^{+} channels, ultimately decreasing intracellular cAMP levels which decreases cell growth [28].

If a patient is deemed too high-risk for surgery or anesthesia—whether due to age or comorbidities—or if they do not consent to surgery, primary medical therapy may be employed [5]. If a patient has severely anomalous ICA anatomy that precludes a transsphenoidal approach, surgical intervention may be too risky to pursue [25]. Sinus infection may prevent surgical intervention, at least temporarily [25]. Furthermore, if a patient has severe pharyngeal thickness and obstructive sleep apnea, or florid high-output heart failure, preoperative SRL therapy may be necessary to reduce surgical risk [12].

Some tumors—such as macroadenomas that have low likelihood of surgical cure and no significant mass effect symptoms—may be substantially shrunken with preoperative SRL therapy, making resection easier [29]. However, just as preoperative SRL therapy can make resection more effective, resection can also make postoperative medical therapy more effective. As such, it is theoretically challenging to determine which therapy should come first in these specific cases. Regardless of the theoretical benefits of preoperative medical therapy; however, there is a lack of reliable evidence suggesting a clear benefit to long-term postoperative outcomes, and as such, there is no current standard recommendation to pre-treat with medication.

Additionally, it is important to keep in mind that preoperative SRL therapy may make postoperative hormone level evaluation uninterpretable in some cases. Artificially lowering GH/IGF-1 levels preoperatively can mask residual tumor unintentionally left behind, which makes reoperation decisions challenging. Furthermore, pre-treatment for several months can change tumor anatomy and consistency for the worse. In particular, treatment for too long can begin making the tumor firmer and more fibrous [30], which impairs the ability to easily perform curettage and aspiration of what is typically a gelatinous, soft tumor in acromegalic patients. This can make tumor resection from the cavernous sinus particularly challenging and may lead to subtotal resection that subsequently requires adjunctive radiation therapy.

Operative Details: Transsphenoidal Surgery

Technique

Once surgical resection is deemed necessary, and the preoperative workup is complete, surgical decision-making can begin. This starts prior to reaching the operating room, when decisions about approach and necessary surgical instruments are made. Although a transcranial approach may be resorted to in extreme cases of tumor size or invasion, the vast majority of pituitary adenomas are targeted with a transsphenoidal approach. Both endoscopic and microscopic techniques are effective and dependent upon surgeon preference, but many prefer endoscopic approaches (Fig. 13.2) due to the optimal visualization it provides.

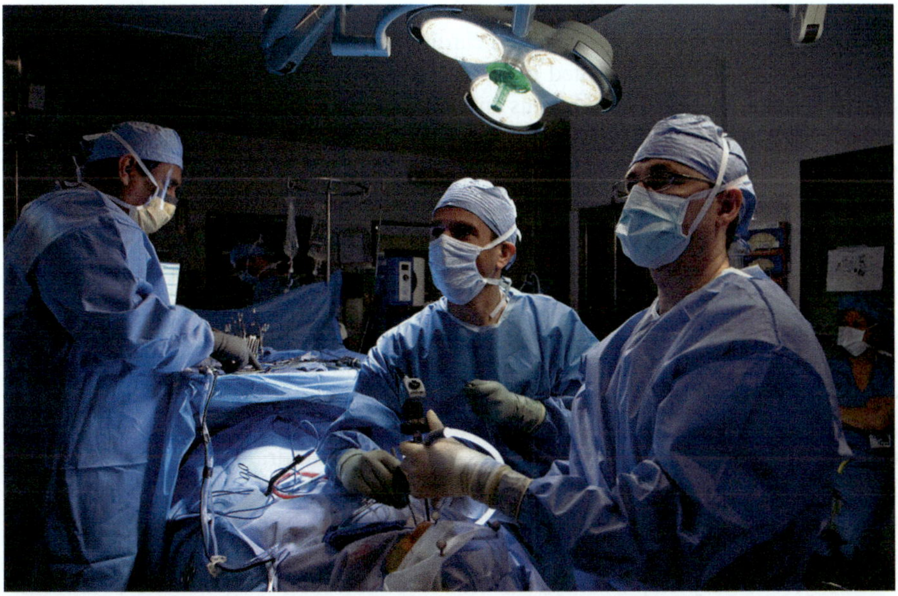

Fig. 13.2 Example of a two-surgeon, endoscopic, transsphenoidal approach for resection of a pituitary adenoma causing acromegaly. The ENT typically holds the endoscope in the right nostril toward the top of the nostril with the neurosurgeon either working across the ENT or besides the ENT, as shown here

Anesthetic Considerations

There are also some intraoperative anesthetic considerations about which the surgeon and anesthesiologist should communicate. Given the potential for mucosal hypertrophy and inflammation and skeletal changes, maintaining open communication between the surgical team and anesthesia remains an important component of care in these patients. The most significant point of communication between the surgical team and anesthesia team is that acromegalics can have difficult airways due to the oropharyngeal soft tissue hypertrophy and edema. The difficulty of acromegalic airways has been shown to correlate with the severity of their IGF-1 elevation [31]. In some cases, the difficulty of the acromegalic airway may lead to a need for videoscopic direct laryngoscopy intubation or awake fiberoptic intubation [32, 33]. Interestingly, this is true even in many patients with Mallampati scores of 1 or 2, suggesting that intubation difficulty must be prepared for, largely irrespective of preoperative anesthetic evaluation [34].

Invasive blood pressure monitoring via an arterial line, if required, may be more dangerous in these patients due to their higher likelihood of carpal tunnel syndrome. This may lead to ulnar artery compression, making them radial-dominant and increasing the risk of radial artery catheterization [35]. In these cases, alternative cannulation sites should be selected. However, invasive blood pressure monitoring is not typically necessary unless patients have poor exercise tolerance, have congestive heart failure, or have documented cardiomyopathy [36].

Additionally, the semi-seated position that some surgeons prefer [37] for these cases can increase the risk of venous air embolism. This can be largely prevented by avoiding a position that is too vertical or only reserving that posture when it is necessary for hemostasis.

Blood glucose should be measured intraoperatively (as well as preoperatively and postoperatively). Although good control of blood glucose is valuable in general, it is more important in the perioperative period to avoid inducing severe hypoglycemia, especially in anesthetized patients who cannot report associated symptoms [36].

Lumbar drains are not typically necessary but may be useful in cases of particularly large adenomas. The surgeon may ask the anesthesiologist to push 10-mL aliquots of saline (or sometimes air) into the lumbar drain at various points in the procedure to facilitate descent of the tumor. This is especially helpful in accessing the suprasellar component of the tumor [38]. If a lumbar drain is deemed necessary, it is usually placed after intubation but prior to positioning. Of note, if air is injected, nitrous oxide administration must be ceased immediately so as to prevent intracranial pressure elevation [36].

Lastly, but very importantly, the choice of anesthetic agents must take into account both the patient's specific comorbidities, as well as the need for rapid emergence postoperatively. These patients have a higher likelihood of hypertension, cardiomyopathy, left ventricular hypertrophy, diastolic dysfunction, and arrhythmias—all of which must be considered when choosing anesthetic agents and doses. Rapid emergence from anesthesia is important for postoperative neurologic exams, including visual exams which could uncover the need for immediate repeat surgical intervention. As such, rapidly metabolized agents or inhalational agents with low blood solubility may be ideal, such as a combination of propofol and remifentanil, or perhaps sevoflurane or desflurane [36]. In patients who are particularly hemodynamically unstable, a combination of an inhalational agent and remifentanil may be effective [39].

Positioning

There are various positioning options for transsphenoidal procedures. One common variant is placing the patient in a supine position in reverse Trendelenburg, with slight head rotation toward the surgeons. Slight neck flexion can facilitate access to tumors that extend particularly inferiorly, while extension can make suprasellar extensions more accessible. Another option is tilting the head toward the left, with the left ear toward the left shoulder, followed by rotating the operating table to the right and elevating the head of bed 25–30° [40, 41]. These positioning decisions should be case-specific and should take into account the tumor's directional extensions, the patient's body habitus, and the surgeon's posture and comfort.

Typical Surgical Steps

First, if needed, the abdomen or thigh should be prepared for a potential fat graft. Our otolaryngology (ear, nose, and throat or ENT) colleagues typically perform an endoscopic approach; this is particularly helpful with acromegalic patients, given that their excess GH and IGF-1 may lead to hypertrophied turbinates (Fig. 13.1c); thickened mucous membranes; significant mucosal inflammation—including polyposis; and septal deviation or spurs which are challenging to navigate [26, 42]. Additionally, these patients often have sinonasal pathologies such as adenoid hyperplasia (Fig. 13.1a) that may need tissue sampling by the ENT surgeon. Although cooperating with an ENT colleague makes this portion of the case safer and easier, it does come with logistical considerations in terms of case scheduling. If a microscopic approach is chosen, the acromegalic nasal speculum may be needed for patients with enlarged nasal passageways.

Once the anterior aspect of the sphenoid sinus is visualized, the sphenoid ostium must be localized. Neuronavigation or fluoroscopy may be of significant value here. At this stage, a sphenoidotomy is made. It is often recommended to extensively drill so as to expose the whole sellar floor [43]. Some surgeons resect all mucosa in the sphenoid sinus, but others attempt to preserve and simply spread the sphenoid mucosa, which is put back together at the conclusion of the case. This more conservative method is more suitable for small tumors. Once again, neuronavigation or fluoroscopy can be helpful to navigate the relatively large septal bony compartments in the sphenoid sinus that can be found in acromegalic patients.

Once the sellar floor is well-visualized, it can be opened with a bayoneted chisel or high-speed diamond burr [44]. It should be opened in the exact midline, using the superior rostrum of the sphenoid sinus as a landmark (other landmarks, such as the sphenoid sinus septum, can be unreliable midline markers). Reliance of navigation can lead to devastating complications if the navigation is inaccurate. Kerrison rongeurs can be used to expand this opening. While one should open as widely as possible, typically from the medial cavernous sinus wall on both sides, it is important to avoid breaching the cavernous sinus as this leads to unnecessary blood loss and risks injury to the ICA.

Once the bone is removed and the dura is visualized, the ICAs can be identified prior to dural incision using micro-Doppler. A dural incision is typically made in a cruciate fashion, and any bleeding can be coagulated with straight- or right-angle bipolar cautery. Again, it is important to expose as widely as possible here—laterally from cavernous sinus wall to cavernous sinus wall and vertically from the tuberculum to the sella-clivus junction [45]. This wide exposure should not be understated; a common cause of postoperative hemorrhage is subtotal resection, and the most common cause of subtotal resection/residual tumor and need for repeat surgery is inadequate exposure [46].

Once the dura is opened, some tumors will immediately come into view, while others will be covered by a rim of normal gland that must be elevated off the tumor. Pituitary adenomas can be relatively easy to distinguish from normal pituitary;

normal anterior pituitary is yellowish and has fine, superficial vasculature, whereas pituitary adenomas tend to be white in color and soft, gelatinous, or flaky. However, as mentioned above, patients who have had more than a few months of preoperative medical therapy with SRLs may have tumors that are firmer and more fibrous and more difficult to dissect and resect.

It is becoming increasingly recognized that pituitary microadenomas should be resected en bloc via pseudocapsular dissection if possible [47, 48]. As such, it is very important to attempt to find the pseudocapsule plane and stay in this plane while dissecting the tumor from the normal pituitary gland. It may be necessary to cut through a small amount of normal pituitary to access the pseudocapsule, and it may also be necessary to take a thin margin of normal pituitary deep to the pseudocapsule as well to facilitate this type of resection. Microadenomas that are not readily visible may require some level of intraoperative exploration. This is typically carried out through a series of vertical incisions in the pituitary gland (so as to avoid as much of the vertically oriented pituitary vasculature as possible) [49]. Each incision is made about 2 mm apart and 1 mm deep, followed by increasing depth, but stopping by the time the intermediate lobe or anterior aspect of the neurohypophysis is found. If there is dural involvement, the involved dura should be radically resected as well, although this is relatively uncommon.

While performing these resections, the main two priorities are complete resection and hemostasis. Given that these are hormone-secreting tumors, gross total resection is key for preventing sequelae. This means that more aggressive maneuvers may be taken than might be necessary for nonfunctional tumors for which the priority may simply be debulking. As such, it is common to pursue resection of tumor that has invaded the cavernous sinus, especially since somatotroph adenomas are typically soft and easily aspirated. However, with tumor components that are too far lateral to the ICAs, or too firm and fibrous, it is often safest to avoid overly aggressive resection and instead leave those remaining portions for stereotactic radiosurgery or radiation therapy postoperatively.

Closure details are dependent on the defects caused by each particular case. In the absence of a readily identifiable cerebrospinal fluid (CSF) leak, the sella can be packed with fat, and the sellar floor can be reconstructed with a well-tailored prosthesis sheet [46]. The sphenoid sinus is rarely packed, and the nares are infrequently packed as well. As always, adequate hemostasis should be ensured upon closure.

Morbidity of Transsphenoidal Surgery for Acromegaly

Transsphenoidal surgery has become incredibly safe in recent years, particularly in the hands of experienced surgeons. Mortality rates are below 0.4% [50], and although short-term morbidity can surpass 30% in some series due to temporary endocrine disturbances [50, 51], overall complication rates in the hands of experienced surgeons are as low as 3% [52]. Some morbidities that can arise from transsphenoidal pituitary adenoma resection become more common in patients who have acromegaly, underscoring the importance of relying on experienced surgeons.

Vascular Complications

While rare, vascular complications are among the most important to consider in acromegalic patients. Extradurally, the posterior nasal septal arteries—branches off of the respective sphenopalatine arteries—are of particular concern during the sphenoidotomy. In an untreated, hypervascular or mucosally inflamed patient, the potential to injure these arteries and place the nasal septal flaps at risks is increased to slightly more than the 3% rate with which this injury occurs after all pituitary surgeries [53]. The posterior nasal septal arteries are found at the inferolateral aspect of the sphenoidotomy and are especially at risk when using electrocautery near the sphenoid ostium or when dividing and manipulating the middle turbinate in an attempt to improve exposure [44]. Partial injury without proper treatment can lead to postoperative epistaxis that can vary from a mild nuisance to the patient to more severe blood loss requiring hospitalization. Careful hemostasis during opening and closure are crucial to reduce the risk of postoperative epistaxis. In rare cases where a patient develops postoperative epistaxis and presents to the clinic or emergency room, nasal packing will usually tamponade the bleeding, with bedside cautery or return to the OR for cautery rarely needed.

ICA injury is a very rare complication, occurring in 0.2–1% of cases [54]. However, it is potentially devastating. Careful interpretation of preoperative imaging is key in charting the courses of these arteries. In some rare cases, especially in acromegalic patients, their courses may preclude the option of transsphenoidal approaches altogether. However, in most cases, ICA anatomy allows for this approach, and they can be charted intraoperatively with micro-Doppler so they can be avoided or safely manipulated. If they are breached, often due to instrumentation in the lateral sella or cavernous sinus, torrential bleeding can ensue. This can be addressed with swift but gentle packing with cottonoid patties [46]. Overly aggressive packing can exacerbate the hemorrhage. Once hemostasis is achieved, some surgeons opt to conclude the procedure immediately to obtain an angiogram. However, in cases in which hemostasis is readily achieved, the patient is stable, and more resection of the tumor is deemed critical, it may be reasonable to proceed with resection and obtain an angiogram afterward. Given collateral blood supply as well as improved management methods, the rates of mortality and severe neurologic complications are both roughly 10% for this complication [55].

Intercavernous sinus bleeding can typically be well-managed with cottonoids, Gelfoam, and bone wax [56]. Excessive cavernous sinus bleeding can be managed with thrombin-soaked Gelfoam, tamponade, and sometimes head elevation [46]. However, head elevation carries the risk of air embolism, which must be considered before employing this technique to decrease bleeding.

CSF Leak

Intraoperative CSF leaks can occur during resection of large adenomas relatively often, with rates surpassing 60% [57]. However, thanks to modern repair techniques such as nasoseptal flaps, the rate of postoperative CSF leaks has declined from ~20% to 8%, thus preventing the need for a substantial amount of repeat surgery [58]. Unfortunately, there is insufficient literature describing CSF leak rates in acromegalic patients after nasoseptal flaps, but it may be similar to the overall rate of those undergoing transsphenoidal surgery for other pituitary adenomas.

When postoperative CSF leak does occur, it is managed as quickly as possible by returning the patient to the operating room. Of course, large tumors and large diaphragmatic/dural defects are associated with increased risk of CSF leak. Any conditions causing elevated intracranial pressure such as obesity can increase the risk of a postoperative CSF leakage requiring repair.

For simple cases in which there is minimal CSF leakage, the typical closure consists of an autologous fat graft placed into the sella or sphenoid sinus. More tissue may have to be placed for bigger leaks, but it is important to avoid overpacking, as this could lead to mass effect similar to that of the tumor itself [59]. Mucosal grafts can be placed so as to cover the sella, and this is an effective and fast-healing option. Some surgeons also use bone or absorbable plates to fasten grafts into place, which is a very effective but slightly riskier closure option. Vascularized flaps, such as nasoseptal flaps, can be phenomenal resources for large defects or anticipated high-flow CSF leaks [59]. This is yet another reason why vasculature such as the sphenopalatine arteries must be preserved during the operation. Given that more intensive closure methods are reserved for cases in which more significant CSF leaks are expected, it is difficult to objectively compare the effectiveness of all these closure options. However, this decision is always one that should be made thoughtfully, taking into account not only the defect but also several patient characteristics, as failed closure is a common reason for repeat surgery and infection.

Adenohypophysis Hormonal Deficits

Rates of new hormonal deficits of the anterior pituitary are as low as 8% after transsphenoidal surgery [60]. This risk is substantially increased in large tumors that significantly compress the pituitary gland or in cases in which a significant portion of the pituitary must be resected. However, it is important to keep in mind that a similar percentage of patients actually gain function of the anterior pituitary postoperatively, which is a benefit that should be weighed against the risk of decreased function. Hormone assessment (e.g., cortisol and electrolyte levels) and thorough exams should be performed to evaluate for this complication.

Diabetes Insipidus and SIADH

Diabetes insipidus (DI) and the syndrome of inappropriate antidiuretic hormone secretion (SIADH) occurring after 2–10% of transsphenoidal surgeries [61, 62]. Although these conditions can be mild and transient if well-managed, poor management can lead to devastating sequelae. Strict intakes and outputs must be monitored, patients must be precisely weighed, sodium should be measured every 6 h in the early postoperative stage, and several hormones (e.g., cortisol) must be closely monitored. Desmopressin, while essential in some cases, must not be overdosed. Often, if these steps are followed and if patients drink to thirst (but do not drink excessively), DI will self-resolve rather quickly.

SIADH tends to occur slightly later in the recovery course, typically just under 1 week after surgery. It can be very challenging to predict which patients will go on to develop this condition. Similarly to the workup and management of DI, patients should be closely monitored while inpatient, and then their labs should again be drawn at one postoperative week to evaluate for this complication [35]. Fluid restriction is typically sufficient to rehabilitate these patients.

Biochemical Outcomes and Management of Residual Tumor

Postoperatively, GH may decline quickly, but IGF-1 can decline at a slow rate. Even with rapid biochemical (GH) and radiologic evidence of surgical success, it takes an average of 10 months for IGF-1 to normalize, although the majority of patients will experience IGF-1 normalization within 3 months (range of 3 days to 57 months) [63]. As such, IGF-1 levels should be checked about 3 months postoperatively, at which time a definitive postoperative MRI can also be obtained [64]. The criteria for remission and cure are regularly changing, and standards have dramatically increased over the past several decades. Originally, a postoperative GH level of <5 μg/L was considered a desirable outcome, but criteria have become more stringent. We now seek a random sensitive GH level of <1 μg/L, a normal IGF-1 level (adjusted for patient characteristics), and an OGTT demonstrating a GH of <0.4 μg/L. However, given that an OGTT can be an inconvenient test, our practice is to simply get a postoperative morning GH level (with a level of <1 μg/L predicting cure) and follow IGF-1 over time to confirm normalization. Increasingly stringent remission/cure criteria may cause postoperative biochemical control rates to artificially decline, but they are still quite impressive, especially for tumors that are confined to the sella. Surgical success for microadenomas is roughly 80% and can be up to 95% for particularly simple cases. Macroadenomas respond very well to surgical intervention 50–60% of the time and even more often if not invasive [65–67].

Although surgical success is common, there may be persistent sequelae from longstanding GH and IGF-1 excess. Fortunately, many acromegaly-induced conditions, such as myocardial fibrosis and early-stage cardiomyopathy (concentric biventricular hypertrophy) [68, 69], significantly improve after treatment. Indeed, improvements such as this largely explain the substantial mortality benefit of treatment. However, some stigmata of acromegaly persist indefinitely and can lead to significant morbidity. For example, hypertension—which is strongly associated with acromegaly—often remains after treatment [70]. Coronary artery disease also often remains a high risk [71]. Furthermore, although cardiac function—such as diastolic filling—often improves, some valvular disease involving aortic root dilation may be irreversible [72]. Diabetes mellitus is another important consideration, as it has several cardiovascular implications. Some evidence suggests that glucose homeostasis and insulin sensitivity are largely stabilized, even with treatment that is only moderately successful [73, 74]. However, other reports find persistently higher rates of diabetes mellitus postoperatively than in the overall population [75]. As such, it is important to screen for this condition even with adequate GH and IGF-1 control. Two other conditions that can dramatically impact patient quality of life after treatment are arthropathy and physical appearance. If treatment is successful in early-stage arthropathy, when there is only cartilage hypertrophy and ligament laxity, it may be reversible. However, after joint degeneration begins, it may become an irreversible, lifelong complaint [71]. Acromegalic changes to physical appearance also continue to bother many patients. We have found that skull deformities such as frontal bossing (Fig. 13.1b) and cranial thickening fail to naturally regress after cure [76]. It is important to note, however, that perceived body image actually tends to be more closely associated with depressive symptoms in these patients than objective acromegalic facial/body changes [77]. As such, proper screening for and treatment of depression and other psychological and cognitive complaints are key in optimizing outcomes.

In instances in which biochemical remission is not attained postoperatively, there are several avenues that can be pursued. Often, stereotactic radiosurgery can precisely target residual tumor and can be so effective that intraoperative resection aggression can be decreased. Medical therapy is also often turned to in order to attain biochemical control postoperatively. In many instances, it is more effective in debulked tumors anyways and can be guided by the pathology specimen from surgery. For example, pathological analysis of tumor cell somatostatin receptor (SSTR) expression (including SSTR density, specific receptor(s) expressed (SSTR 1–5), and receptor splice variant) can predict which somatostatin receptor ligand therapies, if any, are valid and promising options [78]. For many patients, repeat surgery can also be a viable option and is sometimes favored over medial therapy or radiation therapy given that it may obviate the need for lifelong treatment or some lifelong side effects. This is a nuanced, multidisciplinary decision that should be made on an individual basis.

References

1. Ezzat S, Asa SL, Couldwell WT, Barr CE, Dodge WE, Vance ML, McCutcheon IE. The prevalence of pituitary adenomas: a systematic review. Cancer. 2004;101:613–9.
2. Vilar L, Vilar CF, Lyra R, Lyra R, Naves LA. Acromegaly: clinical features at diagnosis. Pituitary. 2017;20:22–32.
3. Lonser RR, Kindzelski BA, Mehta GU, Jane JA Jr, Oldfield EH. Acromegaly without imaging evidence of pituitary adenoma. J Clin Endocrinol Metab. 2010;95:4192–6.
4. Gadelha MR, Kasuki L, Lim DST, Fleseriu M. Systemic complications of acromegaly and the impact of the current treatment landscape: an update. Endocr Rev. 2019;40:268–332.
5. Melmed S, Bronstein MD, Chanson P, Klibanski A, Casanueva FF, Wass JAH, Strasburger CJ, Luger A, Clemmons DR, Giustina A. A consensus statement on acromegaly therapeutic outcomes. Nat Rev Endocrinol. 2018;14:552–61.
6. Keskin FE, Yetkin DO, Ozkaya HM, Haliloglu O, Sadri S, Gazioglu N, Tanrıover N, Ak H, Hatipoglu E, Kadıoglu P. The problem of unrecognized acromegaly: surgeries patients undergo prior to diagnosis of acromegaly. J Endocrinol Invest. 2015;38:695–700.
7. Bolfi F, Neves AF, Boguszewski CL, Nunes-Nogueira VS. Mortality in acromegaly decreased in the last decade: a systematic review and meta-analysis. Eur J Endocrinol. 2018;179:59–71.
8. Gu J, Xiang S, He M, Wang M, Gu Y, Li L, Yin Z. Quality of life in patients with acromegaly before and after transsphenoidal surgical resection. Int J Endocrinol. 2020;2020:5363849.
9. Caton R. Notes of a case of acromegaly treated by operation. Br Med J. 1893;2:1421–3.
10. Cohen-Gadol AA, Liu JK, Laws ER Jr. Cushing's first case of transsphenoidal surgery: the launch of the pituitary surgery era. J Neurosurg. 2005;103:570–4.
11. Reid TJ, Post KD, Bruce JN, Nabi Kanibir M, Reyes-Vidal CM, Freda PU. Features at diagnosis of 324 patients with acromegaly did not change from 1981 to 2006: acromegaly remains under-recognized and under-diagnosed. Clin Endocrinol. 2010;72:203–8.
12. Katznelson L, Laws ER Jr, Melmed S, Molitch ME, Murad MH, Utz A, JAH W, Endocrine Society. Acromegaly: an endocrine society clinical practice guideline. J Clin Endocrinol Metab. 2014;99:3933–51.
13. Oldfield EH, Jane JA Jr, Thorner MO, Pledger CL, Sheehan JP, Vance ML. Correlation between GH and IGF-1 during treatment for acromegaly. J Neurosurg. 2017;126:1959–66.
14. Hage M, Kamenický P, Chanson P. Growth hormone response to oral glucose load: from normal to pathological conditions. Neuroendocrinology. 2019;108:244–55.
15. Melmed S. Acromegaly pathogenesis and treatment. J Clin Invest. 2009;119:3189–202.
16. Lugo G, Pena L, Cordido F. Clinical manifestations and diagnosis of acromegaly. Int J Endocrinol. 2012;2012:540398.
17. Pokrajac A, Wark G, Ellis AR, Wear J, Wieringa GE, Trainer PJ. Variation in GH and IGF-I assays limits the applicability of international consensus criteria to local practice. Clin Endocrinol. 2007;67:65–70.
18. Clemmons DR. Consensus statement on the standardization and evaluation of growth hormone and insulin-like growth factor assays. Clin Chem. 2011;57:555–9.
19. Casanueva FF, Barkan AL, Buchfelder M, et al. Criteria for the definition of Pituitary Tumor Centers of Excellence (PTCOE): a Pituitary Society statement. Pituitary. 2017;20:489–98.
20. Varrassi M, Cobianchi Bellisari F, Bruno F, et al. High-resolution magnetic resonance imaging at 3T of pituitary gland: advantages and pitfalls. Gland Surg. 2019;8:S208–15.
21. Ghazi AA, Amirbaigloo A, Dezfooli AA, et al. Ectopic acromegaly due to growth hormone releasing hormone. Endocrine. 2013;43:293–302.
22. Raymond J, Hardy J, Czepko R, Roy D. Arterial injuries in transsphenoidal surgery for pituitary adenoma; the role of angiography and endovascular treatment. AJNR Am J Neuroradiol. 1997;18:655–65.
23. Laws ER Jr. Vascular complications of transsphenoidal surgery. Pituitary. 1999;2:163–70.

24. Ebner FH, Kuerschner V, Dietz K, Bueltmann E, Naegele T, Honegger J. Reduced intercarotid artery distance in acromegaly: pathophysiologic considerations and implications for transsphenoidal surgery. Surg Neurol. 2009;72:456–60; discussion 460.
25. Laws ER Jr, Cohen-Gadol AA, Schwartz TH, Sheehan JP. Transsphenoidal surgery complication avoidance and management techniques. Cham: Springer; 2017.
26. Ebner FH, Kürschner V, Dietz K, Bültmann E, Nägele T, Honegger J. Craniometric changes in patients with acromegaly from a surgical perspective. Neurosurg Focus. 2010;29:E3.
27. Rajagopal N, Thakar S, Hegde V, Aryan S, Hegde AS. Morphometric alterations of the sphenoid ostium and other landmarks in acromegaly: anatomical considerations and implications in endoscopic pituitary surgery. Neurol India. 2020;68:573–8.
28. Gadelha MR, Wildemberg LE, Bronstein MD, Gatto F, Ferone D. Somatostatin receptor ligands in the treatment of acromegaly. Pituitary. 2017;20:100–8.
29. Fleseriu M, Hoffman AR, Katznelson L, AACE Neuroendocrine and Pituitary Scientific Committee. American Association of Clinical Endocrinologists and American College of Endocrinology disease state clinical review: management of acromegaly patients: what is the role of pre-operative medical therapy? Endocr Pract. 2015;21:668–73.
30. Plöckinger U. Medical therapy of acromegaly. Int J Endocrinol. 2012;2012:268957.
31. Zhang Y, Guo X, Pei L, Zhang Z, Tan G, Xing B. High levels of IGF-1 predict difficult intubation of patients with acromegaly. Endocrine. 2017;57:326–34.
32. Friedel ME, Johnston DR, Singhal S, Al Khalili K, Farrell CJ, Evans JJ, Nyquist GG, Rosen MR. Airway management and perioperative concerns in acromegaly patients undergoing endoscopic transsphenoidal surgery for pituitary tumors. Otolaryngol Head Neck Surg. 2013;149:840–4.
33. Lim M, Williams D, Maartens N. Anaesthesia for pituitary surgery. J Clin Neurosci. 2006;13:413–8.
34. Bindra A, Prabhakar H, Bithal PK, Singh GP, Chowdhury T. Predicting difficult laryngoscopy in acromegalic patients undergoing surgery for excision of pituitary tumors: a comparison of extended Mallampati score with modified Mallampati classification. J Anaesthesiol Clin Pharmacol. 2013;29:187–90.
35. Dunn LK, Nemergut EC. Anesthesia for transsphenoidal pituitary surgery. Curr Opin Anaesthesiol. 2013;26:549–54.
36. Burton CM, Nemergut EC. Anesthetic and critical care management of patients undergoing pituitary surgery. Front Horm Res. 2006;34:236–55.
37. Buchfelder M, Schlaffer S-M. The surgical treatment of acromegaly. Pituitary. 2017;20:76–83.
38. Smith M, Hirsch NP. Pituitary disease and anaesthesia. Br J Anaesth. 2000;85:3–14.
39. Gemma M, Tommasino C, Cozzi S, Narcisi S, Mortini P, Losa M, Soldarini A. Remifentanil provides hemodynamic stability and faster awakening time in transsphenoidal surgery. Anesth Analg. 2002;94:163–8, table of contents.
40. Chaichana KL, Quiñones-Hinojosa A. Transnasal transsphenoidal approach to sellar and suprasellar lesions. In: Core techniques in operative neurosurgery; 2011. p. 53–9.
41. Dunn IF, Laws ER. Transsphenoidal approaches: microscopic. In: Cranial, craniofacial and skull base surgery. Milan: Springer; 2010. p. 225–38.
42. Cappabianca P, Cavallo LM, Solari D, di Somma A. Endoscopic transsphenoidal surgery: anatomy, instrumentation, and technique. In: Transsphenoidal surgery. Cham: Springer; 2017. p. 213–31.
43. Laws ER, Cote DJ, Iuliano S. Transsphenoidal surgery for acromegaly. In: Laws Jr RE, Cohen-Gadol AA, Schwartz TH, Sheehan JP, editors. Transsphenoidal surgery: complication avoidance and management techniques. Cham: Springer; 2017. p. 441–56.
44. Bakhsheshian J, Zada G. Transsphenoidal surgery for recurrent pituitary disease. In: Laws Jr RE, Cohen-Gadol AA, Schwartz TH, Sheehan JP, editors. Transsphenoidal surgery: complication avoidance and management techniques. Cham: Springer; 2017. p. 383–402.
45. Zada G, Agarwalla PK, Mukundan S Jr, Dunn I, Golby AJ, Laws ER Jr. The neurosurgical anatomy of the sphenoid sinus and sellar floor in endoscopic transsphenoidal surgery. J Neurosurg. 2011;114:1319–30.

46. Hendricks B, Cohen-Gadol A. Pituitary adenoma: diagnosis and operative considerations. Neurosurgical Atlas; 2016. https://doi.org/10.18791/nsatlas.v4.ch04.1.1.
47. Taylor DG, Jane JA, Oldfield EH. Resection of pituitary macroadenomas via the pseudocapsule along the posterior tumor margin: a cohort study and technical note. J Neurosurg. 2018;128:422–8.
48. Kim EH, Ku CR, Lee EJ, Kim SH. Extracapsular en bloc resection in pituitary adenoma surgery. Pituitary. 2015;18:397–404.
49. Oldfield EH. Surgical management of Cushing's disease: a personal perspective. Clin Neurosurg. 2011;58:13–26.
50. Asemota AO, Gallia GL. Impact of frailty on short-term outcomes in patients undergoing transsphenoidal pituitary surgery. J Neurosurg. 2019;132:360–70.
51. Wilson D, Jin DL, Wen T, Carmichael JD, Cen S, Mack WJ, Zada G. Demographic factors, outcomes, and patient access to transsphenoidal surgery for Cushing's disease: analysis of the Nationwide Inpatient Sample from 2002 to 2010. Neurosurg Focus. 2015;38:E2.
52. Younus I, Gerges MM, Uribe-Cardenas R, Morgenstern P, Kacker A, Tabaee A, Anand VK, Schwartz TH. The slope of the learning curve in 600 consecutive endoscopic transsphenoidal pituitary surgeries. Acta Neurochir. 2020;162:2361–70.
53. De Los Reyes KM, Gross BA, Frerichs KU, Dunn IF, Lin N, Rincon-Torroella J, Annino DJ, Laws ER. Incidence, risk factors and management of severe post-transsphenoidal epistaxis. J Clin Neurosci. 2015;22:116–22.
54. Griauzde J, Gemmete JJ, Pandey AS, McKean EL, Sullivan SE, Chaudhary N. Emergency reconstructive endovascular management of intraoperative complications involving the internal carotid artery from trans-sphenoidal surgery. J Neurointerv Surg. 2015;7:67–71.
55. Barkhoudarian G, Kelly DF. Complications with transsphenoidal surgery: a review. In: Laws Jr RE, Cohen-Gadol AA, Schwartz TH, Sheehan JP, editors. Transsphenoidal surgery: complication avoidance and management techniques. Cham: Springer; 2017. p. 315–43.
56. Foxx K, Sandwell S, Silberstein H, Vates GE, Miller M, Shafiq I, Manuylova E, Calvi L. Transsphenoidal surgery for craniopharyngiomas. In: Laws Jr RE, Cohen-Gadol AA, Schwartz TH, Sheehan JP, editors. Transsphenoidal surgery: complication avoidance and management techniques. Cham: Springer; 2017. p. 403–25.
57. Ivan ME, Iorgulescu JB, El-Sayed I, McDermott MW, Parsa AT, Pletcher SD, Jahangiri A, Wagner J, Aghi MK. Risk factors for postoperative cerebrospinal fluid leak and meningitis after expanded endoscopic endonasal surgery. J Clin Neurosci. 2015;22:48–54.
58. Gruss CL, Al Komser M, Aghi MK, Pletcher SD, Goldberg AN, McDermott M, El-Sayed IH. Risk factors for cerebrospinal leak after endoscopic skull base reconstruction with nasoseptal flap. Otolaryngol Head Neck Surg. 2014;151:516–21.
59. Gardner PA, Snyderman CH, Fernandez-Miranda JC, Wang EW. Closure methods following transsphenoidal surgery. In: Laws Jr RE, Cohen-Gadol AA, Schwartz TH, Sheehan JP, editors. Transsphenoidal surgery: complication avoidance and management techniques. Cham: Springer; 2017. p. 303–14.
60. Jahangiri A, Wagner J, Han SW, et al. Morbidity of repeat transsphenoidal surgery assessed in more than 1000 operations. J Neurosurg. 2014;121:67–74.
61. Nemergut EC, Zuo Z, Jane JA Jr, Laws ER Jr. Predictors of diabetes insipidus after transsphenoidal surgery: a review of 881 patients. J Neurosurg. 2005;103:448–54.
62. Barber SM, Liebelt BD, Baskin DS. Incidence, etiology and outcomes of hyponatremia after transsphenoidal surgery: experience with 344 consecutive patients at a single tertiary center. J Clin Med Res. 2014;3:1199–219.
63. Shin M-S, Yu JH, Choi JH, Jung CH, Hwang JY, Cho YH, Kim CJ, Kim M-S. Long-term changes in serum IGF-1 levels after successful surgical treatment of growth hormone-secreting pituitary adenoma. Neurosurgery. 2013;73:473–9; quiz 479.
64. Feelders RA, Bidlingmaier M, Strasburger CJ, Janssen JAM, Uitterlinden P, Hofland LJ, Lamberts SWJ, van der Lely AJ, de Herder WW. Postoperative evaluation of patients with acromegaly: clinical significance and timing of oral glucose tolerance testing and measure-

ment of (free) insulin-like growth factor I, acid-labile subunit, and growth hormone-binding protein levels. J Clin Endocrinol Metab. 2005;90:6480–9.
65. Jane JA Jr, Starke RM, Elzoghby MA, Reames DL, Payne SC, Thorner MO, Marshall JC, Laws ER Jr, Vance ML. Endoscopic transsphenoidal surgery for acromegaly: remission using modern criteria, complications, and predictors of outcome. J Clin Endocrinol Metab. 2011;96:2732–40.
66. Dallapiazza RF, Jane JA Jr. Outcomes of endoscopic transsphenoidal pituitary surgery. Endocrinol Metab Clin North Am. 2015;44:105–15.
67. Sarkar S, Jacob KS, Pratheesh R, Chacko AG. Transsphenoidal surgery for acromegaly: predicting remission with early postoperative growth hormone assays. Acta Neurochir. 2014;156:1379–87; discussion 1387.
68. Ciulla MM, Epaminonda P, Paliotti R, et al. Evaluation of cardiac structure by echoreflectivity analysis in acromegaly: effects of treatment. Eur J Endocrinol. 2004;151:179–86.
69. Colao A, Marzullo P, Cuocolo A, Spinelli L, Pivonello R, Bonaduce D, Salvatore M, Lombardi G. Reversal of acromegalic cardiomyopathy in young but not in middle-aged patients after 12 months of treatment with the depot long-acting somatostatin analogue octreotide. Clin Endocrinol. 2003;58:169–76.
70. Maison P, Tropeano A-I, Macquin-Mavier I, Giustina A, Chanson P. Impact of somatostatin analogs on the heart in acromegaly: a metaanalysis. J Clin Endocrinol Metab. 2007;92:1743–7.
71. Claessen KM, Pereira AM, Biermasz NR. Outcome of complications in acromegaly patients after long-term disease remission. Expert Rev Endocrinol Metab. 2015;10:499–510.
72. van der Klaauw AA, Bax JJ, Smit JWA, Holman ER, Delgado V, Bleeker GB, Biermasz NR, Roelfsema F, Romijn JA, Pereira AM. Increased aortic root diameters in patients with acromegaly. Eur J Endocrinol. 2008;159:97–103.
73. Jaffrain-Rea M-L, Minniti G, Moroni C, Esposito V, Ferretti E, Santoro A, Infusino T, Tamburrano G, Cantore G, Cassone R. Impact of successful transsphenoidal surgery on cardiovascular risk factors in acromegaly. Eur J Endocrinol. 2003;148:193–201.
74. Stelmachowska-Banaś M, Zieliński G, Zdunowski P, Podgórski J, Zgliczyński W. The impact of transsphenoidal surgery on glucose homeostasis and insulin resistance in acromegaly. Neurol Neurochir Pol. 2011;45:328–34.
75. Rochette C, Graillon T, Albarel F, Morange I, Dufour H, Brue T, Castinetti F. Increased risk of persistent glucose disorders after control of acromegaly. J Endocr Soc. 2017;1:1531–9.
76. Rick JW, Jahangiri A, Flanigan PM, Aghi MK. Patients cured of acromegaly do not experience improvement of their skull deformities. Pituitary. 2017;20:292–4.
77. Dimopoulou C, Leistner SM, Ising M, Schneider HJ, Schopohl J, Rutz S, Kosilek R, Frohner R, Stalla GK, Sievers C. Body image perception in acromegaly is not associated with objective acromegalic changes but depends on depressive symptoms. Neuroendocrinology. 2017;105:115–22.
78. Paragliola RM, Salvatori R. Novel somatostatin receptor ligands therapies for acromegaly. Front Endocrinol. 2018;9:78.

Chapter 14
Stereotactic Radiosurgery and Radiation Therapy for Acromegaly

Adomas Bunevicius, Daniel Trifiletti, and Jason Sheehan

Introduction

Acromegaly is most commonly caused by a growth hormone (GH)-secreting pituitary adenoma [1]. Excessive and unopposed GH secretion causes raised levels of insulin-like growth factor 1 (IGF-1). Acromegaly is considered a relatively rare disorder with incidence rate of approximately 3 cases per one million population [2] and with estimated prevalence rates ranging from 8 to 42 cases per million population per year [3–5]. However, acromegaly remains under or undiagnosed and often untreated. For example, in a study in unselected sample of adult primary care patients, it was discovered that 125 out of 6773 screened patients (1.8%) had elevated IGF-1 levels corresponding to a prevalence of 1034 per million patients [6]. Acromegaly is often underestimated in patients with diabetes mellitus or glucose intolerance [7].

GH hypersecretion can damage numerous organ systems with varying levels of severity, and this can consequentially result in variable clinical manifestations of acromegaly that may range from soft tissue swelling, acral enlargement, and visceromegaly to life-threatening somatic complications, such as diabetes, hypertension, and respiratory and cardiac failure [1, 8]. Acromegaly patients are at 1.48-fold increased mortality risk when compared to the general population with hypertension, diabetes, hypopituitarism, and cardiomyopathy being the most important

A. Bunevicius
Department of Neurosurgery, University of Virginia, Charlottesville, VA, USA

D. Trifiletti · J. Sheehan (✉)
Department of Radiation Oncology, Mayo Clinic, Jacksonville, FL, USA
e-mail: Trifiletti.daniel@mayo.edu; jsheehan@virginia.edu

L. S. Blevins Jr., M. K. Aghi (eds.), *Acromegaly*, Contemporary Endocrinology,
https://doi.org/10.1007/978-3-031-16258-9_14

contributing factors [9, 10]. In young patients, GH hypersecretion before epiphyseal bone closure results in gigantism. Furthermore, compression of the optic chiasm by GH-secreting pituitary macroadenomas and consequential visual dysfunction do occur.

Management of patients with acromegaly remains challenging and requires multidisciplinary expertise that usually includes neurosurgery, neuroendocrinology, radiation oncology, and general medical care. According to the Endocrine Society Clinical Practice Guideline, the goal of acromegaly management is normalization of GH and IGF-1 serum levels [11]. Resection, radiosurgery, radiation therapy, and medical management options should be considered and used as appropriate for management of acromegaly patients (Fig. 14.1). Transsphenoidal resection plays a central role in the management of GH-secreting pituitary tumors as it also allows immediate endocrine control and decompression of neural structures [1, 12]. However, from 20% to 40% of surgically treated acromegaly patients fail to achieve endocrine remission [1, 13, 14]. Medical therapy is used to reduce surgical risk and to improve biochemical control after surgery [11]. Medical therapy can also be used

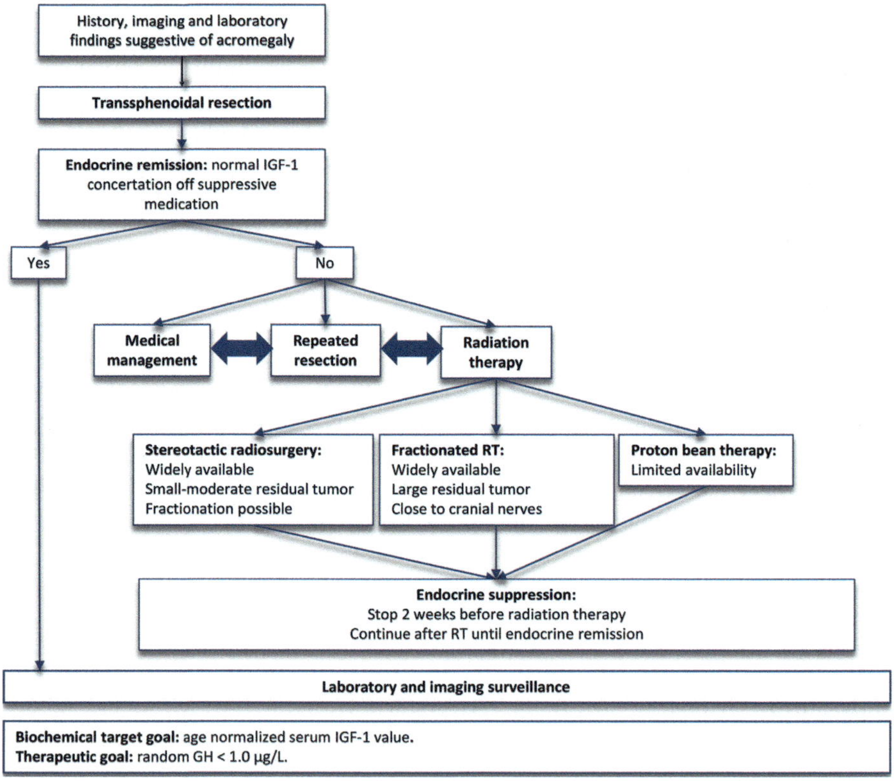

Fig. 14.1 Treatment and follow-up algorithm of acromegaly patients

in patients with persistent disease after surgery, but it usually requires life-long therapy, can be quite expensive, and places patients at risk for side effects [1, 11].

Ionizing radiation in the form of stereotactic radiosurgery (SRS) or fractionated radiotherapy is currently recommended in the treatment of residual GH-secreting pituitary adenomas after attempted incomplete transsphenoidal adenoma resection or if medical therapy is not available, effective, or tolerated [11]. SRS is recommended for many patients with persistent acromegaly, whereas conventional fractionated radiation therapy is often considered for tumors residing in close spatial proximity to critical neural structures, such as the optic nerve or chiasm, or when SRS technology is not available [11].

Historical Perspective

Acromegaly as a clinical entity was first established by Pierre Marie in 1886 [15], and in 1909 Sir Harvey Cushing implicated growth hormone hypersecretion by the pituitary gland as the underlying mechanism of acromegaly. Radiation therapy for treatment of acromegaly was first described in 1909 [16, 17]. Initially, radiation treatment for acromegaly included 200 roentgens delivered to the sella from the oral cavity during twice weekly 1 h sessions over a period of 1 month [18]. Radiation therapy delivery approaches and delivery schedule were subsequently refined, and the dosage of 4000 roentgens was deemed as the most effective for treatment of the pituitary fossa tumors [19, 20].

Stereotactic radiosurgery for treatment of intracranial tumors was introduced by Lars Leksell in 1951 [21]. The Gamma Knife (Elekta AB, Stockholm) was first used to treat a patient with a pituitary adenoma in 1968, and between 1968 and 1982 a total of 27 acromegaly patients were treated using this innovative technique [22]. Around the same time Kjellberg with colleagues described their experience with proton beam hypophysectomy for treatment of acromegaly [23]. More than a decade later Betti and Derechinsky described linear accelerator (LINAC)-based system for SRS that used 10-MV LINAC and targeting based Talairach coordinate system [24].

Brachytherapy is another radiation therapy technique that received attention for treatment of acromegaly. Initial attempts with brachytherapy for pituitary adenomas and other intracranial lesions used radioactive radium needles, also known as the "radium bomb" [25, 26]. In 1961 Joplin with colleagues presented their results of pituitary gland brachytherapy with gold-198 seeds treating of patients with acromegaly [27]. However, brachytherapy is now rarely used for treatment of acromegaly and is now sometimes utilized in the treatment of recurrent craniopharyngiomas [28, 29]. Subsequent technological advancements of Gamma Knife and LINAC-based SRS techniques have substantially improved the efficacy and safety of ionizing radiation delivery to the sella/parasellar region, and this has led to wider adoption of these treatment modalities into everyday clinical practice. Today, SRS plays an important role in the adjuvant treatment of acromegaly.

Stereotactic Radiosurgery for Acromegaly

SRS is used to deliver a high dose of focused radiation with submillimeter spatial accuracy and precision for treatment of small and well-defined intracranial lesion. Steep radiation dose falloff allows highly selective treatment and preservation of the surrounding normal neural tissues from appreciable radiation. Precise and selective treatment is of particular importance for management of intracranial lesions residing in eloquent brain regions surrounded by critical neural and vascular structures. Radiobiological effects underlying therapeutic actions of radiosurgery and radiation therapy include vascular and cytotoxic effects [30]. Ionizing radiation causes biochemical damage of irradiated cells and breakage of single-stranded and double-stranded DNA. This consequentially leads to cell necrosis, apoptosis, or cell survival. Endothelial cell damage of tumor vasculature is considered the dominant cause of cell death from SRS, and the linear quadratic formula is widely used to explain the rationale for the effect of fractionation in radiation therapy. This is relevant as the hypothalamic/pituitary axis is radiosensitive, particularly among normal GH-secreting cells [31].

SRS, in contrast, is usually delivered in a single fraction. However, fractionated SRS treatment (in up to five fractions) can be considered for treatment of large pituitary adenomas and/or tumors that are in close proximity to or encase critical neural structures (such as optic nerves and chiasm) in order to minimize the risk of inadvertent radiation injury to normal tissues. There are three main current approaches to deliver SRS: (1) GKRS (Elekta Instruments AB, Stockholm, Sweden) using multiple cobalt-60 gamma radiation-emitting radiation beams, (2) Cyberknife Robotic Radiosurgical System (Accuray, Sunnyvale, CA, USA), and (3) linear accelerator-based irradiation.

Patient Selection and Pre-SRS Evaluation

Candidates for SRS procedures should be carefully selected while taking into consideration rigorous clinical, biochemical, and imaging assessment. Comprehensive pre-SRS evaluation should include (1) complete endocrine evaluation (serum concentrations of GH, IGF-1, adrenocorticotropic hormone, cortisol, prolactin, total and free thyroxin, thyroxin-stimulating hormone, luteinizing hormone, follicle-stimulating hormone, and testosterone levels in men) and (2) comprehensive neuroimaging that is used for radiosurgery planning and should include thin-sliced (1 mm sections) T1-weighted contrast-enhanced MRI with and without contrast. Brain computerized tomography (CT) can be considered as alternative option for patients who cannot tolerate MRI or it is contraindicated. Fat saturation MR imaging can be useful for patients with prior resections.

Pre-SRS ophthalmic examination of visual function should also be considered for patients who experience visual dysfunction or have imaging findings suggestive of visual pathway compression, and such evaluation should include assessments of visual acuity and visual fields.

SRS Procedure

For GKRS, a rigid stereotactic frame (Leksell frame; Elekta Instruments AB, Stockholm, Sweden) is commonly used to optimize spatial precision of GKRS procedure. The frame is usually applied under local anesthesia and intravenous sedation in the morning of SRS. The scalp is prepared with alcohol, and areas of pin placement are infiltrated with long-acting local anesthetic. Histories of prior cranial neurosurgical procedures and cranial defects should be considered before pin placement not to cause inadvertent brain damage, and thin-sliced head CT scan should be considered in unclear cases to optimize safety of frame pin placement. Four-pin fixation is typically utilized, but three-pin fixation has been shown to be adequate [32]. As a rule of thumb, stereotactic frame should be placed parallel to the anterior optic apparatus to optimize visualization of the optic apparatus during radiosurgery planning. Frameless SRS using a thermoplastic mask can be considered for patients who are selected for fractionated SRS or when frame application is contraindicated for medical reasons.

Quality imaging is essential for accurate SRS planning and hence optimized efficacy and safety of the procedure. Advancements of imaging techniques have improved spatial resolution and treatment precision. Detailed imaging studies are of paramount importance to delineate residual tumor, its invasiveness, and association with surrounding neurovascular structures and the normal pituitary gland. At the University of Virginia (Charlottesville, Virginia, USA) pre-GKRS treatment planning MRI protocol for pituitary adenoma patients includes pituitary windows of axial and coronal T2w, pre-contrast sagittal T1w, as well as post-contrast axial, sagittal, and coronal T1w series. Thin-sliced (1 mm) planning MRI series include post-contrast T1w axial, sagittal, and coronal series and pre-contrast axial T1w series. Dynamic MRI sequences are also often performed as they are useful to delineate residual tumor remnants and microadenomas. Treatment planning is performed using a computer software called Gamma Plan (Elekta AB). The endocrine remission to complication risk ratio should be carefully balanced when selecting radiosurgical dose. For functional pituitary adenomas, prescription doses of 18 Gy to 30 Gy to prescription isodose line (often around 50% for GKRS) are usually considered reasonable to optimize likelihood of achieving endocrine remission (Fig. 14.2). Close proximity of the adenoma to the surrounding parasellar neural and vascular structures should be carefully considered when planning and deploying radiation therapy. Optic neuropathy is usually avoided by restricting radiation dose to the optic apparatus to less than 8Gy to 12Gy in a single fraction. A minimal distance of at least 3 mm between the lateral edge or rostral extent of the adenoma and optic nerve/chiasm is desirable for single-fraction stereotactic radiosurgery to allow adequate sparing of the optic apparatus. Cranial nerves that run in the cavernous sinus

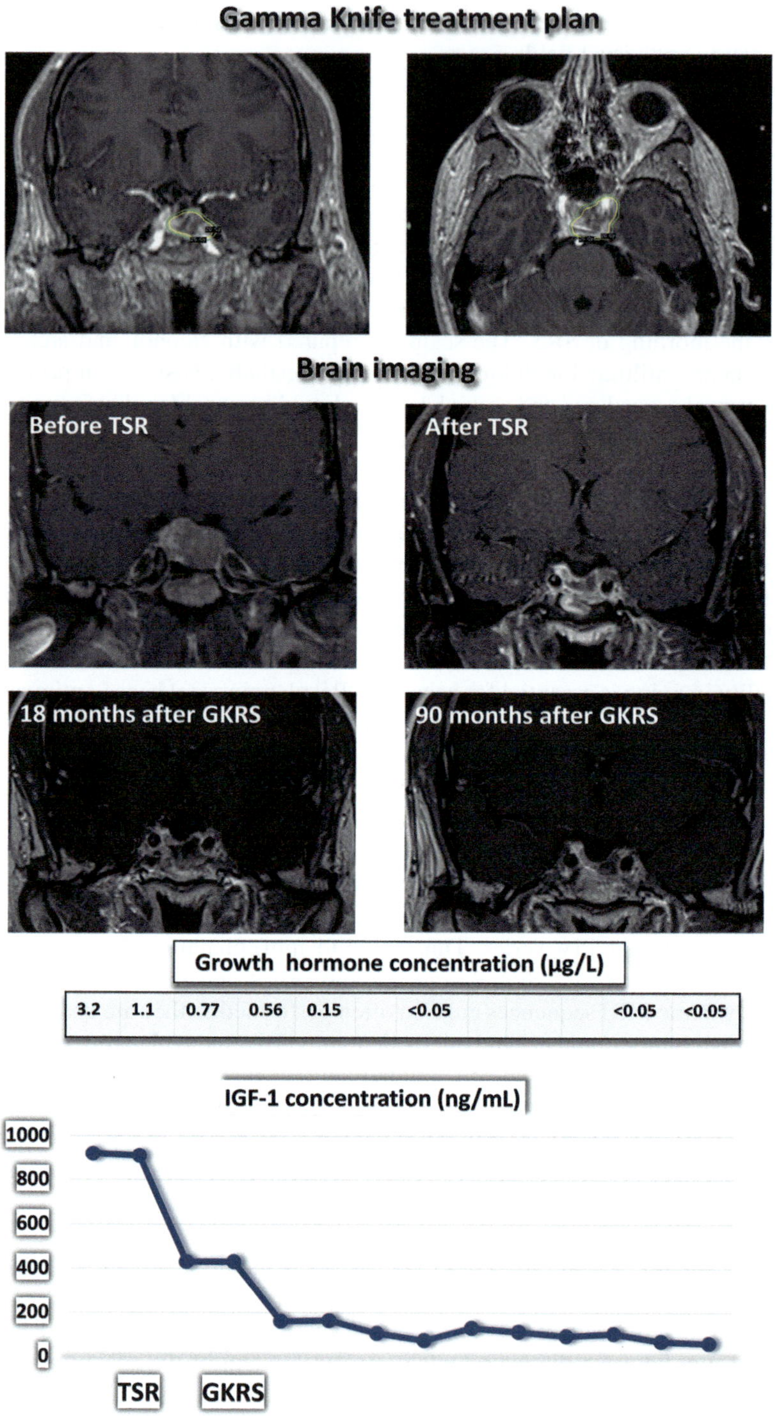
Gamma Knife treatment plan
Brain imaging
Before TSR
After TSR
18 months after GKRS
90 months after GKRS
Growth hormone concentration (µg/L)
3.2
1.1
0.77
0.56
0.15
<0.05
<0.05
<0.05
IGF-1 concentration (ng/mL)
1000
800
600
400
200
0
TSR
GKRS

can typically tolerate substantially larger radiation doses. Radiation-induced injury to the cavernous segment of the internal carotid artery is extremely rare. Nevertheless, care should be taken not to include these neurovascular structures into radiation "hotspots" where the dose may be heterogeneous.

Pituitary adenoma SRS treatment with the Cyberknife Robotic Radiosurgical (CKRS) System (Accuray, Sunnyvale, CA, USA) follows similar steps [33]. Head is immobilized using the aquaplastic mask, i.v. contrast-enhanced head CT is performed, and treatment is planned on the Cyberknife treatment planning workstation. Radiosurgery techniques and procedures using the LINAC-SRS systems depend on the details of the center's technology and workflow but can be employed through a variety of strategies.

Endocrine Control

GKRS is the most widely studied SRS instrument for treatment of GH-secreting tumors, followed by the LINAC-SRS and CKRS (Table 14.1). The majority of published studies are retrospective single-institution series. There are no prospective randomized clinical trials rigorously comparing different SRS delivery methods for the treatment of acromegaly. Also, results of endocrine remission should be interpreted with caution given differences in follow-up duration, definition of endocrine remission, and follow-up protocols between centers and also across studies.

Reported rates of endocrine remission of acromegaly after GKRS range from 17% [39, 53] to over 70% [41, 47]. The largest published series of GKRS for GH-secreting pituitary adenomas to date comes from the International Gamma Knife Research Foundation (IGKRF), an international multi-institutional registry of GKRS centers [13]. They published 10 institution experience with 371 acromegaly patients who were treated with GKRS (mean margin dose: 24.2 Gy) who were followed for 37.7 ± 32.5 months (range: 1–216 months). Fifty-four percent of patients treated with GKRS achieved endocrine remission at a median of 38 months after the GKRS procedure. Endocrine remission was defined according to contemporary criteria as normalization of age- and gender-matched IGF-1 levels while off of all suppressive medication for at least 4–8 weeks. The only independent predictor of durable

Fig. 14.2 41-year-old gentleman presented with clinical features consistent with acromegaly. IGF-1 and GH were elevated at 919 ng/mL and 3.1 ng/mL, respectively. Brain MRI demonstrated pituitary macroadenoma invading left cavernous sinus and surrounding the intracavernous portion of the internal carotid artery and gently elevating of right optic nerve and optic chiasm. He underwent transsphenoidal resection of intra-sellar potion of pituitary adenoma. Pathology documented pituitary adenoma immunoreactive for growth hormone. Postoperative morning growth hormone level dropped to <1 ng/mL after the surgery, and he has had clinical improvement of his symptoms of acromegaly. However, his IGF-1 levels remained elevated, and 4 months later, the patient underwent single-fraction GKRS treating sella and left cavernous sinus with a prescription dose of 25 Gy to the 50% isodose. 7 months after GKRS, his IGF-1 levels normalized, and MRI documented decreased size of treated pituitary adenoma remnants

Table 14.1 Summary of modern series of stereotactic radiosurgery for GH producing pituitary adenomas

Author/country	No. of treated patients	Prescription dose in Gy	Length of follow-up in years	Endocrine remission rate	Time to endocrine remission months	Hypopituitarism	New cranial nerve deficits
Gamma knife radiosurgery							
Ding et al. (2019) [13]/the United States, Taiwan, Czech Republic, Spain, Canada	371	Mean: 24.2 ± 6 Range: 8.8–40	Mean: 5.4	Normal IGF-1: 54%[a]	38 months	26%[b]	4%
Kong et al. (2019) [34]/South Korea	138	Median: 25 Range: 12–35	Mean: 7.1	Normal IGF-1 and GH < 2.5 μg/l: 34.1%[a]	138 months	8.6%[b]	Not reported
Franzin et al. (2012) [35]/Italy	103	Mean: 22.5 ± 0.3 Range: 12–25	Median: 5.9	Normal IGF-1 and GH < 2.5 μg/l: 60.7%[a]	Not reported	7.8%[b]	None
Jezková (2006) [36]/Czech Republic	96	Median: 35 Range: 10–42	Mean: 4.5	Normal IGF-I and GH < 1 μg/l with OGTT: 43%	54 months	27%[b]	None
Castinetti (2005) [37]/France	82	Range: 12–40	Mean: 4.1	Normal IGF-1 and GH < 2 μg/l: 17%	36 months	17%[b]	None
Pai et al. (2019) [38]/Taiwan	76	Median: 15.8 Range: 11.9–22	Median: 6.1	Normal IGF-1 and GH < 1 μg/dL: 24%	63 months	11.8%[b]	None
Vik-Mo et al. (2007) [39]/Norway	61	Mean: 26.5 Range: 12–35	Mean: 5.5	Normal IGF-I and GH < 2.6 mIU/l with OGT: 17%[a]	Not specified	33%[c]	3%
Gutt (2005) [40]/Germany	44	Median: 18 Range: 12–23	Median: 1.9	Normal IGF-1: 48%	Not specified	Not specified	None
Poon et al. (2010) [41]/China	40	Range: 20–35	Mean: 6.2	Normal IGF-1 and GH < 2 μg/dL: 75%	Not specified	Not specified	Not specified

Ronchi (2009) [42]/Italy	35	Median: 20 range: 15–35	Median: 9.5	Normal IGF-1, GH < 2.5 µg/dL and postglucose GH nadir <1 µg/dL: 46%	144 months	50%[b]	None
Liu et al. (2012) [43]/the United States	34	Median: 21 Range 12–30	Median: 6	Normal IGF-1, GH < 2.5 ng/ml: 47.5%[a]	45 months	40%[b]	None
Kim et al. (2018) [44]/Korea	30	Mean: 26.2 Range: 14–35	Median: 3.9	Normal IGF-1 and post-OGTT GH nadir <1 µg/L: 47%[a]	35 months	LH/FSH: 56.6%[b] TSH: 30.2%[b] ACTH: 33.6%[b]	3%
Attanasio (2003) [45]/Italy	30	Mean: 20 Range: 15–35	Mean: 3.8	Normal IGF-1 and safe GH: 23%[a]	Not specified	7%[b]	None
Erdur (2011) [46]/Turkey	22	Mean: 23.8 Range: 18–28	Median: 5	Normal IGF-1 and post-OGTT GH nadir <1 ng/dL: 54.5%[a]	28 months	28.6%[b]	None
Sims-Williams et al. (2019) [47]/the United Kingdom	20[d]	Median: 27.5 Range: 17–38	Mean: 13.4	Normal IGF-1 and GH: 71% at 20 years[a]	7.4 years	53%[b]	5%
Fukuoka (2001) [48]/Japan	9	Mean: 20 Range: 18–20	Mean: 3.5	Normal IGF-1 and GH: 50% at 3 yrs	31 months	None	None
CyberKnife radiosurgery							
Sala et al. (2018) [49]/the United States[e]	22	Median: 24 Range: 18–30	Mean: 3.6	Normal IGF-1 and GH <1 mcg/L: 41%[a]	50 months	27%[b]	None
Roberts et al. (2007) [33]/the United States[e]	9	Mean: 21 Range: 18–24	Mean: 2.1	Normal IGF-1: 44%[a]	12 months	33%[b]	None

(continued)

Table 14.1 (continued)

Author/country	No. of treated patients	Prescription dose in Gy	Length of follow-up in years	Endocrine remission rate	Time to endocrine remission months	Hypopituitarism	New cranial nerve deficits
Linear accelerator							
Wilson et al. (2013) [50]/ Australia	86	Median: 20 Range: 14–25	Median: 5.5	Normal IGF-1: 18.6%	26 months	19.8%[b]	1%
Voges et al. (2006) [51]/ Germany	64	Mean: 16.5	Mean: 6.8	Normal IGF-1 and GH < 2 ng/mL: 37.5%	Not specified	Not specified	Not specified
Yan et al. [52] (2013)/ Taiwan	22	Mean: 23	Median: 7.9	Normal IGF-1 and GH <2.5 ng/mL: 68.2%	53 months	23%	None

CKRS CyberKnife radiosurgery; *GKRS* Gamma Knife radiosurgery
[a]Off suppressive medication
[b]New onset after radiosurgery
[c]Pre- and postirradiation combined
[d]Primary treatment
[e]Report from the same center with overlap of patient inclusion periods

endocrine remission was cessation of IGF-1 suppressing medication around the time of GKRS. Another multicentered retrospective series from South Korea, which included 138 acromegaly patients treated with GKRS and with a median follow-up of 85.2 months, reported that 34% of patients achieved endocrine remission [34]. Female gender, low IGF-1 level (≤ twofold of the maximal age- and sex-matched level), and use of GKRS as adjuvant treatment were independent predictors of endocrine remission. A study from Italy of 103 patients with acromegaly and median follow-up of 75 months reported that 61% of patients achieved endocrine remission after treatment with GKRS [35]. Jezkova with colleagues reported that 44% of 43 patients at risk achieved endocrine remission (GH < 1 µg/l in oGTT and normal IGF-I) 54 months after treatment. Castinetti reported that 17% out of 82 GKRS-treated acromegaly patients achieved endocrine remission during a mean follow-up of 49.5 months [53]. Higher levels of GH and IGF-I before GKRS were associated with decreased likelihood of endocrine remission after GKRS [53]. Pai with colleagues reported that low-dose GKRS (margin dose <25 Gy; median dose, 15.8 Gy; range, 11.9–22 Gy) resulted in endocrine remission in 43% of their patients during a median follow-up of 6 years. Absence of cavernous sinus invasion and lower pre-GKRS IGF-1 concentration were independent predictors of biochemical remission [38]. Vik-Mo with colleagues reported that 9 out of 53 (17%) of patients treated with GKRS for GH-secreting pituitary adenomas achieved endocrine remission [54]) during a median follow-up period of 5.5 years [39]. Smaller (<50 patients) contemporary series of acromegaly patients treated with GKRS reported comparable success rates (see Table 14.1). Higher preoperative endocrine burden [13, 34, 38, 53] and the use of suppressive medication around the radiosurgical procedure [13] were commonly shown to be associated with a reduced likelihood to achieve endocrine remission after the GKRS procedure.

Published experience with CKRS for treatment of GH-secreting pituitary adenomas is more limited when compared to GKRS (Table 14.1) [33, 49]. A group from Stanford used a median prescription dose to GH-secreting pituitary adenomas of 24 Gy that ranged from 18 to 30 Gy. They reported during a mean of 3.6 years of follow-up, 41% of their patients experienced endocrine "cure" defined as normal gender and age standardized serum IGF-1 levels, random GH concentration < 1mcg/L without used of medical therapy for at least 12 weeks [49]. Higher biologically effective dose (BED) was associated with remission, suggesting that the highest safest dose of radiation should be delivered to maximize treatment success; however, this should be interpreted with caution given small sample size [49]. Groups from Japan [55] and South Korea [56] also presented their experience with CKRS system for treatment of pituitary adenomas that also included acromegaly patients; however, treatment regiments, outcomes, and safety profile of a subgroup of patients with acromegaly were not specified.

LINAC systems are also used for radiosurgery of GH-producing pituitary adenomas albeit published experience is more limited when compared to GKRS. Wilson with colleagues published the largest series of acromegaly patients (n = 86) treated with the LINAC-SRS using the BRW head ring [50]. Median prescription dose was 20 Gy (range: 14–25 Gy), and median follow-up duration was 5.5 years. Fourteen percent of patients achieved endocrine remission defined as fasting GH concentration of <2.5 ng/mL, and 18.6% of patients achieved age and gender-matched target IGF-1 levels. A group from Germany reported that 24 out of 64 (37.5%) patients treated with LINAC-SRS achieved endocrine remission during a mean follow-up of almost 7 years [51]. A group from Taiwan reported their experience with 22 patients treated with LINAC SRS and using the Cosman-Roberts-Wells stereotactic frame system between 1994 and 2004 for intractable acromegaly [52]. During a median follow-up period of 94.7 months that ranged from 36 to 161 months, 68.2% and 27.3% of patients achieved that was defined as fasting GH concentration of <2.5 ng/mL and <1 ng/mL, respectively (the proportion of patients taking suppressive medication was not specified). Higher GH levels at diagnosis and before SRS were associated with longer time to endocrine remission.

Complications from SRS

SRS for GH-secreting pituitary adenomas has acceptable safety profile. The most common complication after SRS for a pituitary adenoma is new onset pituitary deficiency that usually affect up to one third of treated patients. Pituitary hormone deficiencies can be readily diagnosed via endocrine surveillance and can be well managed with hormone replacement therapy. The incidence rate of SRS-induced cranial nerve neuropathy is substantially lower and is usually well below 4%.

In GKRS series, the incidence of new hypopituitarism and cranial nerve neuropathy was 8–50% and less than 4%, respectively (Table 14.1). The largest series of GH-secreting pituitary adenomas treated with GKRS reported the incidence rate of new post-GKRS hypopituitarism and cranial deficit at 26% and 4%, respectively. Among acromegaly patients treated with CKRS, approximately one third experienced some degree of new hypopituitarism [33, 49]. Patients with preexisting pituitary dysfunction were more likely to develop new pituitary deficit(s). In LINAC-SRS series, approximately 20% of acromegaly patients experienced some degree of new hypopituitarism, while the risk of new cranial nerve neuropathy was minimal [50, 52].

Careful selection of patients for SRS procedures and optimal SRS techniques and meticulous SRS planning are critical for optimized outcomes and safety profile of SRS procedures. Ongoing technological advancements of neuroimaging techniques, radiosurgical planning algorithms, and radiation delivery are expected to continue to improve precision and accuracy of radiation delivery and hence contribute to improved safety profile of SRS.

Repeated GKRS

Repeated GKRS can be considered for patients who experience disease recurrence after prior surgery and radiosurgery [57]. A multi-institutional series of 21 acromegalic patients who were retreated with repeated GKRS at a median of 5 years after initial GKRS found that 83% and 43% of patients had adequate tumor control and achieved endocrine remission, respectively. Four (19%) patients experienced adverse events after their second GKRS, and they included new cranial neuropathy ($n = 3$) and some degree of new pituitary dysfunction ($n = 1$). While repeated SRS can place patients at increased risk for radiation-induced cranial nerve damage, it can be a reasonable alternative that can be considered for treatment of persistent acromegaly in these challenging clinical scenarios after failure of first-line resection, medical management, and prior SRS. Repeated GKRS can be an appealing treatment option for patients with persistent acromegaly who cannot tolerate medical treatment and for patients deemed unfit surgical candidates due to size and/or location of residual/recurrent pituitary adenoma or poor surgical candidates due to medical comorbidities.

Brief Cessation of Antisecretory Medication around the Time of SRS

Accumulating evidence suggests that cessation of antisecretory medication before the SRS procedure may improve endocrine control rates and reduce time interval to achieve endocrine remission [13, 58, 59].

In IGKRF series of 371 acromegalic patients, 132 patients were taking antisecretory medication prior to SRS. Medical therapy was intentionally held in 74 patients (56%) in the time period around the SRS procedure. In multivariate regression analyses, temporary cessation of IGF-1-lowering medication prior to SRS was independently associated with initial endocrine remission, and it was a significant independent predictor of durable endocrine remission (HR = 2.49, 95% CI: 1.21–5.11; $P = 0.01$) [13]. Similar findings were reported by a group from Switzerland in a study of 31 patients who were treated with GKRS for recurrent and persistent acromegaly after adenoma resection surgery [58]. They found that patients who were not taking octreotide at the time of GKRS reached normal levels of GH and IGF-1 significantly faster when compared to patients taking the drug. Another retrospective series from Mayo Clinic of 46 consecutive acromegaly patients treated by radiosurgery between 1991 and 2004 also found that absence of pituitary suppressive medication at the time of radiosurgery was associated with fourfold increased odds for biochemical remission [59]. On the other hand, a study in 82 acromegaly patients with 49.5 months of follow-up did not find that discontinuation of suppressive medication increased the likelihood of endocrine remission after GKRS [53]. Nevertheless, when feasible, a brief cessation of pituitary adenoma suppressive medication around the time of SRS seems prudent. Given possible radioresistance-inducing effect of somatostatin analogues in the setting of GH-producing pituitary adenomas, we generally recommend that our patients have a brief cessation of suppressive therapy around an SRS procedure.

Fractionated Radiation Therapy for Acromegaly

Endocrine Control

Conventional fractionated radiation therapy (FRT) has been used for over 50 years for irradiation of GH-secreting pituitary adenomas. It continues to be used especially in centers where SRS is not available. FRT should also be considered for adenomas compressing the anterior optic apparatus (not amenable to decompression) in order optimize safety and reduce risk of radiation-induced neuropathy (Fig. 14.3). Summary of studies that reported FRT treatment results for treatment of GH induced pituitary adenomas is presented in Table 14.2. Series that reported combined cohorts of acromegaly patients treated using both FRT and SRS were not included.

The largest published series of FST for GH-secreting pituitary tumors comes from a registry in the United Kingdom that includes retrospectively and prospectively collected data of 884 patients treated at 14 centers during a period from 1970 to 2004 [60]. Patients who received pituitary radiotherapy before tumor resection surgery were treated with irradiation on more than one occasion or received SRS or brachytherapy with yttrium implants excluded, leaving a total sample of 656 acromegaly patients. Radiation therapy was delivered via three-field technique with median administered dose of 45 Gy in 25 fractions (1.8 Gy per fraction). Median duration of follow-up was 7 years (interquartile range, 3–13 year). At 10 years 60% of patients at risk achieved GH levels of <2.5 ng/ml, and 63% had normal IGF-1 levels. Higher pre-irradiation GH levels were associated with longer interval to achieve GH normalization.

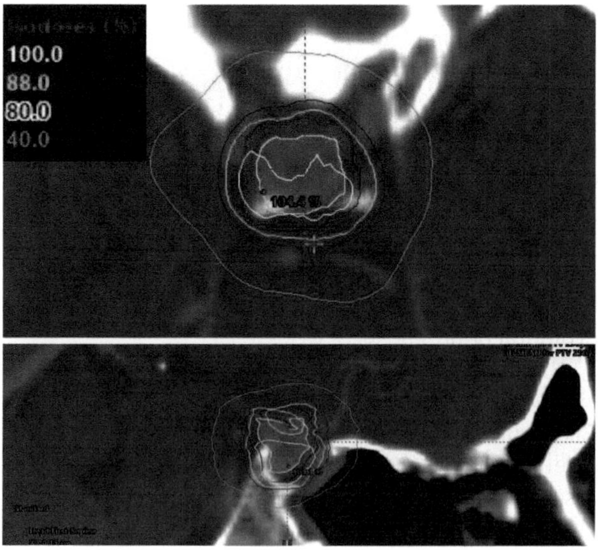

Fig. 14.3 A patient with a recurrent pituitary adenoma who received fractionated radiotherapy. Note that the IMRT inverse planning algorithm allows for "dose painting" or intensification of dose within certain components of the tumor

Table 14.2 Studies of fractionated radiation therapy for acromegaly

Authors, year/country	No. of patients	Technique	Mean dose in Gy (range)	No. of fractions	Mean dose per fraction in Gy	Length of follow-up (years)	Endocrine remission criteria: rate in %	Time to endocrine remission	Hypopituitarism	New cranial nerve deficits
Jenkins et al. (2006) [60]/the United Kingdom	656	Variety of techniques	45 (10–55)	25	1.8	Median: 7	GH < 2.5 ng/ml at 10 years: 60%[a] Normal IGF-1 at 10 years: 63%[a]	Not specified	10 years follow-up: LH/FSH: 18%[b] ACTH: 15%[b] TSH: 27%[b]	None
Barrande et al. (2000) [61]/France	128	Variety of techniques	52	–	1.8	Mean: 11.5 ± 8.5	GH < 5 μg/L at 15 years: 79%[a] GH < 2.5 μg/L at 15 years: 66%[a] Normal IGF-I at 15 years: 79%[a] GH suppression with OGTT: 61%[a]	Not specified	LH/FSH: 80%[c] TSH: 78%[c] ACTH: 82%[c]	3%
Gonzales-Virla et al. (2019) [62]/Mexico	94	TrueBeam and Versa HD systems	52 (52–57)	20–25	Range: 2–2.5	Mean: 12.9 ± 7.3	IGF-1 < 1.2 × UNL at 10 years: 66%[a] GH < 1 ng/mL: 44%[a]	Not specified	10 years follow-up: LH/FSH: 38%[c] TSH: 64% [C] ACTH: 53%[c]	1%
Epaminonda et al. (2001) [63]/Italy	67	Not specified	53.6 (40–75)	30–35	1.5	Mean: 11 ± 6	Normal IGF-1 and GH: 55%[d]	Not specified	60%[c]	None
Cozzi et al. (2001) [64]	49	Variety of techniques	45.08	22.4	2	Median: 14	Normal IGF-1: 16%[d] GH < 2.5 μg/L: 12%	Not specified	8%[b]	8%

(continued)

Table 14.2 (continued)

Authors, year/ country	No. of patients	Technique	Mean dose in Gy (range)	No. of fractions	Mean dose per fraction in Gy	Length of follow-up (years)	Endocrine remission criteria: rate in %	Time to endocrine remission	Hypopituitarism	New cranial nerve deficits
Minniti et al. (2005) [65]/ Italy	47	Not specified	Range: 45–50	25–28	1.8	Median: 12	Basal GH < 2.5 μg/l at 10 years: 55% Normal IGF-1 at 10 years: 42% GH suppression with OGTT: 52%	Not specified	78% at 10 years[c]	2%
Diallo et al. (2015) [66]/ France	34	Clinac-Exactrac and Novalis Tx	50	27	1.85	Mean: 12.6	Normal IGF-1: 38.2%[d]	62 months	39%[b]	None
Roug et al. (2010) [67]/ Denmark	34	Not specified	54	27–30	Not reported	Mean: 3.75	Normal IGF-1 and GH suppression with OGTT: 50% (on suppressive therapy) and 29% (off suppressive therapy)	30 months	97%[c]	Not reported
Powell et al. (2000) [68]/ the United States	32	Not specified	47.4 (45–54)	25–30	1.8	Mean: 5.6	IGF-1 normalization: 43.7%	Not specified	31.7%[b]	None
Patt et al. (2016) [69]	36	High-precision 3D	45	25	Not reported	Mean: 4.7	Normal of GH and IGF1: 55%	63 months	33%[b]	None

GH growth hormone, *IGF-1* insulin-like growth factor-1, *OGTT* oral glucose tolerance test
[a]Not reported if suppressive medication were discontinued
[b]New hypopituitarism
[c]Pre- and postirradiation combined
[d]Off suppressive medication

Another large single-institution series reported experience with 128 acromegaly patients who were followed for 11.5 ± 8.5 years after FST that was administered in daily fractions of 1.8 Gy (mean dose: 52 ± 8.5 Gy) [61]. GH levels of <2.5 μg/L were reached in 66% of patient at 15 years, and suppression of GH during OGTT was seen in 61% of patients at 15 years. 79% of patients had normal IGF-I levels. Higher pre-irradiation GH levels predicted longer time to endocrine remission.

A recent study from Mexico of 94 acromegaly patients treated with FRT and followed for 12.9 ± 7.3 years reported that at 10 years after FRT, 66% of treated patients achieved IGF-1 levels of <1.2× the upper limit of normal, and 44% of patients had basal GH levels <1 ng/mL [62].

Another study of 67 acromegaly patients treated with FRT with mean follow-up of 11 ± 6 years reported that 55% of patients achieved normal IGF-1 levels, 58% patients achieved GH levels <2.5 μg/L, and 55% of patients achieved both criteria [63].

Smaller institutional series that reported their experience with less than 50 acromegaly patients irradiated with FRT reported endocrine remission rates ranging from 12% [64] to 55% [65]. Large variations of endocrine remission rates across series can be attributed to varying lengths of endocrine follow-up and different criteria used to define endocrine remission. Specifically, mean or median follow-up duration across series ranged from 45 months [67] to almost 13 years [62]. Endocrine remission criteria were also variable and include normalization of IGF-1 and/or GH levels. GH suppression with OGTT test was employed by some studies [61, 65]. Furthermore, the use of suppressive medication use was reported by some studies [63, 66, 68].

Complications Following FRT

As with SRS, new onset hypopituitarism or decline in normal pituitary function is the most common side effect of FRT. Reported rates of some degree of pituitary dysfunction of acromegaly patients treated with FRT approached 80% in some series that combined pre-FRT with post-FRT pituitary dysfunction (Table 14.2) [61, 65]. New onset post-FRT pituitary dysfunction occurs in approximately one third of patients [66, 68, 69]. The risk of FRT-induced radiation neuropathy is low with reported incidence rates ranging from 1% [62] to 8% [64].

Other reported complications of FRT include radiation necrosis, radiation-induced intracranial neoplasms, and stroke. For example, in one series 3% of patients presented with neurological event after FRT and were diagnosed with cerebral necrosis on brain imaging that occurred 10–19 years after irradiation [61]. Others reported two cases of temporal region radiation necrosis 4 and 10 years after FRT [65]. Kim with colleagues detected radiation necrosis in 13.8% of treated patients [44]. Reported cases of presumably FRT-induced tumors include meningiomas (five reported cases) [62–64] and one pineal tumor [63].

Proton Beam Irradiation

Proton beam radiation therapy and radiosurgery have been used for irradiation of the pituitary gland for pituitary adenomas since 1960s [23, 70–72]. However, technological advancements of photon irradiation (like intensity modulated radiation therapy, IMRT) methods have called into question the therapeutic benefit of proton beam irradiation. Nevertheless, proton beam radiotherapy is an effective modality, and the number of proton beam centers in the United States has grown, and today there are 30 proton beam centers in the United States. European and Asian countries have also witnessed gradual increases of proton beam centers. Hence, it can be expected that the number of acromegaly patients treated with proton beam radiotherapy will grow. However, the role of proton beam radiosurgery is still to be defined, as current physical uncertainties with small volume proton beam irradiation limit its applicability to tumors under 1–2 cm.

In 1968 Kjellberg and colleagues presented treatment results of 22 acromegalic patients treated with 160-million-electron-volt (Mev) Harvard Cyclotron between 1963 and 1967 [23]. They followed 14 of the treated patients for 2 to 36 months after the procedure and found that levels of GH fell in 8 patients and glucose tolerance curves improved to normal in three patients. There have been no deaths associated with the procedure, and three patients reported intermittent mild diplopia.

More recently, a group from the Massachusetts General Hospital presented their experience with proton therapy in 165 functioning pituitary adenomas that included 50 acromegaly patients treated between 1992 and 2012 [73]. They found that 26% of acromegaly patients achieved endocrine remission, and median time to achieve endocrine remission was 62 months. Endocrine remission was defined as age and sex-appropriate IGF-1 levels, supported by a normal oral glucose tolerance test result in some cases. Time to achieve remission was the longest in patients with acromegaly when compared to patients harboring other types of pituitary adenomas. Of 127 patients treated with proton beam therapy and at risk for new post-procedural pituitary deficiency, actuarial 3-year and 5-year rates of new deficiency requiring hormone replacement therapy were 45% and 62%, respectively. Median time to hypopituitarism was 40 months. One acromegaly patients experienced temporal lobe seizures associated with imaging changes. Another acromegaly patient who received proton beam therapy after external beam irradiation experienced osteonecrosis of the ethmoid sinus that was associated with a chronic fungal infection.

Conclusions

Stereotactic radiosurgery and fractionated radiation therapy play important roles in the contemporary management of GH-producing pituitary adenomas. Pituitary tumor irradiation should be considered after unsuccessful adenoma resection surgery or when suppressive therapy is not tolerated. SRS is the most commonly used method as it allows spatially precise irradiation of recurring, persistent, and/or invading adenoma tissue. Fractionated radiation therapy is also effective treatment method that is associated with acceptable safety profile and is used in centers without SRS availability. Proton therapy is another alternative however with more limited availability. Delayed postradiation therapy hypopituitarism is the most common complication that should be monitored and appropriately managed. Cranial nerve damage and other serious, irreversible complications are rare.

References

1. Melmed S. Medical progress: acromegaly. N Engl J Med. 2006;355:2558–73.
2. Holdaway IM, Rajasoorya C. Epidemiology of acromegaly. Pituitary. 1999;2:29–41.
3. Chanson P, Salenave S. Acromegaly. Orphanet J Rare Dis. 2008;3:17.
4. Hoskuldsdottir GT, Fjalldal SB, Sigurjonsdottir HA. The incidence and prevalence of acromegaly, a nationwide study from 1955 through 2013. Pituitary. 2015;18:803–7.
5. Placzek H, Xu Y, Mu Y, Begelman SM, Fisher M. Clinical and economic burden of commercially insured patients with acromegaly in the United States: a retrospective analysis. J Manag Care Spec Pharm. 2015;21:1106–12.
6. Schneider HJ, Sievers C, Saller B, Wittchen HU, Stalla GK. High prevalence of biochemical acromegaly in primary care patients with elevated IGF-1 levels. Clin Endocrinol. 2008;69:432–5.
7. Rosario PW. Frequency of acromegaly in adults with diabetes or glucose intolerance and estimated prevalence in the general population. Pituitary. 2011;14:217–21.
8. Giustina A, Barkan A, Beckers A, et al. A consensus on the diagnosis and treatment of acromegaly comorbidities: an update. J Clin Endocrinol Metab. 2019;105(4):dgz096. https://doi.org/10.1210/clinem/dgz096.
9. Holdaway IM, Rajasoorya RC, Gamble GD. Factors influencing mortality in acromegaly. J Clin Endocrinol Metab. 2004;89:667–74.
10. Kauppinen-Mäkelin R, Sane T, Reunanen A, et al. A nationwide survey of mortality in acromegaly. J Clin Endocrinol Metab. 2005;90:4081–6.
11. Katznelson L, Laws ER, Melmed S, Molitch ME, Murad MH, Utz A, Wass JAH, Endocrine Society. Acromegaly: an endocrine society clinical practice guideline. J Clin Endocrinol Metab. 2014;99:3933–51.
12. Katznelson L, Atkinson JLD, Cook DM, Ezzat SZ, Hamrahian AH, Miller KK, American Association of Clinical Endocrinologists. American Association of Clinical Endocrinologists medical guidelines for clinical practice for the diagnosis and treatment of acromegaly--2011 update. Endocr Pract Off J Am Coll Endocrinol Am Assoc Clin Endocrinol. 2011;17(Suppl 4):1–44.
13. Ding D, Mehta GU, Patibandla MR, et al. Stereotactic radiosurgery for acromegaly: an international multicenter retrospective cohort study. Neurosurgery. 2019;84:717–25.
14. Giustina A, Chanson P, Bronstein MD, et al. A consensus on criteria for cure of acromegaly. J Clin Endocrinol Metab. 2010;95:3141–8.
15. Mammis A, Eloy JA, Liu JK. Early descriptions of acromegaly and gigantism and their historical evolution as clinical entities. Neurosurg Focus. 2010;29:E1.
16. Beclere. The radiotherapeutic treatment of tumours of the hypophysis, gigantism and acromegaly. Arch Roentgen Ray. 1909;111:114.
17. Sheaves R. A history of acromegaly. Pituitary. 1999;2:7–28.

18. Adler JR, Altenau L, Barani IJ, Barbaro NM, Barnett GH, Baxi N. Stereotactic radiosurgery for pituitary adenomas. Intracran Stereotact Radiosurg. 2016. https://doi.org/10.1055/b-0035-122550.
19. Bachman AL, Harris W. Roentgen therapy for pituitary adenoma; correlation of tumor dose with response in 64 cases. Radiology. 1949;53:331–41.
20. Sheline GE, Goldberg MB, Feldman R. Pituitary irradiation for acromegaly. Radiology. 1961;76:70–5.
21. Leksell L. The stereotaxic method and radiosurgery of the brain. Acta Chir Scand. 1951;102:316–9.
22. Leksell L. Stereotactic radiosurgery. J Neurol Neurosurg Psychiatry. 1983;46:797–803.
23. Kjellberg RN, Shintani A, Frantz AG, Kliman B. Proton-beam therapy in acromegaly. N Engl J Med. 1968;278:689–95.
24. Betti O, Derechinsky V. Multiple-beam stereotaxic irradiation. Neurochirurgie. 1983;29:295–8.
25. Hirsch. Die operative Behandlung von Hypophysistumoren nach endonasalen Methoden. Arch Laryngol Rhinol. 1912:529–686.
26. Schulder M, Loeffler JS, Howes AE, Alexander E, Black PM. The radium bomb: Harvey Cushing and the interstitial irradiation of gliomas. J Neurosurg. 1996;84:530–2.
27. Joplin GF, Fraser R, Steiner R, Laws J, Jones E. Partial pituitary ablation by needle implantation of gold-198 seeds for acromegaly and Cushing's disease. Lancet Lond Engl. 1961;2:1277–80.
28. Di Mambro A, Giuliani C, Ammannati F, et al. A single-institution retrospective experience of brachytherapy in the treatment of pituitary tumors: transsphenoidal approach combined with (192)Ir-after loading catheters. J Endocrinol Investig. 2010;33:455–60.
29. Julow JV. Intracystic irradiation for craniopharyngiomas. Pituitary. 2013;16:34–45.
30. Garcia-Barros M, Paris F, Cordon-Cardo C, Lyden D, Rafii S, Haimovitz-Friedman A, Fuks Z, Kolesnick R. Tumor response to radiotherapy regulated by endothelial cell apoptosis. Science. 2003;300:1155–9.
31. Laughton SJ, Merchant TE, Sklar CA, et al. Endocrine outcomes for children with embryonal brain tumors after risk-adapted craniospinal and conformal primary-site irradiation and high-dose chemotherapy with stem-cell rescue on the SJMB-96 trial. J Clin Oncol Off J Am Soc Clin Oncol. 2008;26:1112–8.
32. Ho JC, Luo D, Guha-Thakurta N, Ferguson SD, Ghia AJ, Yang JN, Brown PD, Voong KR. Gamma knife stereotactic radiosurgery for brain metastases using only 3 pins. Neurosurgery. 2016;78:877–82.
33. Roberts BK, Ouyang DL, Lad SP, Chang SD, Harsh GR, Adler JR, Soltys SG, Gibbs IC, Remedios L, Katznelson L. Efficacy and safety of CyberKnife radiosurgery for acromegaly. Pituitary. 2007;10:19–25.
34. Kong D-S, Kim Y-H, Kim YH, Hur KY, Kim JH, Kim M-S, Paek SH, Kwon D-H, Kim D-K, Lee J-I. Long-term efficacy and tolerability of gamma knife radiosurgery for growth hormone-secreting adenoma: a retrospective multicenter study (MERGE-001). World Neurosurg. 2019;122:e1291–9.
35. Franzin A, Spatola G, Losa M, Picozzi P, Mortini P. Results of gamma knife radiosurgery in acromegaly. Int J Endocrinol. 2012;2012:342034.
36. Jezková. 2006. https://onlinelibrary.wiley.com/doi/abs/10.1111/j.1365-2265.2006.02513.x.
37. Castinetti. 2005. https://academic.oup.com/jcem/article/90/8/4483/3058880.
38. Pai F-Y, Chen C-J, Wang W-H, et al. Low-dose gamma knife radiosurgery for acromegaly. Neurosurgery. 2019;85:E20–30.
39. Vik-Mo EO, Oksnes M, Pedersen P-H, Wentzel-Larsen T, Rødahl E, Thorsen F, Schreiner T, Aanderud S, Lund-Johansen M. Gamma knife stereotactic radiosurgery for acromegaly. Eur J Endocrinol. 2007;157:255–63.
40. Gutt. 2005. https://www.thieme-connect.com/products/ejournals/abstract/10.1055/s-2005-837552.
41. Poon TL, Leung SCL, Poon CYF, Yu CP. Predictors of outcome following Gamma Knife surgery for acromegaly. J Neurosurg. 2010;113(Suppl):149–52.

42. Ronchi. 2009. https://www.researchgate.net/profile/Sabrina-Corbetta/publication/24262686_Prevalence_of_GH_deficiency_in_cured_acromegalic_patients_Impact_of_different_previous_treatments/links/564db6c008aefe619b0e10d4/Prevalenceof-GH-deficiency-in-cured-acromegalic-patients-Impact-of-different-previous-treatments.pdf.
43. Liu et al. 2012. https://link.springer.com/article/10.1007/s11060-012-0862-z.
44. Kim EH, Oh MC, Chang JH, Moon JH, Ku CR, Chang W-S, Lee EJ, Kim SH. Postoperative gamma knife radiosurgery for cavernous sinus-invading growth hormone-secreting pituitary adenomas. World Neurosurg. 2018;110:e534–45.
45. Attanasio. 2003. https://scholar.google.com/scholar_url?url=https://academic.oup.com/jcem/article/88/7/3105/2845265&hl=en&sa=X&ei=XhIpY96nAYvGsQL685eIDA&scisig=AAGBfm10aVLIDROybZQgZ5JtSnniE1LrHw&oi=scholarr.
46. Erdur. 2011. https://www.researchgate.net/profile/Fatih-Erdur/publication/306367581_Gamma-Knife_Radiosurgery_in_Acromegaly_Patients/links/58b5376a92851cf7ae957262/Gamma-Knife-Radiosurgery-in-Acromegaly-Patients.pdf.
47. Sims-Williams HP, Rajapaksa K, Sinha S, Radatz M, Walton L, Yianni J, Newell-Price J. Radiosurgery as primary management for acromegaly. Clin Endocrinol. 2019;90:114–21.
48. Fukuoka. 2001. https://www.karger.com/Article/Abstract/66721.
49. Sala E, Moore JM, Amorin A, Martinez H, Bhowmik AC, Lamsam L, Chang S, Soltys SG, Katznelson L, Harsh GR. CyberKnife robotic radiosurgery in the multimodal management of acromegaly patients with invasive macroadenoma: a single center's experience. J Neuro-Oncol. 2018;138:291–8.
50. Wilson PJ, De-Loyde KJ, Williams JR, Smee RI. Acromegaly: a single centre's experience of stereotactic radiosurgery and radiotherapy for growth hormone secreting pituitary tumours with the linear accelerator. J Clin Neurosci Off J Neurosurg Soc Australas. 2013;20:1506–13.
51. Voges J, Kocher M, Runge M, et al. Linear accelerator radiosurgery for pituitary macroadenomas. Cancer. 2006;107:1355–64.
52. Yan J-L, Chang C-N, Chuang C-C, Hsu P-W, Lin J-D, Wei K-C, Lee S-T, Tseng J-K, Pai P-C, Chen Y-L. Long-term follow-up of patients with surgical intractable acromegaly after linear accelerator radiosurgery. J Formos Med Assoc Taiwan Yi Zhi. 2013;112:416–20.
53. Castinetti F, Nagai M, Morange I, et al. Long-term results of stereotactic radiosurgery in secretory pituitary adenomas. J Clin Endocrinol Metab. 2009;94:3400–7.
54. Giustina A, Barkan A, Casanueva FF, Cavagnini F, Frohman L, Ho K, Veldhuis J, Wass J, Von Werder K, Melmed S. Criteria for cure of acromegaly: a consensus statement. J Clin Endocrinol Metab. 2000;85:526–9.
55. Kajiwara K, Saito K, Yoshikawa K, Kato S, Akimura T, Nomura S, Ishihara H, Suzuki M. Image-guided stereotactic radiosurgery with the CyberKnife for pituitary adenomas. Minim Invasive Neurosurg MIN. 2005;48:91–6.
56. Cho CB, Park HK, Joo WI, Chough CK, Lee KJ, Rha HK. Stereotactic radiosurgery with the CyberKnife for pituitary adenomas. J Korean Neurosurg Soc. 2009;45:157–63.
57. Alonso CE, Bunevicius A, Trifiletti DM, et al. Safety and efficacy of repeat radiosurgery for acromegaly: an International Multi-Institutional Study. J Neuro-Oncol. 2019;145:301–7.
58. Landolt AM, Haller D, Lomax N, Scheib S, Schubiger O, Siegfried J, Wellis G. Octreotide may act as a radioprotective agent in acromegaly. J Clin Endocrinol Metab. 2000;85:1287–9.
59. Pollock BE, Jacob JT, Brown PD, Nippoldt TB. Radiosurgery of growth hormone-producing pituitary adenomas: factors associated with biochemical remission. J Neurosurg. 2007;106:833–8.
60. Jenkins PJ, Bates P, Carson MN, Stewart PM, Wass JAH. Conventional pituitary irradiation is effective in lowering serum growth hormone and insulin-like growth factor-I in patients with acromegaly. J Clin Endocrinol Metab. 2006;91:1239–45.
61. Barrande G, Pittino-Lungo M, Coste J, Ponvert D, Bertagna X, Luton JP, Bertherat J. Hormonal and metabolic effects of radiotherapy in acromegaly: long-term results in 128 patients followed in a single center. J Clin Endocrinol Metab. 2000;85:3779–85.

62. Gonzales-Virla B, Vargas-Ortega G, Martínez-Vázquez K-B, de Lo Monteros ALE, Sosa-Erosa E, López-Félix B, Mendoza-Zubieta V, Mercado M. Efficacy and safety of fractionated conformal radiation therapy in acromegaly: a long-term follow-up study. Endocrine. 2019;65:386–92.
63. Epaminonda P, Porretti S, Cappiello V, Beck-Peccoz P, Faglia G, Arosio M. Efficacy of radiotherapy in normalizing serum IGF-I, acid-labile subunit (ALS) and IGFBP-3 levels in acromegaly. Clin Endocrinol. 2001;55:183–9.
64. Cozzi R, Barausse M, Asnaghi D, Dallabonzana D, Lodrini S, Attanasio R. Failure of radiotherapy in acromegaly. Eur J Endocrinol. 2001;145:717–26.
65. Minniti G, Jaffrain-Rea M-L, Osti M, Esposito V, Santoro A, Solda F, Gargiulo P, Tamburrano G, Enrici RM. The long-term efficacy of conventional radiotherapy in patients with GH-secreting pituitary adenomas. Clin Endocrinol. 2005;62:210–6.
66. Diallo AM, Colin P, Litre CF, Diallo MM, Decoudier B, Bertoin F, Higel B, Patey M, Rousseaux P, Delemer B. Long-term results of fractionated stereotactic radiotherapy as third-line treatment in acromegaly. Endocrine. 2015;50:741–8.
67. Roug S, Rasmussen AK, Juhler M, Kosteljanetz M, Poulsgaard L, Heebøll H, Roed H, Feldt-Rasmussen U. Fractionated stereotactic radiotherapy in patients with acromegaly: an interim single-Centre audit. Eur J Endocrinol. 2010;162:685–94.
68. Powell JS, Wardlaw SL, Post KD, Freda PU. Outcome of radiotherapy for acromegaly using normalization of insulin-like growth factor I to define cure. J Clin Endocrinol Metab. 2000;85:2068–71.
69. Patt H, Jalali R, Yerawar C, Khare S, Gupta T, Goel A, Lila A, Bandgar T, Shah NS. High-precision conformal fractionated radiotherapy is effective in achieving remission in patients with acromegaly after failed transsphenoidal surgery. Endocr Pract Off J Am Coll Endocrinol Am Assoc Clin Endocrinol. 2016;22:162–72.
70. Hockaday TD, Laing AH, Welbourn RB, Hartog M. Letter: proton beam therapy for acromegaly. Br Med J. 1975;1:457.
71. Kjellberg RN, Kliman B. Bragg peak proton treatment for pituitary-related conditions. Proc R Soc Med. 1974;67:32–3.
72. Levy RP, Fabrikant JI, Frankel KA, Phillips MH, Lyman JT, Lawrence JH, Tobias CA. Heavy-charged-particle radiosurgery of the pituitary gland: clinical results of 840 patients. Stereotact Funct Neurosurg. 1991;57:22–35.
73. Wattson DA, Tanguturi SK, Spiegel DY, et al. Outcomes of proton therapy for patients with functional pituitary adenomas. Int J Radiat Oncol Biol Phys. 2014;90:532–9.

Chapter 15
Challenging Questions in the Management of Acromegaly in the Young

Nancy Youssef and Kevin C. J. Yuen

Introduction

Acromegaly is a rare systemic disorder characterized by persistent hypersecretion of growth hormone (GH), mostly due to a pituitary GH-secreting pituitary adenoma [1], that can lead to excess morbidity and mortality if not adequately treated [2–4]. Appropriate and effective treatment regimens to achieve long-term disease remission frequently require multimodal treatment approaches including surgery, medical therapy, and radiotherapy [5]. Previous consensus guidelines have proposed that the objectives of effective acromegaly treatment should include normalization of serum insulin-like growth factor-I (IGF-1) levels, reduction of serum GH levels <1.0 μg/L, reduction of tumor volume, improvement of clinical symptoms, and preservation of pituitary function [6–8].

Transsphenoidal surgery is the first-line treatment for most patients [9, 10] and is effective when performed in experienced centers with biochemical remission rates in excess of 80%. However, because most patients present with macroadenomas, the remission rates after surgery are lower, and a significant number of patients often require medical therapy [8]. Additionally, there are cases where patients who may be ineligible for surgery due to their tumor being technically difficult to resect and/or other concurrent comorbid conditions, and primary medical therapy has been shown to induce disease remission in such patients [11]. Currently, there are three different classes of drugs available: somatostatin

N. Youssef · K. C. J. Yuen (✉)
Department of Neuroendocrinology and Neurosurgery, Barrow Pituitary Center, Barrow Neurological Institute, University of Arizona College of Medicine and Creighton School of Medicine, Phoenix, AZ, USA
e-mail: nancy.youssef@dignityhealth.org; kevin.yuen@dignityhealth.org

L. S. Blevins Jr., M. K. Aghi (eds.), *Acromegaly*, Contemporary Endocrinology,
https://doi.org/10.1007/978-3-031-16258-9_15

receptor ligands (SRLs), dopamine agonists (DAs), and the GH receptor antagonist (GHRA) pegvisomant (PegV). First-generation SRLs, such as octreotide, octreotide LAR (long-acting release) and lanreotide, are recommended in patients with persistent disease after surgery and as first-line treatment for those ineligible for surgery, whereas their role in neoadjuvant settings is still debatable [8]. In 2014, pasireotide long-acting release (LAR) was approved by the US Food and Drug Administration (FDA) and the European Medicines Agency (EMA) for treatment of patients with acromegaly who failed surgery and for patients in whom surgery is not an option (Signifor LAR). Pasireotide LAR is a somatostatin multireceptor ligand that exhibits higher binding affinities to somatostatin receptor subtypes 5 (SSTR5) and a lesser extent to SSTR2, SSTR3, and SSTR1 [12]. Because of its broader SSTR-binding profile, pasireotide LAR has been suggested to have greater clinical efficacy in acromegaly than first-generation SRLs. The Acromegaly Consensus Group in 2017 recommended medical therapy with first-generation SRLs, DAs, or the GHRA PegV for patients who have failed surgery and for patients in whom surgery is not an option and pasireotide LAR monotherapy as second-line therapy [8]. In June 2020, the FDA approved the use of oral octreotide capsules (OOC) for long-term maintenance of acromegaly patients who have responded to and tolerated treatment with injectable octreotide and lanreotide [13]. By contrast, radiotherapy is generally reserved as third-line therapy in patients with persistent disease or tumor growth after surgery or while on medical therapy [14, 15]. When surgery fails to induce disease remission, treatment decisions at this stage (e.g., repeat surgery or medical therapy or medical therapy followed by radiotherapy) can be challenging and are determined by multiple factors, including visibility of the adenoma on MRI, patient age, underlying patient comorbidities, patient preference, patient tolerability to the adverse effects of each treatment modality, and whether surgical remission is achievable safely without compromising pituitary function.

In this chapter, we present a young patient with acromegaly who had failed multiple transsphenoidal surgeries despite being operated on by an experienced surgeon and discuss the challenging management issues that arose over time that shaped our medical decision-making in treating this patient. While the goal of this chapter is to provide clinical guidance for the approach and treatment to a young patient with aggressive acromegaly, it is our strong opinion that patients with this rare disorder should be managed at expert centers, consisting of a multidisciplinary team (endocrinologists, neurosurgeons, radiation oncologists, neurologists, neuro-ophthalmologists, pathologists, and genetic counsellors) experienced and dedicated to the care for patients with complex pituitary disorders. In addition to providing clinical care to such patients, the expert multidisciplinary teams establish recurring tumor board review which provides a platform for the exchange of clinical experience among various medical specialties, scientific knowledge, coordination of clinical trials, and translational research activities.

Case Presentation

On November 11, 2012, a 16-year-old female, who at that time was living in New Hampshire, presented to her endocrinologist in Massachusetts with a 16-month history of secondary amenorrhea, fatigue, and frontal headaches. Laboratory tests revealed prolactin 31.5 ng/mL, IGF-I 1085 ng/mL (reference range: 185–551 ng/mL), 8 AM GH 7.5 ng/mL, TSH 1.04 mU/L, free T4 1.1 ng/dL, 8 AM cortisol 10.2 μg/dL, and 8 AM ACTH 23 pg/mL. A pituitary-dedicated magnetic resonance imaging (MRI) showed a pituitary macroadenoma measuring 2.0 × 2.3 × 1.8 cm invading down into the sphenoid sinus and extending superiorly compressing the optic chiasm with no invasion into the cavernous sinuses. She underwent her first transsphenoidal surgery with an experienced neurosurgeon in Massachusetts on December 19, 2012. Pathologic findings revealed strong GH and prolactin positivity on immunohistochemistry. Postoperatively, she developed secondary hypothyroidism, but remission from acromegaly was not achieved with postoperative IGF-I levels in the range of 600–800 ng/mL and an oral glucose tolerance test nadir GH level of 3.7 ng/mL. She continued to report symptoms of headache, fatigue, and increased perspiration. A 3-month postoperative MRI revealed postsurgical changes with notable residual tumor measuring 2 mm inferior to the pituitary gland. Based on this result, she was commenced on lanreotide injections 60 mg every 28 days, and her dose was gradually increased to 90 mg and eventually 120 mg every 28 days over 6 months. However, with each injection of lanreotide, she experienced nausea and diarrhea for 2–3 days before these symptoms resolved spontaneously. She was able to escalate her dose of lanreotide up to 120 mg every 28 days, but her IGF-I levels remained persistently elevated above 600 ng/mL. Another MRI performed on December 4, 2014, revealed interval enlargement of the residual tumor measuring 4 mm inferior to the normal gland and IGF-I remained elevated at 742 ng/mL. Because of lack of normalization of IGF-I levels and side effects associated with lanreotide, the decision at this point was made to undergo a second transsphenoidal surgery with the same surgeon in Massachusetts. The surgery took place on January 13, 2015, and her postoperative IGF-I and 8 AM GH in April 2015 remained elevated at 577 ng/mL and 7.4 ng/mL, respectively. Lanreotide was resumed but she could only tolerate 90 mg every 28 days. Pathologic findings revealed similar findings to those after her first surgery of GH and prolactin positivity on immunohistochemistry. Postoperative MRI on May 12, 2015, revealed postsurgical changes with stable residual tumor measuring 3 mm inferior to the pituitary gland. The patient then relocated to Montana to stay with her mother on June 10, 2015, and presented to me for the first time in Washington on June 16, 2015, with increasing fatigue, sweaty palms, body odor, central weight gain, arthralgias, frontal headaches, and persistent amenorrhea. Laboratory testing confirmed secondary adrenal insufficiency, secondary hypothyroidism, secondary hypogonadism, and central diabetes insipidus, and she was started on hydrocortisone 15 mg in the morning and 5 mg at noon, levothyroxine 75 μg a day, Orsythia® (levonorgestrel and ethinyl estradiol) tablets, and desmopressin tablets 0.05 mg twice a day, respectively. Because her IGF-I remained elevated at 658 ng/mL (reference range: 185–551 ng/mL) and her previous intolerance and lack of IGF-I normalization with lanreotide, the decision was made to switch her to PegV 20 mg 3 days a week. While on PegV, she reported improvement in her arthralgias and headaches, and her dose of PegV was eventually decreased to 20 mg 2 days a week on February 8, 2016, based on her IGF-I levels. Sleep study excluded sleep apnea and colonoscopy revealed two colonic polyps that were successfully excised. However, surveillance MRI on February 8, 2016, showed that the previously noted in the sella cavity has now filled with a heterogeneous mass extending into the suprasellar cistern measuring 1.5 × 1.4 × 1.3 cm and almost contacting the underside of the optic chiasm (Fig. 15.1). Because the recurrent mass was sufficiently close to the optic chiasm, the decision was made for the patient to undergo her third transsphenoidal surgery in Washington on March 15, 2016, to allow the administration of a single full dose of 24 Gy to the 50% isodense line Gamma Knife radiosurgery on May 13, 2016. Pathologic findings indicated sparsely granulated GH cell type and focal prolactin staining with strong diffuse bodies on CAM5.2 stain, Ki-67 5%, and weak P53 immunostaining 4%. Genetic testing on June 22, 2016, revealed heterozygosity for the aryl hydrocarbon receptor-interacting peptide (*AIP*) missense mutation on exon 6. Further genetic testing of

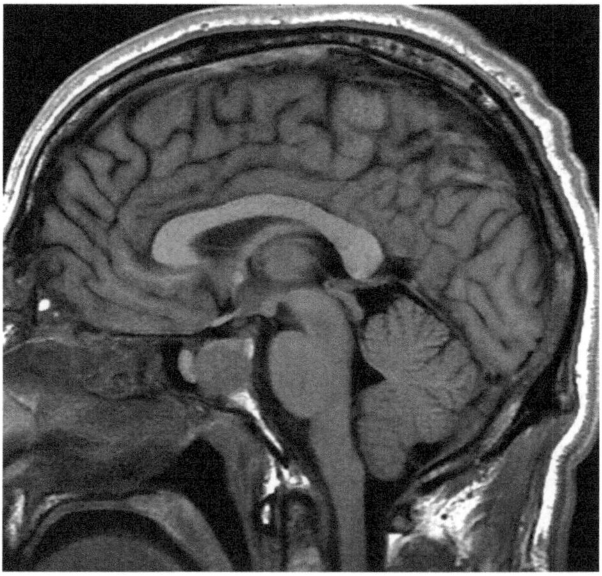

Fig. 15.1 MRI images before the patient's third transsphenoidal surgery

her parents was negative of the any *AIP* mutations. Postoperatively, her IGF-I continued to be mildly elevated at 451 ng/mL (reference range: 85–370 ng/mL) on June 15, 2016, so she was restarted on PegV 10 mg 3 days a week. She continued to report of sporadic headaches, and after consultation with neurology, she was treated with subcutaneous (sc) octreotide 100 μg injections no more than three injections a day on an "as required basis," and she found that these injections were effective in relieving her headaches. Since her third transsphenoidal surgery, surveillance MRIs from 2016 to 2020 revealed postsurgical changes in the pituitary fossa and no evidence of recurrence of the pituitary mass. Her dose of PegV was adjusted further down to 20 mg once a week when her results on June 7, 2017, showed an IGF-I level of 287 ng/mL (reference range: 85–370 ng/mL), and the patient continues to obtain relief from her arthralgic pains. On March 21, 2018, surveillance MRI revealed a partially empty sella, resolving enhancement of the pituitary stalk now positioned midline, and new downward traction upon the optic chiasm possibly representing developing optic chiasm herniation in the setting of an empty sella. In addition, there was interval decrease in the extent of migrated fat packing material throughout the ventricular system. Because her IGF-I on July 19, 2019, had decreased to 74 ng/mL (reference range: 85–370 ng/mL), the possibility of developing adult GH deficiency following three transsphenoidal surgeries and Gamma Knife radiosurgery was considered, and PegV was discontinued at this time. The patient saw a reproductive endocrinologist in Montana on January 2, 2020, to discuss about the prospects of future fertility, and laboratory tests revealed prolactin 11.8 ng/mL, IGF-I 103 ng/mL (reference range: 73–320 ng/mL), TSH 0.33 mU/L, free T4 1.0 ng/dL, FSH 0.3 mIU/mL, LH < 0.3 mIU/mL, estradiol <5.0 pg/mL, and anti-Mullerian hormone 2.6 (reference range: 0.9–9.5 ng/mL). She was commenced on transdermal estrogen patch twice a week and progesterone 10 days every 3 months to induce withdrawal bleed. Surveillance MRI on August 19, 2020, revealed postsurgical changes in the pituitary fossa, no evidence of recurrence of pituitary mass, and slight increase in soft tissue change extending into the ventral clivus likely mucosal regeneration, whereas bone densitometry scan revealed osteopenia in her proximal femur and osteoporosis in her lumbar spine that had worsened since her previous study on February 6, 2019. Although she denies any history of previous fractures, the patient is concerned of the worsening osteoporosis. On July 14, 2020, laboratory tests revealed IGF-I 122 ng/mL (reference range: 73–320 ng/mL), FSH < 0.3 mIU/mL, LH < 0.3 mIU/mL, prolactin 53.6 ng/mL, TSH 0.62 mU/L, free T4 0.8 ng/dL, procollagen type I N propeptide (PINP) 65 μg/L (reference range: 19–83 μg/L), and C-terminal telopeptide of type I collagen (CTX-I) 434 pg/mL (reference range: 25–573 pg/mL), while thoracolumbar spine X-ray revealed no evidence of fractures. In order to address her bone health, she was started on calcium supplements 1200 mg a day and vitamin D 2000 IU a day and advised to remain on estradiol patch 0.075 mg twice a week. She eventually agreed to consider GH replacement therapy based on her having panhypopituitarism and an IGF-I in the lower half of the reference range; hence a low dose of GH replacement therapy of 0.2 mg a day was

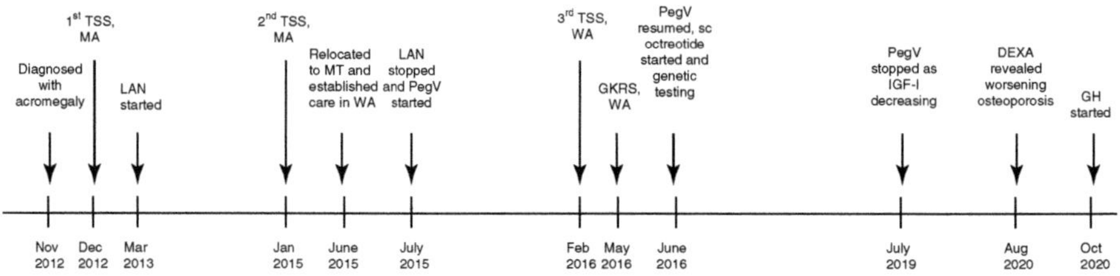

Fig. 15.2 Timelines of significant events and treatment milestones of the patient. *Aug* August, *Dec* December, *DEXA* dual energy X-ray absorptiometry, *Feb* February, *GH* growth hormone, *GKRS* Gamma Knife radiosurgery, *IGF-I* insulin-like growth factor-I, *Jan* January, *LAN* lanreotide, *MA* Massachusetts; *Mar* March, *Nov* November, *Oct* October *PegV* pegvisomant, *TSS* transsphenoidal surgery, *MT* Montana, *sc* subcutaneous, *WA* Washington

commenced on October 1, 2020. Figure 15.2 illustrates the timelines of important treatment milestones in our patient.

Challenging Clinical Management Questions

Question 1

If this patient was tested earlier after her first transsphenoidal surgery and found to be AIP mutation positive, should she have been managed differently?

Mutations in the *AIP* gene account for the largest proportion of genetic/inheritable forms of acromegaly. Among unselected acromegaly populations, 0–4% of patients have *AIP* mutations/deletions, which rises in more focused groups such as familial isolated pituitary adenoma kindreds and young patients [16]. These patients harbor adenomas that consist of more than 80% of GH-secreting or prolactin-secreting or mixed GH and prolactin or silent GH/prolactin-producing types with no apparent family history [17].

AIP mutations confer important aggressive and treatment-resistant characteristics in acromegaly. Compared with non-mutated acromegaly patients, those with AIP mutations present at a younger age at onset (peak age of onset during the 2nd and 3rd decades of life, with 65% of patients developing symptoms aged ≤18 years and 87% by theage of 30 years) [17], larger tumors, more susceptible to apoplexy [18], and more frequently consisting of sparsely granulated adenomas [19], a subtype which has been previously suggested to respond less well to first-generation SRLs (octreotide and lanreotide) [20]. A greater need for reoperation/s after initial surgery and of multiple therapies, including radiotherapy [17], has also been described. Conversely, postoperative use of adjuvant PegV has been shown to be effective in inducing biochemical remission by normalizing serum IGF-I levels children with sporadic GH-secreting pituitary macroadenomas due to *AIP* mutations [21].

The aggressive nature of pituitary adenomas in those with *AIP* mutations raises a number of challenges for clinical management. As tumors are often large and invasive at diagnosis, primary neurosurgical cure is, unfortunately, the exception, as is with our patient. Furthermore, unlike in acromegaly in general where it is usually helpful, surgical debulking in *AIP*-mutated acromegaly cases is not guaranteed to increase control with postoperative SRLs [22, 23]. Use of PegV in combination with first-generation SRLs has proven effective in young *AIP*-mutated patients [21, 24]. For our patient, if she had been found to be *AIP* mutation positive soon after her first transsphenoidal surgery, proceeding with radiation therapy followed by PegV therapy would have been reasonable. As a high percentage of young-onset GH-secreting adenomas show mutations in the *AIP* gene [22], earlier referral to genetic counselling would have also benefitted this patient as she could have been offered screening for *AIP* mutations sooner. Some investigators have recommended that *AIP* mutation screening be routinely conducted in patients diagnosed with a GH- or prolactin-secreting macroadenomas before the age of 30 years [25]. The patient's parents were *AIP*-negative and had a normal MRI, so we have no plans to follow up her parents in the future. As for the patient, we are following her in clinic every 6 to 9 months and performing surveillance MRIs at 12- to 18-month intervals.

Question 2

Would treating this patient with pasireotide have been more effective than lanreotide in this patient?

The underlying explanation for the relative resistance to first-generation SRLs may occur via Gai proteins or ZAC1, which themselves are important mediators of SST2 actions [26, 27]. Given the relatively poor results achieved with first-generation SRLs in patients with *AIP* mutations, the role of pasireotide has been considered [21, 28]. Because of the broader binding SSTR profile, pasireotide LAR has been suggested to have greater clinical efficacy in acromegaly than first-generation SRLs [29, 30].

Where surgery has failed to control the GH hypersecretion, there is some evidence that pasireotide may be more effective than the first-generation SRLs in reducing the IGF-I burden in *AIP* mutation positive patients, especially tumors that express SSTR5 [28]. Pasireotide monotherapy has been recommended by Coopmans et al. [31] as a second-line therapy for young patients who show tumor growth during first-generation SRL therapy and combination therapy of pasireotide and PegV as a third-line treatment option in patients with tumor growth or symptoms of active acromegaly during first-generation SRL and PegV combination therapy. In some cases, more aggressive treatment regimens may even be necessary. For example, in the youngest known case of 4 years of age, surgery followed by first-generation SRL, temozolomide, bevacizumab, radiotherapy, PegV, Gamma Knife therapy, and SRL combined with increasing dose of PegV was required to induce biochemical remission and stabilization of further tumor growth [32].

Question 3

Why was PegV effective in normalizing this patient's serum IGF-I levels?

Pegvisomant is a direct GH receptor antagonist that antagonizes endogenous GH binding at its receptor and inhibits IGF-I synthesis [33]. However, because GH levels increase due to the negative feedback from the antagonistic effects of PegV on GH receptors, measuring IGF-I, and not GH levels, best monitors treatment efficacy [33]. Pegvisomant has been shown to be effective in adult trials of acromegaly with control rates exceeding 60% after 5 years use [34, 35], but data in pediatric patients are limited [21, 36]. Combined PegV with SRLs and DAs in pituitary gigantism has reported control in 53.5% cases [37], but there remains a theoretical concern of its effects in causing tumor regrowth, although the data in adults to date remains reassuring [38–40].

Question 4

How should acromegaly headaches be managed?

In acromegaly, headache is a prominent and disabling symptom frequently reported, regardless if the tumor is a macroadenoma or a microadenoma [41]. The pathophysiology remains uncertain but likely multifactorial and may be related to dural stretch, changes in skull structure, invasion of the cavernous sinus, functional disturbance within the hypothalamo-pituitary axis, or secondary to concurrent sleep apnea. Rarely, increased ventricular pressure due to large adenomas as well as pituitary apoplexy may be involved, but patients tend to present with acute rather than chronic headaches [42, 43].

Early studies have shown that transsphenoidal surgery improves headaches in 75–100% of patients [44, 45] that was not correlated with biochemical remission of acromegaly, whereas data are limited on the effects of radiosurgery on headaches. SRLs have been reported to be effective in the treatment of primary headache [46] due to the distribution of SSTR2 within the central nervous system [47], and the analgesic effect of SRLs, especially sc octreotide, is well recognized [48, 49] that is unrelated to either GH suppression or tumor shrinkage. Subsequent reports have indicated several important features of the effects of octreotide in acromegaly headache: rapidity of onset (and offset) of the effect of the sc formulation [50], greater analgesic potency vs the other clinically available SRL lanreotide SR [51, 52], and persistency during time of the analgesic effect of octreotide also with the LAR formulation in most patients (without the rebound effect seen with the sc formulation) [51]. Our patient developed chronic headaches that persisted after her transsphenoidal surgeries and only found relief with sc octreotide and not lanreotide injections suggesting a direct and more potent (but short lived) analgesic effect of sc octreotide.

If our patient had failed to find relief from her headaches with sc octreotide, pasireotide would be the next alternative that we would have considered for her. Two small studies have reported that after failing octreotide LAR therapy, three young women with acromegaly between the ages of 21 to 33 experienced resolution of her intractable headaches within a month of first receiving pasireotide treatment without achieving biochemical control [53, 54], raising the possibility of a direct analgesic and/or anti-inflammatory effect mediated via SSTRs, in particular SSTR1, SSTR4, and SSTR5 [55, 56]. More studies are needed to further elucidate the effects of pasireotide in alleviation of headaches, particularly in patients with persistently elevated GH levels, despite surgery and other interventions.

Question 5

Is there a possibility for this patient to get pregnant?

This patient developed panhypopituitarism with hypothalamic amenorrhea and secondary hypoestrogenemia, making her chances of getting pregnant very slim. She consulted a reproductive endocrinologist and was recommended for now to remain estrogen and cyclic or continuous progesterone replacement to ensure a healthy endometrial lining free of endometrial hyperplasia. When she is ready to get pregnant, she will be considered for gonadotropin induction of ovulation. Because of her headaches and her family beliefs of being on oral contraceptives for an unmarried female, she was commenced on transdermal estrogen (Vivelle Dot 0.5 mg twice weekly) and cyclic progesterone replacement therapy. Currently she is not on any medications for acromegaly and is on GH replacement therapy, so if she does get pregnant, we will recommend that she discontinue GH as the data for use of GH during pregnancy remains insufficient to recommend its continued use after conception [57], although several studies have demonstrated the safety of GH therapy during pregnancy [58–60]. However, if she was still on any medication/s for acromegaly, then these medication/s should be stopped either before planned conception or immediately after confirming pregnancy [61].

Question 6

Can this patient develop GH deficiency over time, and if so, can she be treated with GH replacement therapy?

In an effort to induce complete biochemical remission in patients with acromegaly, some patients may be overtreated and develop GH deficiency by their different treatment modalities, typically in patients having undergone multiple surgeries and radiotherapy [62]. In some studies, the prevalence of postsurgical GH deficiency was less than 10% [63, 64], whereas others reported greater frequencies exceeding 50% [65]. Differences in the reported rates of severe GHD may be attributable to differences in selection criteria for dynamic testing, tumor size, methods used to evaluate GH secretory function, interval after surgical procedure, metabolic background, and the extent of surgical manipulation of the pituitary adenoma. Growth hormone status evolves with time after cranial radiotherapy and depends on dose, the likelihood of GH deficiency being greater than 50% if the biological effective dose is greater than 40 Gy [66]. In our patient, her age, longer interval after radiotherapy, and higher radiation dose were all risk factors of developing GH deficiency after irradiation. The persistently low IGF-I after PegV was discontinued in our patient with underlying panhypopituitarism strongly indicated the diagnosis of GH deficiency without the need to undergo any GH stimulation tests [57].

Patients with acromegaly have an excess burden of comorbidities (e.g., cardiomyopathy, hypertension, diabetes mellitus, sleep apnea, and osteoarthropathy) which leads to the impairment of quality of life and premature mortality [3, 4, 6, 67]. Adult GH deficiency is also associated with high cardiometabolic risk owing to alterations in body composition, lipid profile, fibrinolytic activity, endothelial function, impaired quality of life, osteoporosis, and increased mortality [68–71]. Therefore, transition from active acromegaly to GHD may affect several target organs, such as the cardiovascular system and the skeleton, with consequent worsening of some clinical complications already caused by chronic GH excess. Hypertension and insulin resistance may be persistent in some patients with acromegaly even after adequate biochemical control of GH hypersecretion [72, 73]. In this specific clinical context, it is expected that the development of GH deficiency, with consequent negative effects on body composition and endothelial function, worsens hypertension and insulin resistance. Growth hormone excess and deficiency may have opposite effects on bone health, leading both to skeletal fragility and increased risk of vertebral fractures [74, 75], whereas increased body fat and visceral adipose tissue in acromegaly patients with GH deficiency may result in persistent glucose intolerance and dyslipidemia [65].

Studies of acromegaly patients with GH deficiency of short- or long-term GH therapy have generated inconsistent results. In a sub-analysis of the KIMS database, 6-month GH therapy determined no improvement in quality of life, BMI, waist circumference, and blood pressure [76]. In a subsequent 6-month prospective study on 15 patients randomized to GH compared with 15 patients randomized to placebo, reductions in body fat mass, visceral and sc abdominal adipose tissue, an increase in fat-free mass, and an improvement in quality of life were observed [77]. Similar favorable effects of GH therapy on quality of life were found in a group of women with GHD with prior acromegaly [78]. Conversely, a 1-year open-label prospective study found that replacement with GH therapy neither echocardiographic parameters nor any of the cardiovascular risk factors and quality of life parameters changed significantly during GH treatment but did show changes in bone turnover markers without changes in lumbar spine bone mineral density (BMD) [79]. In a another study of KIMS data on 115 acromegaly patients with GH deficiency patients treated for up to 5 years with GH, a significant reduction of total and LDL cholesterol levels, as well as a significant improvement of HDL cholesterol levels and quality of life, was reported [80]. In this analysis, the change in lipids was not associated with changes in BMI or body adiposity, supporting a beneficial role of GH therapy on lipoprotein kinetics. Collectively, current data seem to suggest that long-term GH treatment might be needed to achieve improvements in body composition, lipid profile, and quality of life in acromegaly patients with GH deficiency.

Side effects of GH therapy are infrequent, mild, and comparable between the GH-treated and placebo groups or other reference groups (76–78). Nonetheless, safety issues have been raised in prospective and long-term retrospective intervention studies on GH therapy concerning cardio- and cerebrovascular safety and mortality [76, 80]. On the basis of these data, we adopted a conservative approach in considering GH therapy for our patient mainly to capitalize on the positive effects of GH therapy on BMD and reduction of future cardiovascular risk factors. Because the neoplastic risk is intrinsically increased in acromegaly, we plan to closely assess the neoplastic risk of our patient in the future, e.g., breast and colon cancer.

Question 7
Given her young age, how should her worsening BMD be managed?

Most patients with acromegaly show normal or even increased BMD at various skeletal sites, and osteopenia and osteoporosis are not common features [81–84]. However, when concurrent hypogonadism is present [81, 85, 86], BMD was low at the lumbar spine and, to a lesser extent at the femoral neck [87], consistent with the concept that loss of sex steroids increases bone turnover at the trabecular level, which is predominant in the spine. Moreover, the differences between lumbar spine and femoral neck BMD may be also influenced by the activity of acromegaly, reflecting the different effects of GH excess on trabecular and cortical bone [87]. Vertebral fractures are slightly more frequent in males as compared with females and more common in hypogonadal compared with eugonadal patients [84, 88–90]. These fractures occur more frequently at the thoracic spine and are commonly anterior wedge fractures [90]. Because there is consistent evidence that acromegaly causes deterioration of bone microstructure leading to high risk of vertebral fractures, development of panhypopituitarism with secondary hypogonadism, and worsening BMD in our patient, we assessed her vertebral morphometry with thoracic and lumbar spine X-rays and bone turnover markers PINP and CTX. We found that PINP and CTX were normal and that there was no evidence of vertebral fractures on the X-rays. Thus, we started her on calcium supplements 1200 mg a day and vitamin D 2000 IU a day and advised her to remain on estradiol patch 0.075 mg twice a week. She also agreed to consider GH replacement therapy, and we started her on low dose of GH 0.2 mg a day and plan to repeat her bone densitometry scan after 18 months of GH therapy. Conversely, had she demonstrated evidence of vertebral fractures and increased bone turnover markers, we would have then considered oral or intravenous bisphosphonate therapy despite data of its use in premenopausal women being scarce. The duration of bisphosphonate therapy will depend on the response of BMD, and we would plan to treat her with bisphosphonate therapy for 2–3 years before considering discontinuation, with the notion that combined bisphosphonates with GH therapy might synergistically improve and maintain her BMD for several years to come.

Conclusions

Due to the aggressive nature of the disease, young acromegaly patients often require careful and thoughtful diagnostic work-up that includes genetic testing and multimodal treatment involving a multidisciplinary team. For our patient, although we were able to control tumor growth after her third transsphenoidal surgery followed by radiotherapy, the biochemical effects of excess GH secretion was only effectively controlled by PegV. Coupled with recent advances in the genetic underpinnings of the disease, the standardization and multidisciplinary approach to clinical care of young acromegaly patients provide an opportunity toward personalized management and improved outcomes. While centralization and expert-based care for patients with rare disease, such as acromegaly, are an essential requirement toward progress, the scarcity of expert programs and long travel distances in many cases preclude patients from seeking care at centers of excellence with expertise in management of patients with complex pituitary disorders. Fortunately, our patient and her mother were proactive in seeking follow-up care of her disease after she relocated back to Montana. In the era of the expanding informational technology and development of telemedicine practices, efforts should be placed toward expert-guided local care where local medical providers collaborate with the multidisciplinary expert teams to provide excellent and up-to date care for patients with complex acromegaly presentations.

Author Disclosure Summary Nancy Youssef has nothing to disclose. Kevin C. J. Yuen has served on advisory boards for Ipsen, Chiasma, Crinetics, and Novartis.

Funding/Support Kevin C. J. Yuen has received research grants to Barrow Neurological Institute from Novartis, Ionis and Chiasma.

References

1. Melmed S. Acromegaly pathogenesis and treatment. J Clin Invest. 2009;119(11):3189–202.
2. Arosio M, Reimondo G, Malchiodi E, Berchialla P, Borraccino A, De Marinis L, et al. Predictors of morbidity and mortality in acromegaly: an Italian survey. Eur J Endocrinol. 2012;167(2):189–98.
3. Dekkers OM, Biermasz NR, Pereira AM, Romijn JA, Vandenbroucke JP. Mortality in acromegaly: a metaanalysis. J Clin Endocrinol Metab. 2008;93(1):61–7.
4. Ritvonen E, Loyttyniemi E, Jaatinen P, Ebeling T, Moilanen L, Nuutila P, et al. Mortality in acromegaly: a 20-year follow-up study. Endocr Relat Cancer. 2016;23(6):469–80.
5. Giustina A, Barkhoudarian G, Beckers A, Ben-Shlomo A, Biermasz N, Biller B, et al. Multidisciplinary management of acromegaly: a consensus. Rev Endocr Metab Disord. 2020;21(4):667–78.
6. Giustina A, Barkan A, Beckers A, Biermasz N, Biller BMK, Boguszewski C, et al. A consensus on the diagnosis and treatment of acromegaly comorbidities: an update. J Clin Endocrinol Metab. 2020;105(4):dgz096.
7. Katznelson L, Laws ER Jr, Melmed S, Molitch ME, Murad MH, Utz A, et al. Acromegaly: an endocrine society clinical practice guideline. J Clin Endocrinol Metab. 2014;99(11):3933–51.
8. Melmed S, Bronstein MD, Chanson P, Klibanski A, Casanueva FF, Wass JAH, et al. A consensus statement on acromegaly therapeutic outcomes. Nat Rev Endocrinol. 2018;14(9):552–61.
9. Fahlbusch R, Honegger J, Buchfelder M. Surgical management of acromegaly. Endocrinol Metab Clin N Am. 1992;21(3):669–92.
10. Ross DA, Wilson CB. Results of transsphenoidal microsurgery for growth hormone-secreting pituitary adenoma in a series of 214 patients. J Neurosurg. 1988;68(6):854–67.
11. Carlsen SM, Svartberg J, Schreiner T, Aanderud S, Johannesen O, Skeie S, et al. Six-month preoperative octreotide treatment in unselected, de novo patients with acromegaly: effect on biochemistry, tumour volume, and postoperative cure. Clin Endocrinol. 2011;74(6):736–43.
12. Schmid HA. Pasireotide (SOM230): development, mechanism of action and potential applications. Mol Cell Endocrinol. 2008;286(1–2):69–74.

13. Food and Drug Administration. 2020. https://www.medscape.com/viewarticle/933087. Accessed 12 Nov 2020.
14. Abu Dabrh A, Asi N, Farah W, Mohammed K, Wang Z, Farah M, et al. Radiotherapy vs. radiosurgery in treating patients with acromegaly: systematic review and meta-analysis. Endocr Pract. 2015:1–33.
15. Hannon MJ, Barkan AL, Drake WM. The role of radiotherapy in acromegaly. Neuroendocrinology. 2016;103(1):42–9.
16. Daly AF, Beckers A. Familial isolated pituitary adenomas (FIPA) and mutations in the aryl hydrocarbon receptor interacting protein (AIP) gene. Endocrinol Metab Clin N Am. 2015;44(1):19–25.
17. Marques P, Caimari F, Hernandez-Ramirez LC, Collier D, Iacovazzo D, Ronaldson A, et al. Significant benefits of AIP testing and clinical screening in familial isolated and young-onset pituitary tumors. J Clin Endocrinol Metab. 2020;105(6):e2247–60.
18. Hernandez-Ramirez LC, Gabrovska P, Denes J, Stals K, Trivellin G, Tilley D, et al. Landscape of familial isolated and young-onset pituitary adenomas: prospective diagnosis in AIP mutation carriers. J Clin Endocrinol Metab. 2015;100(9):E1242–54.
19. Chahal HS, Chapple JP, Frohman LA, Grossman AB, Korbonits M. Clinical, genetic and molecular characterization of patients with familial isolated pituitary adenomas (FIPA). Trends Endocrinol Metab. 2010;21(7):419–27.
20. Bhayana S, Booth GL, Asa SL, Kovacs K, Ezzat S. The implication of somatotroph adenoma phenotype to somatostatin analog responsiveness in acromegaly. J Clin Endocrinol Metab. 2005;90(11):6290–5.
21. Joshi K, Daly AF, Beckers A, Zacharin M. Resistant paediatric somatotropinomas due to AIP mutations: role of pegvisomant. Horm Res Paediatr. 2018;90(3):196–202.
22. Daly AF, Tichomirowa MA, Petrossians P, Heliovaara E, Jaffrain-Rea ML, Barlier A, et al. Clinical characteristics and therapeutic responses in patients with germ-line AIP mutations and pituitary adenomas: an international collaborative study. J Clin Endocrinol Metab. 2010;95(11):E373–83.
23. Petrossians P, Borges-Martins L, Espinoza C, Daly A, Betea D, Valdes-Socin H, et al. Gross total resection or debulking of pituitary adenomas improves hormonal control of acromegaly by somatostatin analogs. Eur J Endocrinol. 2005;152(1):61–6.
24. Mangupli R, Rostomyan L, Castermans E, Caberg JH, Camperos P, Krivoy J, et al. Combined treatment with octreotide LAR and pegvisomant in patients with pituitary gigantism: clinical evaluation and genetic screening. Pituitary. 2016;19(5):507–14.
25. Korbonits M, Storr H, Kumar AV. Familial pituitary adenomas - who should be tested for AIP mutations? Clin Endocrinol. 2012;77(3):351–6.
26. Chahal HS, Trivellin G, Leontiou CA, Alband N, Fowkes RC, Tahir A, et al. Somatostatin analogs modulate AIP in somatotroph adenomas: the role of the ZAC1 pathway. J Clin Endocrinol Metab. 2012;97(8):E1411–20.
27. Tuominen I, Heliovaara E, Raitila A, Rautiainen MR, Mehine M, Katainen R, et al. AIP inactivation leads to pituitary tumorigenesis through defective Galphai-cAMP signaling. Oncogene. 2015;34(9):1174–84.
28. Daly AF, Rostomyan L, Betea D, Bonneville JF, Villa C, Pellegata NS, et al. AIP-mutated acromegaly resistant to first-generation somatostatin analogs: long-term control with pasireotide LAR in two patients. Endocr Connect. 2019;8(4):367–77.
29. Bronstein MD, Fleseriu M, Neggers S, Colao A, Sheppard M, Gu F, et al. Switching patients with acromegaly from octreotide to pasireotide improves biochemical control: crossover extension to a randomized, double-blind, Phase III study. BMC Endocr Disord. 2016;16:16.
30. Shimon I, Saeger W, Wildemberg LE, Gadelha MR. Somatotropinomas inadequately controlled with octreotide may over-respond to pasireotide: the importance of dose adjustment to achieve long-term biochemical control. Hormones (Athens). 2017;16(1):84–91.
31. Coopmans EC, van Meyel SWF, van der Lely AJ, Neggers S. The position of combined medical treatment in acromegaly. Arch Endocrinol Metab. 2019;63(6):646–52.

32. Dutta P, Reddy KS, Rai A, Madugundu AK, Solanki HS, Bhansali A, et al. Surgery, octreotide, temozolomide, bevacizumab, radiotherapy, and pegvisomant treatment of an *AIP* mutation positive child. J Clin Endocrinol Metab. 2019;104(8):3539–44.
33. Giustina A, Arnaldi G, Bogazzi F, Cannavo S, Colao A, De Marinis L, et al. Pegvisomant in acromegaly: an update. J Endocrinol Investig. 2017;40(6):577–89.
34. Higham CE, Chung TT, Lawrance J, Drake WM, Trainer PJ. Long-term experience of pegvisomant therapy as a treatment for acromegaly. Clin Endocrinol. 2009;71(1):86–91.
35. van der Lely AJ, Hutson RK, Trainer PJ, Besser GM, Barkan AL, Katznelson L, et al. Long-term treatment of acromegaly with pegvisomant, a growth hormone receptor antagonist. Lancet. 2001;358(9295):1754–9.
36. Bergamaschi S, Ronchi CL, Giavoli C, Ferrante E, Verrua E, Ferrari DI, et al. Eight-year follow-up of a child with a GH/prolactin-secreting adenoma: efficacy of pegvisomant therapy. Horm Res Paediatr. 2010;73(1):74–9.
37. Rostomyan L, Daly AF, Petrossians P, Nachev E, Lila AR, Lecoq AL, et al. Clinical and genetic characterization of pituitary gigantism: an international collaborative study in 208 patients. Endocr Relat Cancer. 2015;22(5):745–57.
38. Cuny T, Zeiller C, Bidlingmaier M, Defilles C, Roche C, Blanchard MP, et al. In vitro impact of pegvisomant on growth hormone-secreting pituitary adenoma cells. Endocr Relat Cancer. 2016;23(7):509–19.
39. Freda PU, Gordon MB, Kelepouris N, Jonsson P, Koltowska-Haggstrom M, van der Lely AJ. Long-term treatment with pegvisomant as monotherapy in patients with acromegaly: experience from ACROSTUDY. Endocr Pract. 2015;21(3):264–74.
40. Marazuela M, Paniagua AE, Gahete MD, Lucas T, Alvarez-Escola C, Manzanares R, et al. Somatotroph tumor progression during pegvisomant therapy: a clinical and molecular study. J Clin Endocrinol Metab. 2011;96(2):E251–9.
41. Forsyth PA, Posner JB. Headaches in patients with brain tumors: a study of 111 patients. Neurology. 1993;43(9):1678–83.
42. Dubuisson AS, Beckers A, Stevenaert A. Classical pituitary tumour apoplexy: clinical features, management and outcomes in a series of 24 patients. Clin Neurol Neurosurg. 2007;109(1):63–70.
43. Gondim JA, Tella OI Jr, Schops M. Intrasellar pressure and tumor volume in pituitary tumor: relation study. Arq Neuropsiquiatr. 2006;64(4):971–5.
44. Giustina A, Gola M, Colao A, De Marinis L, Losa M, Sicolo N, et al. The management of the patient with acromegaly and headache: a still open clinical challenge. J Endocrinol Investig. 2008;31(10):919–24.
45. Wolf A, Goncalves S, Salehi F, Bird J, Cooper P, Van Uum S, et al. Quantitative evaluation of headache severity before and after endoscopic transsphenoidal surgery for pituitary adenoma. J Neurosurg. 2016;124(6):1627–33.
46. Kapicioglu S, Gokce E, Kapicioglu Z, Ovali E. Treatment of migraine attacks with a long-acting somatostatin analogue (octreotide, SMS 201-995). Cephalalgia. 1997;17(1):27–30.
47. Giustina A, Veldhuis JD. Pathophysiology of the neuroregulation of growth hormone secretion in experimental animals and the human. Endocr Rev. 1998;19(6):717–97.
48. Sicolo N, Martini C, Ferla S, Roggenkamp J, Vettor R, De Palo C, et al. Analgesic effect of Sandostatin (SMS 201-995) in acromegaly headache. Minerva Endocrinol. 1990;15(1):37–42.
49. Williams G, Ball JA, Lawson RA, Joplin GF, Bloom SR, Maskill MR. Analgesic effect of somatostatin analogue (octreotide) in headache associated with pituitary tumours. Br Med J (Clin Res Ed). 1987;295(6592):247–8.
50. Musolino NR, Marino Junior R, Bronstein MD. Headache in acromegaly: dramatic improvement with the somatostatin analogue SMS 201-995. Clin J Pain. 1990;6(3):243–5.
51. Levy MJ, Bejon P, Barakat M, Goadsby PJ, Meeran K. Acromegaly: a unique human headache model. Headache. 2003;43(7):794–7.
52. Maffei P, Martini C, Sicolo N. Incomplete analgesic effect of lanreotide in acromegaly. Headache. 1997;37(5):299–300.

53. Lovato CM, Kapsner PL. Analgesic effect of long-acting somatostatin receptor agonist pasireotide in a patient with acromegaly and intractable headaches. BMJ Case Rep. 2018.
54. Marina D, Burman P, Klose M, Casar-Borota O, Luque RM, Castano JP, et al. Truncated somatostatin receptor 5 may modulate therapy response to somatostatin analogues--Observations in two patients with acromegaly and severe headache. Growth Hormon IGF Res. 2015;25(5):262–7.
55. Imhof AK, Gluck L, Gajda M, Lupp A, Brauer R, Schaible HG, et al. Differential antiinflammatory and antinociceptive effects of the somatostatin analogs octreotide and pasireotide in a mouse model of immune-mediated arthritis. Arthritis Rheum. 2011;63(8):2352–62.
56. Mulak A, Larauche M, Biraud M, Million M, Rivier J, Tache Y. Selective agonists of somatostatin receptor subtype 1 or 2 injected peripherally induce antihyperalgesic effect in two models of visceral hypersensitivity in mice. Peptides. 2015;63:71–80.
57. Yuen KCJ, Biller BMK, Radovick S, Carmichael JD, Jasim S, Pantalone KM, et al. American Association of Clinical Endocrinologists and American College of endocrinology guidelines for management of growth hormone deficiency in adults and patients transitioning from pediatric to adult care. Endocr Pract. 2019;25(11):1191–232.
58. Sakai S, Wakasugi T, Yagi K, Ohnishi A, Ito N, Takeda Y, et al. Successful pregnancy and delivery in a patient with adult GH deficiency: role of GH replacement therapy. Endocr J. 2011;58(1):65–8.
59. Vila G, Akerblad AC, Mattsson AF, Riedl M, Webb SM, Hana V, et al. Pregnancy outcomes in women with growth hormone deficiency. Fertil Steril. 2015;104(5):1210–7 e1.
60. Yoshizawa M, Ieki Y, Takazakura E, Fukuta K, Hidaka T, Wakasugi T, et al. Successful pregnancies and deliveries in a patient with evolving hypopituitarism due to pituitary stalk transection syndrome: role of growth hormone replacement. Intern Med. 2017;56(5):527–30.
61. Abucham J, Bronstein MD, Dias ML. MANAGEMENT OF ENDOCRINE DISEASE: acromegaly and pregnancy: a contemporary review. Eur J Endocrinol. 2017;177(1):R1–R12.
62. Giustina A, Mazziotti G, Fontanella M. Commentary: postsurgical monitoring of acromegaly. Neurosurgery. 2013;73(4):E746–8.
63. Ku CR, Hong JW, Kim EH, Kim SH, Lee EJ. Clinical predictors of GH deficiency in surgically cured acromegalic patients. Eur J Endocrinol. 2014;171(3):379–87.
64. Yamada S, Fukuhara N, Nishioka H, Takeshita A, Suzuki H, Miyakawa M, et al. GH deficiency in patients after cure of acromegaly by surgery alone. Eur J Endocrinol. 2011;165(6):873–9.
65. Ronchi CL, Giavoli C, Ferrante E, Verrua E, Bergamaschi S, Ferrari DI, et al. Prevalence of GH deficiency in cured acromegalic patients: impact of different previous treatments. Eur J Endocrinol. 2009;161(1):37–42.
66. Losa M, Gioia L, Picozzi P, Franzin A, Valle M, Giovanelli M, et al. The role of stereotactic radiotherapy in patients with growth hormone-secreting pituitary adenoma. J Clin Endocrinol Metab. 2008;93(7):2546–52.
67. Holdaway IM, Rajasoorya RC, Gamble GD. Factors influencing mortality in acromegaly. J Clin Endocrinol Metab. 2004;89(2):667–74.
68. Di Somma C, Pivonello R, Pizza G, De Rosa A, Lombardi G, Colao A, et al. Prevalence of the metabolic syndrome in moderately-severely obese subjects with and without growth hormone deficiency. J Endocrinol Investig. 2010;33(3):171–7.
69. Pappachan JM, Raskauskiene D, Kutty VR, Clayton RN. Excess mortality associated with hypopituitarism in adults: a meta-analysis of observational studies. J Clin Endocrinol Metab. 2015;100(4):1405–11.
70. Stochholm K, Gravholt CH, Laursen T, Laurberg P, Andersen M, Kristensen LO, et al. Mortality and GH deficiency: a nationwide study. Eur J Endocrinol. 2007;157(1):9–18.
71. Stochholm K, Laursen T, Green A, Laurberg P, Andersen M, Kristensen LO, et al. Morbidity and GH deficiency: a nationwide study. Eur J Endocrinol. 2008;158(4):447–57.
72. Maison P, Tropeano AI, Macquin-Mavier I, Giustina A, Chanson P. Impact of somatostatin analogs on the heart in acromegaly: a metaanalysis. J Clin Endocrinol Metab. 2007;92(5):1743–7.

73. Mazziotti G, Floriani I, Bonadonna S, Torri V, Chanson P, Giustina A. Effects of somatostatin analogs on glucose homeostasis: a metaanalysis of acromegaly studies. J Clin Endocrinol Metab. 2009;94(5):1500–8.
74. Giustina A, Barkan A, Chanson P, Grossman A, Hoffman A, Ghigo E, et al. Guidelines for the treatment of growth hormone excess and growth hormone deficiency in adults. J Endocrinol Investig. 2008;31(9):820–38.
75. Giustina A, Mazziotti G, Canalis E. Growth hormone, insulin-like growth factors, and the skeleton. Endocr Rev. 2008;29(5):535–59.
76. Feldt-Rasmussen U, Abs R, Bengtsson BA, Bennmarker H, Bramnert M, Hernberg-Stahl E, et al. Growth hormone deficiency and replacement in hypopituitary patients previously treated for acromegaly or Cushing's disease. Eur J Endocrinol. 2002;146(1):67–74.
77. Miller KK, Wexler T, Fazeli P, Gunnell L, Graham GJ, Beauregard C, et al. Growth hormone deficiency after treatment of acromegaly: a randomized, placebo-controlled study of growth hormone replacement. J Clin Endocrinol Metab. 2010;95(2):567–77.
78. Valassi E, Brick DJ, Johnson JC, Biller BM, Klibanski A, Miller KK. Effect of growth hormone replacement therapy on the quality of life in women with growth hormone deficiency who have a history of acromegaly versus other disorders. Endocr Pract. 2012;18(2):209–18.
79. van der Klaauw AA, Bax JJ, Roelfsema F, Stokkel MP, Bleeker GB, Biermasz NR, et al. Limited effects of growth hormone replacement in patients with GH deficiency during long-term cure of acromegaly. Pituitary. 2009;12(4):339–46.
80. Tritos NA, Johannsson G, Korbonits M, Miller KK, Feldt-Rasmussen U, Yuen KC, et al. Effects of long-term growth hormone replacement in adults with growth hormone deficiency following cure of acromegaly: a KIMS analysis. J Clin Endocrinol Metab. 2014;99(6):2018–29.
81. Bolanowski M, Daroszewski J, Medras M, Zadrozna-Sliwka B. Bone mineral density and turnover in patients with acromegaly in relation to sex, disease activity, and gonadal function. J Bone Miner Metab. 2006;24(1):72–8.
82. Kaji H, Sugimoto T, Nakaoka D, Okimura Y, Kaji H, Abe H, et al. Bone metabolism and body composition in Japanese patients with active acromegaly. Clin Endocrinol. 2001;55(2):175–81.
83. Mazziotti G, Biagioli E, Maffezzoni F, Spinello M, Serra V, Maroldi R, et al. Bone turnover, bone mineral density, and fracture risk in acromegaly: a meta-analysis. J Clin Endocrinol Metab. 2015;100(2):384–94.
84. Mazziotti G, Bianchi A, Bonadonna S, Cimino V, Patelli I, Fusco A, et al. Prevalence of vertebral fractures in men with acromegaly. J Clin Endocrinol Metab. 2008;93(12):4649–55.
85. Lesse GP, Fraser WD, Farquharson R, Hipkin L, Vora JP. Gonadal status is an important determinant of bone density in acromegaly. Clin Endocrinol. 1998;48(1):59–65.
86. Zgliczynski W, Kochman M, Misiorowski W, Zdunowski P. In acromegaly, increased bone mineral density (BMD) is determined by GH-excess, gonadal function and gender. Neuro Endocrinol Lett. 2007;28(5):621–8.
87. Claessen KM, Mazziotti G, Biermasz NR, Giustina A. Bone and joint disorders in acromegaly. Neuroendocrinology. 2016;103(1):86–95.
88. Chiloiro S, Mormando M, Bianchi A, Giampietro A, Milardi D, Bima C, et al. Prevalence of morphometric vertebral fractures in "difficult" patients with acromegaly with different biochemical outcomes after multimodal treatment. Endocrine. 2018;59(2):449–53.
89. Madeira M, Neto LV, Torres CH, de Mendonca LM, Gadelha MR, de Farias ML. Vertebral fracture assessment in acromegaly. J Clin Densitom. 2013;16(2):238–43.
90. Wassenaar MJ, Biermasz NR, Hamdy NA, Zillikens MC, van Meurs JB, Rivadeneira F, et al. High prevalence of vertebral fractures despite normal bone mineral density in patients with long-term controlled acromegaly. Eur J Endocrinol. 2011;164(4):475–83.

Chapter 16
Somatostatin Analogues in the Management of Patients with Acromegaly

Lewis S. Blevins Jr.

Somatostatin receptors, types SSTR2 and SSTR5, are expressed in varying degrees on the cell surface membranes of many patients with pituitary adenomas derived from GH-producing cells [1, 2]. Activation of these receptors can lead to inhibition of GH production and release as well as direct and indirect effects that diminish cell proliferation [3]. As a result, somatostatin analogues can be used in the management of some patients with acromegaly.

Octreotide acetate was approved for use in patients with acromegaly in 1988. It is a short-acting analog of somatostatin that must be administered subcutaneously every 6–8 h or even continuously by infusion pump. Typical doses range from 50 mcg every 8 h to 300 mg every 8 h. Approximately 50–60% of patients can be expected to normalize IGF-1 levels. Response rates are greater in those who experience a decline in GH levels in response to a single dose of octreotide and in those with pituitary tumors and positive somatostatin receptor scintigraphy. Due to the advent of several long-acting somatostatin analogues, subcutaneous octreotide is now used mostly to treat headaches in patients with acromegaly and to control acromegaly during pregnancy. The effective dose to treat headaches is 50–100 mcg administered subcutaneously once or twice daily [4].

Three separate long-acting somatostatin analogues have been approved for use in acromegaly by the US FDA [5–7]. These include octreotide LAR, lanreotide depot, and pasireotide LAR. Each is formulated differently to enable a continuous slow release of the analogue from a depot injection. Different injection techniques are required for each. Patients may choose to learn to administer their injections or to receive them from a healthcare professional either in the providers office or at some other location. Most injections are administered every 4 weeks. Lanreotide injections may, however, be administered every 6 to 8 weeks in some patients. Efficacy rates are highly variable from study to study and, in some cases, lead to questions

L. S. Blevins Jr. (✉)
Department of Neurological Surgery, University of California, San Francisco, CA, USA
e-mail: lewis.blevins@ucsf.edu

L. S. Blevins Jr., M. K. Aghi (eds.), *Acromegaly*, Contemporary Endocrinology,
https://doi.org/10.1007/978-3-031-16258-9_16

about bias, preselection, and study design. In my experience, with an intent to treat to optimize therapy, this class of drugs will normalize IGF-1 levels in about 50% of treated patients. Symptomatic improvement often follows reductions in IGF-1. Tumor regression is seen, on average, in a similar number of patients ranging from 30 to 70% across studies [5, 8]. Side-effect profiles are similar and include maldigestion and malabsorption with their attendant symptoms, a spectrum of gall bladder dysfunction, including cholelithiasis, glucose intolerance, diabetes mellitus, bradycardia, and hypothyroidism [5].

I have had considerable experience with this class of drugs. I will share a few caveats and observations that apply to the use of the long-acting injectable preparations.

- Treatment with somatostatin analogues prior to surgery may reduce tumor size. It is not clear, however, whether such reductions improve surgical outcomes.
- Treatment with somatostatin analogues prior to surgery may be reasonable to improve cardiac performance and sleep apnea as well as respiratory compromise thereby decreasing perioperative risks of adverse outcomes because of anesthesia and surgery.
- Pasireotide is more likely to cause diabetes mellitus and glucose intolerance than are other somatostatin analogues.
- Subcutaneous octreotide is useful to manage headaches even in patients who have normalized GH and IGF-1 levels on therapy with other somatostatin analogues.
- Patients are best started on the intermediate doses of these medications. IGF-1 should be checked 2 weeks after the third injection of a dose to assess efficacy.
- For patients with low IGF-1 levels during dose titration, the dose should be lowered to the next lower level.
- For patients with high IGF-1 levels during dose titration, the dose should be raised to the next dose level.
- The dose interval in patients who demonstrate good control on Lanreotide can be extended to 6–8 weeks. Efficacy should be reassessed after three subsequent doses.
- Somatostatin analogues should be withheld for a month before and a few months after planned radiotherapy to the offending tumor. This approach will likely improve the efficacy of radiotherapy.
- In patients who have received radiotherapy, the first sign that they may be responding to radiotherapy and need either a lowering or discontinuance of their dose of somatostatin analogue is a fall of the IGF-1 level within the normal range. In this setting, I discontinue therapy and follow the IGF-1. When retreatment is required, I often start with a dose lower than that used when the IGF-1 level had first declined prompting discontinuance.
- I discontinue treatment in patients who have no biochemical or demonstrable tumor response to therapy.
- I tend to continue treatment in those partial responders who have at least a 40–50% lowering of their IGF-1 levels. A second drug is added to the regimen depending on several different variables.

- I've seen patients affected by one or more of every conceivable side effect of this class of medications. Only two of about ten patients who developed cholelithiasis underwent cholecystectomy due to symptomatic disease. One patient developed hypoglycemia due to presumed inhibition of glucagon secretion. Gastrointestinal side effects often improve over time.
- Patients often fatigue due to the required monthly injections. Though biochemical control may be lost with lapses in injections, it is best to accept that patients simply need drug-free holidays. I've seen too many reasonably compliant patients discharged from practices because they took a break from treatment. Work with patients to find compromises that are acceptable.

An oral form of octreotide was recently approved by the US FDA [9]. The drug is taken twice daily. Slight dietary modifications are required. Patients are candidates for treatment if they experienced normalization of IGF-1 levels in response to treatment with one of the injectable somatostatin analogues. A majority of patients maintain normal IGF-1 levels on treatment. Most patients prefer oral therapy to injectable treatments. In my practice, we inform patients of this suitable alternative when they meet the criteria for treatment.

References

1. Rass L, Rahvar A-H, Matschke J, Saeger W, Renne T, Aberle J, Flitsch J, Rotermund R. Differences in somatostatin receptor subtype expression in patient with acromegaly: new directions for targeted therapy? Hormones. 2022;21:79–89.
2. Kiseljak-Vassiliades K, Xu M, Mills T, Smith EE, Silveira LJ, Lillehei KO, Kerr JM, Kleinschmidt-DeMasters BK, Wierman ME. Differential somatostatin receptor (SSTR) 1-5 expression and downstream effectors in histologic subtypes of growth hormone pituitary tumors. Mol Cell Endocrinol. 2015;417:73–83.
3. Colao AM, Auriemma RS, Pivonello R. The effects of somatostatin analogue therapy on pituitary tumor volume in acromegaly. Pituitary. 2016;19:210–21.
4. Levy M, Bejon P, Barakat M, Goadsby PJ, Meeran K. Acromegaly: a unique human headache model. Headache. 2003;43:794–7.
5. Freda PU. Somatostatin analogues in acromegaly. J Clin Endocrinol Metab. 2002;87:3013–8.
6. Sagvand BT, Khairi S, Haghshenas A, Swearingen B, Tritos NA, Miller KK, Klibanski A, Nachtigall LB. Monotherapy with lanreotide depot for acromegaly: long-term clinical experience in a pituitary center. Pituitary. 2016;19:437–47.
7. Sheppard M, Bronstein MD, Freda P, Serri O, De Marinis L, Naves L, Rozhinskaya L, Resendiz KH, Ruffin M, Chen YM, Colao AM. Pasireotide LAR maintains inhibition of GH and IGF-1 in patients with acromegaly for up to 25 months: results from the blinded extension phase of a randomized, double-blind, multicenter phase III study. Pituitary. 2015;18:385–94.
8. Colao AM, Pivonello R, Auriemma RS, Briganti F, Galdiero M, Tortora F, Caranci F, Cirillo S, Lombardi G. Predictors of tumor shrinkage after primary therapy with somatostatin analogs in acromegaly: a prospective study in 99 patients. J Clin Endocrinol Metab. 2006;91:2112–8.
9. Flesieru M, Dreval A, Bondar I, Vagapova G, Macut D, Pokramovich YG, Molitch ME, Leonova N, Raverot G, Grineva E, Poteshkin YE, Gilgun-Sherki Y, Ludlam WH, Patou G, Haviv A, Gordon MB, Biermasz NR, Melmed S, Strasburger CJ. Maintenance of response to oral octreotide compared with injectable somatostatin receptor ligands in patients with acromegaly: a phase 3, multicenter, randomized controlled trial. Lancet Diabetes Endocrinol. 2022;10:102–11.

Chapter 17
Use of Dopamine Agonists for Acromegaly

Christine E. Chiu and John D. Carmichael

History of Acromegaly Treatment and Use of Dopamine Agonists

Historically, acromegaly was initially treated by pituitary surgery and radiotherapy. The first successful temporal and frontal transcranial surgeries for acromegaly were reported between 1904 and 1906 followed by the reported use of radiotherapy for acromegaly in 1909 [1, 2]. Later around the 1970s, the pathophysiology of acromegaly was better understood, and targeted medical treatments were developed for acromegaly. In the 1970s, bromocriptine was first used to control acromegaly, though future studies have led bromocriptine to fall out of favor due to poor efficacy [3]. Historically, bromocriptine utilized as adjuvant medical therapy in acromegaly has been shown to normalize IGF-1 in only about 10% of patients [4]. Cabergoline later replaced bromocriptine as the dopamine agonist of choice due to improved efficacy and dosing advantages [5]. Of note, while bromocriptine does have FDA approval for an indication of acromegaly, cabergoline does not, though it has been widely studied and accepted for off-label use in acromegaly [6]. Following dopamine agonists, in 1978 somatostatin analogues as therapy for acromegaly were introduced and by 1988 octreotide was registered by the FDA for treatment of acromegaly [7, 8]. Later, GH receptor antagonists were introduced in the early 1990s when pegvisomant proved to be effective medical therapy for acromegaly [9].

C. E. Chiu
Department of Medicine, University of Southern California, LAC+USC Medical Center, Los Angeles, CA, USA
e-mail: Christine.Chiu@med.usc.edu

J. D. Carmichael (✉)
Division of Endocrinology, Diabetes, and Metabolism, Keck School of Medicine of USC, Los Angeles, CA, USA
e-mail: John.Carmichael@med.usc.edu

L. S. Blevins Jr., M. K. Aghi (eds.), *Acromegaly*, Contemporary Endocrinology,
https://doi.org/10.1007/978-3-031-16258-9_17

Mechanism of Action of Dopamine Agonists in Acromegaly

Bromocriptine is an ergot alkaloid derivative dopamine D2 agonist that also is a partial antagonist for D1 dopamine receptors [6]. Similarly, cabergoline is also an ergot derivative but is more selective for the D2 receptor and has a longer duration of action than bromocriptine [10]. Though dopamine and other catecholamines stimulate GH secretion, it has been shown that dopamine agonists paradoxically suppress GH hypersecretion in acromegaly [11–14]. GH-secreting adenomas contain dopamine binding sites, with the D2 receptor as the predominant dopamine receptor subtype in somatotropinomas [15]. Bromocriptine and cabergoline work by binding to these D2 receptors and other dopamine receptor subtypes and thereby suppressing GH hypersecretion. Additionally, it has been shown that D2 receptors and type 5 somatostatin receptors (SSTR5) heterodimerize, leading to a synergistic effect of utilization of both somatostatin receptor ligands and dopamine agonists [16]. Additional in vitro studies have demonstrated that dopamine acting on D2 receptors has anti-proliferation and cell death effects on pituitary tumor cells through oxidative stress pathways [17].

Acromegaly Treatment Algorithm

Primary therapy for acromegaly is transsphenoidal surgery in most patients, with particular emphasis on surgeon experience and a multidisciplinary team to optimize outcomes [18–20]. Occasionally if patients are poor surgical candidates or if the tumor is likely unresectable (i.e., invading the cavernous sinus), surgical management is forgone and primary medical therapy chosen [21–23]. Typically, 12 weeks following surgical resection, an IGF-1 level and GH should be checked to monitor for surgical remission [21, 24, 25]. This timeframe is set to prevent inaccurate values in the immediate postoperative period that may falsely elevate GH in the setting of surgical stress on normal somatotroph function and falsely elevated IGF-1 due to the long half-life of IGF-binding proteins [24–26]. A normal IGF-1 value and low GH signify surgical remission; however, if the GH is detectable, measurement of the GH nadir after a glucose load may be done for confirmation, with a GH nadir <0.4 μg/L as a marker of postsurgical remission now given ultrasensitive GH assays [27, 28]. In most cases, assessment of surgical success can be made with IGF-I alone, with OGTT used for confirmation with borderline or abnormal IGF-I results. Additionally, postoperative MRI of the pituitary should also be performed at 12 weeks postoperatively as a new baseline image [21, 29]. If persistent disease is noted, patients should undergo adjuvant medical therapy. Different medical therapies are employed based on the degree of residual disease, both in terms of biochemical disease activity and visible residual tumor. If patients demonstrate significant persistent disease, a somatostatin receptor ligand or pegvisomant (human GH receptor antagonist) is typically chosen as the initial adjuvant medical therapy. If there is only mild or modest elevation of IGF-1 and mild clinical symptoms, cabergoline may be employed instead. Furthermore, if patients are still uncontrolled despite single-agent adjuvant therapy, combination medical therapy is typically employed [21]. For this review, we will focus our discussion on the use of cabergoline alone or in combination with other therapies.

Dopamine Agonist Dosing in Acromegaly

Dopamine agonist dosing is variable, and typically up-titrated to reach therapeutic goal. Jackson et al. performed a preliminary dose finding study with cabergoline in the treatment of acromegaly [30]. During this study, cabergoline dose was escalated on a monthly basis for 4 months with the goal of reaching biochemical remission as defined as serum GH <5 mU/l. All ten patients showed maximum GH response at a dose of 0.5 mg daily with maximum suppression of GH achieved within the dose range of 1 mg twice weekly to 0.5 mg daily.

Dopamine Agonists as Monotherapy

Integrated data regarding efficacy of dopamine agonists in acromegaly comes from a meta-analysis of 15 studies (237 total patients included) performed by Sandret et al. [31]. Among the 10 trials (160 patients) including cabergoline monotherapy, normalization of IGF-1 levels was achieved in 34% of patients. Other parameters studied in this meta-analysis demonstrated a mean reduction of IGF-1 by 33% and a mean reduction of GH levels by 47%. Likelihood of IGF-1 normalization was related to the baseline IGF-1 concentration, with lower baseline IGF-1 elevation more likely to result in normalization of IGF-1. This meta-analysis demonstrated that the likelihood of normalizing IGF-1 improved to 50% if the IGF-1 level was less than 150% of the ULN, as compared to only 30% if over 150% of the ULN. Radiotherapy was also shown to be associated with efficacy of cabergoline, though notably could be related to lower baseline IGF-1 levels at time of initiation of medical therapy. Additionally, hyperprolactinemia demonstrated a trend toward a relationship with efficacy of cabergoline, though not statistically significant in this meta-analysis. Within this meta-analysis, cabergoline dose ranged from 0.5 mg to 7 mg/week with only a statistical trend toward a relationship between cabergoline dose and decline in IGF-1, though a statistically significant relationship was noted for decrease in GH. The mean cabergoline dose was 2.5 mg/week in patients who achieved normal IGF-1 levels. The mean duration of treatment was 15 months in those who achieved normal IGF-1 levels. Tumor shrinkage was noted with about one third of patients who received cabergoline [31]. Of note, among studies included in this meta-analysis, Abs et al. performed the largest (64 patients) retrospective study investigating the efficacy of cabergoline, which demonstrated decrease in IGF-1 levels in 39% of patients, defined as a decline to less than 300 ng/ml. This study also demonstrated that efficacy of cabergoline was associated with hyperprolactinemia and low pretreatment plasma IGF-1 below 750 ug/L [5]. This finding of association between prolactin co-secretion and favorable treatment outcomes has not been independently validated.

Additional studies performed after the publishing of the meta-analysis by Sandret et al. have produced variable results. For example, a single-center retrospective study of 82 patients in Brazil demonstrated short-term disease control (defined as random GH <1.0 μg/L and normal age-matched IGF-1 level after 3–6 months of treatment) in only 21% of patients who received cabergoline monotherapy with PRL level noted as a predictive factor for treatment response [32]. The UK Acromegaly Register demonstrated normalization of IGF-1 in 36% of patients on cabergoline [33]. Retrospective analysis of data from the Bulgarian Acromegaly Database (between the years of 1980 and 2012) demonstrated disease control in 18.8% of patients treated with bromocriptine and 31.4% treated with cabergoline, which decreased to 16.3% and 18.2%, respectively, when including only patients without prior radiotherapy [34]. From the other end of the spectrum, there have been case reports of remission of acromegaly following long-term cabergoline monotherapy, in which patients maintained normal GH and IGF-1 levels 2.5–5.5 years after discontinuation of cabergoline [35].

Despite the wide variation of results of cabergoline monotherapy across different studies, generally cabergoline therapy is thought to be less effective than other medical therapies, specifically somatostatin analogues, which are generally considered the initial choice by many for medical therapy. A recent review comparing efficacy of medical treatment for acromegaly noted control of acromegaly in about 40% of patients on somatostatin analogue monotherapy and normalization of IGF-1 levels in about 80% of patients on pegvisomant monotherapy [36].

Dopamine Agonists as Combination Therapy

Dopamine Agonists and Somatostatin Analogues

In the meta-analysis conducted by Sandret et al., combination therapy with somatostatin receptor ligands and cabergoline normalized IGF-1 levels in 52% of patients whose levels were unable to be normalized with a somatostatin receptor ligand alone. Addition of cabergoline led to a further 22% decrease in IGF-1 level as compared to SRL alone. This decrease in IGF-1 also showed a statistically significant correlation with baseline IGF-1 concentration, with a lower IGF-1 level associated with increased cabergoline efficacy. This is the same relationship demonstrated with cabergoline monotherapy [31]. Several studies following publishing of the meta-analysis by Sandret et al. reported slightly lower rates of normalization of IGF-1 between 30% and 40% for patients on combination cabergoline and somatostatin analogue therapy [32, 37–39].

A retrospective single-center study was performed that demonstrated normalization of IGF-1 levels in 58% (75 of 129) of patients when cabergoline was added to SRL treatment. Normalization of IGF-1 levels demonstrated an association with female sex, lack of fibrous bodies in the adenomas, smaller pre- and post-cabergoline tumor size, lower levels of IGF-1 in pre-and postoperative period, and lower levels of IGF-1 in pre-and post-cabergoline treatment. In this study, IGF-1 less than 144% of the ULN and GH level less than 2.35 ng/ml predicted treatment response [40].

Dopamine Agonists and Growth Hormone Receptor Antagonists

Few studies have been performed involving pegvisomant and cabergoline combination therapy. One prospective multicenter trial of 24 patients demonstrated improvement of normalization of IGF-1 from 11% to 68% of patients when pegvisomant was added to cabergoline after 18 weeks of cabergoline monotherapy. Interestingly, after cabergoline was withdrawn, only 26% of patients maintained normalized IGF-1 levels on pegvisomant monotherapy suggesting combination therapy of cabergoline and pegvisomant as more effective than cabergoline or pegvisomant monotherapy alone. Adding cabergoline to pegvisomant has the advantage of potentially lowering pegvisomant doses and thus reducing cost of therapy [41].

Additional studies done include an observational, retrospective, cross-sectional study of 14 patients uncontrolled on a somatostatin analogue alone who were switched to pegvisomant and still had persistent IGF-1 elevation, and then underwent addition of cabergoline, which subsequently normalized IGF-1 in 28% of patients and decreased IGF-1 in 64% of patients. This study demonstrated that lower baseline IGF-1 (less than 160% ULN), female gender, lower body weight, and higher baseline prolactin levels were associated with better response to pegvisomant and cabergoline combination therapy [42]. Additionally, it should be noted that combination therapy with pegvisomant and a somatostatin analogue has demonstrated IGF-1 normalization in 80.6% of patients in a review performed by Grasso et al., ranging from 55.5% to 100% depending on the study [36].

Side Effects of Dopamine Agonists

Side effects of dopamine agonists are typically few and well-tolerated. Some of the most common side effects are headache, nausea, vomiting, dizziness, hypotension, and fatigue with other less common reported side effects of constipation, nasal congestion, Raynaud's phenomenon, psychosis, and fibrosis (pericarditis, pleuropulmonary fibrosis, retroperitoneal fibrosis). Adverse effects typically occur after the initial dose and at each dose increase and typically tolerance develops to the adverse effects [43]. Overall, cabergoline is well-tolerated, and in one meta-analysis, side effects only led to drug interruption in 5.2% of patients with doses ranging between

0.5 and 2 mg/week [31]. Psychosis or exacerbation of preexisting psychosis and impulse control disorders have been associated with bromocriptine and cabergoline in patients with prolactinomas and typically resolve within 72 h of discontinuation of the medication [44–48].

Dopamine agonists have been associated with increased risk of cardiac valve disease when utilized at very high doses (such as daily doses of pergolide or cabergoline at greater than 3 mg) for Parkinson's disease [49, 50]. There have also been studies done investigating whether cabergoline use in acromegaly is associated with cardiac valve disease, especially given the association of acromegaly itself with cardiac valve disease. In a cross-sectional study of cabergoline-treated patients with acromegaly compared to a matched control population of untreated patients, there was no increased risk of cardiac valve regurgitation or remodeling in patients with acromegaly [43, 51].

Side effects are overall less common with cabergoline than with bromocriptine as bromocriptine has a shorter half-life and is less specific for the D2 receptor. Additionally, cabergoline has the benefit of only requiring once- or twice-weekly dosing as compared to daily bromocriptine dosing [43].

Summary

Dopamine agonists remain a choice in the medical treatment of acromegaly, yet their use is often bypassed in favor of other treatment modalities due to a lower efficacy rate in published work. However, meta-analysis suggests a role for use of cabergoline monotherapy in milder disease and as an additional agent in combination with other therapies. We utilize cabergoline monotherapy as an option for those patients with mild elevation of IGF-1 after surgical resection, once it has become clear that the disease is active yet uncontrolled by surgery alone. Additionally, it has been used in combination with SRL therapy and pegvisomant in select patients, some of whom have hyperprolactinemia in addition to GH excess. Rarely, tumor MRI surveillance with cabergoline monotherapy, where slight incremental growth of residual disease has been detected, has prompted a switch to SRL therapy, despite biochemical control. This illustrates the need for comprehensive surveillance with laboratory and radiological data during follow-up observation.

Generally, cabergoline single-agent adjuvant medical therapy has modest efficacy (about 34% of patients have normalization of IGF-1 levels) in acromegaly. Under the circumstances of postoperative mild-moderate biochemical excess, such as IGF-1 below 150% of ULN, cabergoline may be a reasonable first adjuvant medical therapy, with about 50% of patients achieving a normalized IGF-1. When cabergoline is utilized as an adjunct therapy to somatostatin receptor ligands when biochemical normalization is not yet achieved, about 50% of patients have subsequent normalization of IGF-1 with combination therapy [31].

Some criticisms of cabergoline use for acromegaly have included the lack of randomized-controlled clinical trials and scarcity of evidence of outcomes with cabergoline use in acromegaly as compared with the higher quality evidence and better outcomes (including biochemical outcomes and tumor shrinkage) associated with use of somatostatin analogues and pegvisomant. This lack of evidence and inferior outcomes associated with cabergoline use favors somatostatin analogue use instead as primary medical therapy for acromegaly [52].

However, cabergoline has the benefit of oral administration and lower economic cost as compared to somatostatin analogues and pegvisomant. These factors may lead to improved compliance which is especially beneficial for acromegaly which may require lifelong medical treatment. Cabergoline also has few adverse effects and is generally well-tolerated. Therefore, cabergoline may be most useful as an adjunct in the postoperative setting when there are mild or moderate elevations of GH and IGF-1 (i.e., <150% of the ULN) [53].

References

1. Horsley V. Address in surgery: delivered at the seventy-fourth annual meeting of the British Medical Association, on the technique of operations on the central nervous system. BMJ. 1906;2(2382):411–23.
2. Gramegna A. Un cas d'acromégalie traité par radiothérapie. Neurol Bull. 1909;17:15–7.
3. Besser GM, Wass JA, Thorner MO. Acromegaly--results of long term treatment with bromocriptine. Acta Endocrinol Suppl (Copenh). 1978;216:187–98.
4. Jaffe CA, Barkan AL. Treatment of acromegaly with dopamine agonists. Endocrinol Metab Clin N Am. 1992;21(3):713–35.
5. Abs R, Verhelst J, Maiter D, Van Acker K, Nobels F, Coolens JL, et al. Cabergoline in the treatment of acromegaly: a study in 64 patients. J Clin Endocrinol Metab. 1998;83(2):374–8.
6. Ozery M, Wadhwa R. Bromocriptine. In: StatPearls [Internet]. Treasure Island, FL: StatPearls Publishing; 2022 [cited 2022 Apr 30]. Available from: http://www.ncbi.nlm.nih.gov/books/NBK555948/.
7. Bauer W, Briner U, Doepfner W, Haller R, Huguenin R, Marbach P, et al. SMS 201–995: a very potent and selective octapeptide analogue of somatostatin with prolonged action. Life Sci. 1982;31(11):1133–40.
8. Lamberts SWJ, van der Lely AJ, de Herder WW, Hofland LJ. Octreotide. N Engl J Med. 1996;334(4):246–54.
9. de Herder WW. The history of acromegaly. Neuroendocrinology. 2016;103(1):7–17.
10. Andreotti AC, Pianezzola E, Persiani S, Pacciarini MA, Strolin Benedetti M, Pontiroli AE. Pharmacokinetics, pharmacodynamics, and tolerability of cabergoline, a prolactin-lowering drug, after administration of increasing oral doses (0.5, 1.0, and 1.5 milligrams) in healthy male volunteers. J Clin Endocrinol Metab. 1995;80(3):841–5.
11. Giustina A, Veldhuis JD. Pathophysiology of the neuroregulation of growth hormone secretion in experimental animals and the human. Endocr Rev. 1998;19(6):717–97.
12. Chiodini PG, Liuzzi A, Botalla L, Cremascoli G, Silvestrini F. Inhibitory effect of dopaminergic stimulation on GH release in acromegaly. J Clin Endocrinol Metab. 1974;38(2):200–6.
13. Liuzzi A, Chiodini PG, Botalla L, Cremascoli G, Silvestrini F. Inhibitory effect of L-dopa on GH release in acromegalic patients. J Clin Endocrinol Metab. 1972;35(6):941–3.
14. Mims RB, Stein RB, Bethune JE. The effect of a single dose of L-dopa on pituitary hormones in acromegaly, obesity and in normal subjects. J Clin Endocrinol Metab. 1973;37(1):34–9.
15. Neto LV, de O Machado E, Luque RM, Taboada GF, Marcondes JB, Chimelli LMC, et al. Expression analysis of dopamine receptor subtypes in normal human pituitaries, nonfunc-

tioning pituitary adenomas and somatotropinomas, and the association between dopamine and somatostatin receptors with clinical response to octreotide-LAR in acromegaly. J Clin Endocrinol Metab. 2009;94(6):1931–7.
16. Rocheville M, Lange DC, Kumar U, Patel SC, Patel RC, Patel YC. Receptors for dopamine and somatostatin: formation of hetero-oligomers with enhanced functional activity. Science. 2000;288(5463):154–7.
17. An JJ, Cho SR, Jeong DW, Park KW, Ahn YS, Baik JH. Anti-proliferative effects and cell death mediated by two isoforms of dopamine D2 receptors in pituitary tumor cells. Mol Cell Endocrinol. 2003;206(1–2):49–62.
18. Jane JA, Starke RM, Elzoghby MA, Reames DL, Payne SC, Thorner MO, et al. Endoscopic transsphenoidal surgery for acromegaly: remission using modern criteria, complications, and predictors of outcome. J Clin Endocrinol Metab. 2011;96(9):2732–40.
19. McLaughlin N, Laws ER, Oyesiku NM, Katznelson L, Kelly DF. Pituitary centers of excellence. Neurosurgery. 2012;71(5):916–26.
20. Wass JAH, Turner HE, Adams CBT. The importance of locating a good pituitary surgeon. Pituitary. 1999;2(1):51–4.
21. Katznelson L, Laws ER, Melmed S, Molitch ME, Murad MH, Utz A, et al. Acromegaly: an endocrine society clinical practice guideline. J Clin Endocrinol Metab. 2014;99(11):3933–51.
22. Nomikos P, Buchfelder M, Fahlbusch R. The outcome of surgery in 668 patients with acromegaly using current criteria of biochemical 'cure'. Eur J Endocrinol. 2005;152(3):379–87.
23. Petrossians P, Borges-Martins L, Espinoza C, Daly A, Betea D, Valdes-Socin H, et al. Gross total resection or debulking of pituitary adenomas improves hormonal control of acromegaly by somatostatin analogs. Eur J Endocrinol. 2005;152(1):61–6.
24. Freda PU. Monitoring of acromegaly: what should be performed when GH and IGF-1 levels are discrepant? Clin Endocrinol. 2009;71(2):166–70.
25. Freda PU, Nuruzzaman AT, Reyes CM, Sundeen RE, Post KD. Significance of "abnormal" nadir growth hormone levels after oral glucose in postoperative patients with acromegaly in remission with normal insulin-like growth factor-I levels. J Clin Endocrinol Metab. 2004;89(2):495–500.
26. Krieger MD, Couldwell WT, Weiss MH. Assessment of long-term remission of acromegaly following surgery. J Neurosurg. 2003;98(4):719–24.
27. Kim EH, Oh MC, Lee EJ, Kim SH. Predicting long-term remission by measuring immediate postoperative growth hormone levels and oral glucose tolerance test in acromegaly. Neurosurgery. 2012;70(5):1106–13.
28. Giustina A, Barkhoudarian G, Beckers A, Ben-Shlomo A, Biermasz N, Biller B, et al. Multidisciplinary management of acromegaly: a consensus. Rev Endocr Metab Disord. 2020;21(4):667–78.
29. Dina TS, Feaster SH, Laws ER, Davis DO. MR of the pituitary gland postsurgery: serial MR studies following transsphenoidal resection. AJNR Am J Neuroradiol. 1993;14(3):763–9.
30. Jackson SNJ, Fowler J, Howlett TA. Cabergoline treatment of acromegaly: a preliminary dose finding study. Clin Endocrinol. 1997;46(6):745–9.
31. Sandret L, Maison P, Chanson P. Place of cabergoline in acromegaly: a meta-analysis. J Clin Endocrinol Metab. 2011;96(5):1327–35.
32. Kasuki L, Dalmolin MD, Wildemberg LE, Gadelha MR. Treatment escape reduces the effectiveness of cabergoline during long-term treatment of acromegaly in monotherapy or in association with first-generation somatostatin receptor ligands. Clin Endocrinol. 2018;88(6):889–95.
33. Howlett TA, Willis D, Walker G, Wass JAH, Trainer PJ, UK Acromegaly Register Study Group (UKAR-3). Control of growth hormone and IGF1 in patients with acromegaly in the UK: responses to medical treatment with somatostatin analogues and dopamine agonists. Clin Endocrinol. 2013;79(5):689–99.
34. Vandeva S, Elenkova A, Natchev E, Kirilov G, Tcharaktchiev D, Yaneva M, et al. Treatment outcome results from the Bulgarian acromegaly database: adjuvant dopamine agonist therapy is efficient in less than one fifth of non-irradiated patients. Exp Clin Endocrinol Diabetes. 2015;123(01):66–71.

35. Verhelst JA, Abrams PJ, Abs R. Remission of acromegaly following long-term therapy with cabergoline: report of two cases. Pituitary. 2008;11(1):103–7.
36. Grasso LFS, Auriemma RS, Pivonello R, Colao A. Somatostatin analogs, cabergoline and pegvisomant: comparing the efficacy of medical treatment for acromegaly. Expert Rev Endocrinol Metab. 2017;12(1):73–85.
37. Mattar P, Alves Martins MR, Abucham J. Short- and long-term efficacy of combined cabergoline and octreotide treatment in controlling IGF-I levels in acromegaly. Neuroendocrinology. 2010;92(2):120–7.
38. Vilar L, Azevedo MF, Naves LA, Casulari LA, Albuquerque JL, Montenegro RM, et al. Role of the addition of cabergoline to the management of acromegalic patients resistant to longterm treatment with octreotide LAR. Pituitary. 2011;14(2):148–56.
39. Suda K, Inoshita N, Iguchi G, Fukuoka H, Takahashi M, Nishizawa H, et al. Efficacy of combined octreotide and cabergoline treatment in patients with acromegaly: a retrospective clinical study and review of the literature. Endocr J. 2013;60(4):507–15.
40. Sahin S, Fidan MC, Korkmaz OP, Durcan E, Ozkaya HM, Kadioglu P. Effectiveness of cabergoline treatment in patients with acromegaly uncontrolled with SSAs: experience of a single tertiary center. Exp Clin Endocrinol Diabetes. 2021;129(09):644–50.
41. Higham CE, Atkinson AB, Aylwin S, Bidlingmaier M, Drake WM, Lewis A, et al. Effective combination treatment with cabergoline and low-dose pegvisomant in active acromegaly: a prospective clinical trial. J Clin Endocrinol Metab. 2012;97(4):1187–93.
42. Bernabeu I, Alvarez-Escolá C, Paniagua AE, Lucas T, Pavón I, Cabezas-Agrícola JM, et al. Pegvisomant and cabergoline combination therapy in acromegaly. Pituitary. 2013;16(1):101–8.
43. Kuhn E, Chanson P. Cabergoline in acromegaly. Pituitary. 2017;20(1):121–8.
44. Boyd A. Bromocriptine and psychosis: a literature review. Psychiatry Q. 1995;66(1):87–95.
45. Bancos I, Nannenga MR, Bostwick JM, Silber MH, Erickson D, Nippoldt TB. Impulse control disorders in patients with dopamine agonist-treated prolactinomas and nonfunctioning pituitary adenomas: a case-control study. Clin Endocrinol. 2014;80(6):863–8.
46. Noronha S, Stokes V, Karavitaki N, Grossman A. Treating prolactinomas with dopamine agonists: always worth the gamble? Endocrine. 2016;51(2):205–10.
47. Barake M, Evins AE, Stoeckel L, Pachas GN, Nachtigall LB, Miller KK, et al. Investigation of impulsivity in patients on dopamine agonist therapy for hyperprolactinemia: a pilot study. Pituitary. 2014;17(2):150–6.
48. Moore TJ, Glenmullen J, Mattison DR. Reports of pathological gambling, hypersexuality, and compulsive shopping associated with dopamine receptor agonist drugs. JAMA Intern Med. 2014;174(12):1930–3.
49. Schade R, Andersohn F, Suissa S, Haverkamp W, Garbe E. Dopamine agonists and the risk of cardiac-valve regurgitation. N Engl J Med. 2007;356(1):29–38.
50. Zanettini R, Antonini A, Gatto G, Gentile R, Tesei S, Pezzoli G. Valvular heart disease and the use of dopamine agonists for Parkinson's disease. N Engl J Med. 2007;356(1):39–46.
51. Maione L, Garcia C, Bouchachi A, Kallel N, Maison P, Salenave S, et al. No evidence of a detrimental effect of cabergoline therapy on cardiac valves in patients with acromegaly. J Clin Endocrinol Metab. 2012;97(9):E1714–9.
52. Kasuki L, Vieira Neto L, Gadelha MR. Cabergoline treatment in acromegaly: cons. Endocrine. 2014;46(2):220–5.
53. Marazuela M, Ramos-Leví A, Sampedro-Núñez M, Bernabeu I. Cabergoline treatment in acromegaly: pros. Endocrine. 2014;46(2):215–9.

Chapter 18
Pegvisomant: Lessons Learned After 20 Years and Practical Recommendations of Its Use for the Treatment of Acromegaly

Kevin C. J. Yuen

Introduction

Acromegaly is a chronic, debilitating disease caused by growth hormone (GH) hypersecretion, most often due to a GH-secreting pituitary adenoma [1]. If left untreated, acromegaly results in a significant reduction in quality of life (QoL), with local, systemic, and neuropsychological comorbidities contributing to its excess morbidity and mortality [2–5]. Main treatment goals include biochemical normalization, tumor control, prevention of complications, and improvement of clinical signs and symptoms [6–9]. Surgery is the first-line treatment modality for most patients [8, 9]. However, medical is often considered when surgery is contraindicated or failed to induce remission, when disease recurs after apparent surgical remission, or when the patient is unable or unwilling to undergo surgery [8, 9].

In the USA, there are two classes of medical therapies for treatment of acromegaly approved by the US Food and Drug Administration (FDA): (1) somatostatin receptor ligands (SRLs) including first-generation SRLs (octreotide long-acting release [LAR] and lanreotide autogel) and a multireceptor-targeted SRL (pasireotide LAR) [8] and, recently, oral octreotide capsules and (2) a GH receptor antagonist pegvisomant. Although not approved by the FDA for acromegaly, the dopamine receptor agonist cabergoline is also used in patients with mildly elevated insulin-like growth factor (IGF-I) levels [≤2× upper limit of normal (ULN)] [10–13]. The efficacy rates for these medications range from 18 to 70%, with variable adverse event (AE) rates and profiles (Table 18.1). Additionally, combination therapies have been increasingly proposed to achieve therapeutic goals [28]. Despite these options, acromegaly remains challenging to treat and often requires a multidisciplinary [29]

K. C. J. Yuen (✉)
Department of Neuroendocrinology and Neurosurgery, Barrow Pituitary Center, Barrow Neurological Institute, University of Arizona College of Medicine and Creighton School of Medicine, Phoenix, AZ, USA
e-mail: kevin.yuen@dignityhealth.org

L. S. Blevins Jr., M. K. Aghi (eds.), *Acromegaly*, Contemporary Endocrinology,
https://doi.org/10.1007/978-3-031-16258-9_18

Table 18.1 Medical therapies currently available in the USA for the treatment of acromegaly

Drug	Mechanism of action	Dose and route of administration	Biochemical efficacy (%)	Patients with ≥20% tumor volume reduction (%)	Major adverse events
Octreotide long-acting release [14–17]	SRL (greater SSTR2 affinity)	10–40 mg/month, IM	30–50	73–80	Gastrointestinal, injection-site reactions
Lanreotide autogel [15–18]	SRL (greater SSTR2 affinity)	60–120 mg/month, deep SC	40–50	63–79	Gastrointestinal, injection-site reactions
Pasireotide long-acting release [15, 16, 19, 20]	SRL (multireceptor ligand greatest SSTR5 and SSTR2 affinity)	40–60 mg/month, IM	25–54	81	Hyperglycemia, gastrointestinal, injection-site reactions
Oral octreotide capsules [21–23]	SRL (greater SSTR2 affinity)	40–80/day, PO containing transient permeability enhancer formulation	58–65	Unknown	Gastrointestinal
Pegvisomant [24–26]	GHR antagonist	10–30 mg/day, SC	70	No effect in majority	Injection-site reactions, liver transaminitis
Cabergoline[a] [11, 27]	D2R agonist	1–3.5 mg/week, PO	18	~33[b]	Gastrointestinal, nasal congestion, orthostatic hypotension, headaches

D2R dopamine 2 receptor, *FDA* US Food and Drug Administration, *GHR* growth hormone receptor, *IM* intramuscular, *NA* not available, *PO* by mouth, *SC* subcutaneous, *SRL* somatostatin receptor ligand, *SSTR* somatostatin receptor

[a]Not FDA approved

[b]Threshold for percentage reduction in tumor size not noted

and personalized approach [30–33]. Current therapeutic options leave room for improvement as full biochemical and symptomatic control are often not achieved [34] and AEs can limit use, decrease treatment adherence, and can lead to treatment cessation (Table 18.1).

Currently, the most effective treatment for biochemical control is pegvisomant [35–37]. Approved in the USA in 2003 [38] and Europe in 2002 [39], general indications for treatment with pegvisomant include inadequate biochemical control after pituitary surgery, radiotherapy, and inadequate control or intolerance to long-acting SRLs [7–9]. In recent years, pegvisomant has mostly been used as an adjuvant in either monotherapy [40–42] or combined with SRLs [24, 28, 43, 44] and cabergoline [45, 46], although its use as first-line therapy after surgery has been proposed [42, 47]. Herein, we review lessons learned from published clinical trial data and experience of pegvisomant use after 20 years and provide recommendations for its optimal use in treating patients with acromegaly.

Data from Clinical Studies of Pegvisomant

Pegvisomant is a recombinant, bioengineered 191 amino acid GH analog, which carries a glycine to lysine mutation (residue 120) as well as 8 additional amino acid substitutions intended to enhance the binding affinity of pegvisomant over that of the native GH molecule, but does not activate the GH receptor [48]. Several polyethylene glycol chains are covalently attached to the pegvisomant backbone, leading to the prolongation of its half-life in comparison to native GH from 15 min to 6 days [48, 49]. Following subcutaneous administration, pegvisomant effectively decreased IGF-I levels in healthy volunteers [50]. In a subsequent proof-of-concept study, IGF-I levels decreased by 31 % in patients with acromegaly with pegvisomant therapy at a dose of 80 mg weekly over 6 weeks [48]. In a pivotal phase III, double-blind, placebo-controlled study, 112 patients with acromegaly were randomly allocated to 1 of 3 daily doses of pegvisomant or placebo [36]. Serum IGF-I level normalization was reported in 54, 81, and 89 % of patients treated with pegvisomant at 10, 15, or 20 mg daily, respectively, for up to 12 weeks, and symptoms (e.g., fatigue, headache, arthralgias, edema, and excess sweating) and signs (ring size) associated with GH excess improved. In an open-label extension study of 160 patients, pegvisomant therapy at a higher dose of 40 mg daily for 18 months normalized IGF-I levels in up to 97 % of patients [51]. Improvement in QoL was further demonstrated in a prospective, double-blind, placebo-controlled, crossover study involving 20 acromegaly patients without significant change in IGF-I levels after adding 40 mg pegvisomant weekly to SRL therapy in patients who had normalized IGF-I levels on SRL monotherapy, suggesting added benefits of pegvisomant on QoL without correlation to IGF-I levels [52].

However, data from a large pharmacoepidemiological surveillance database (ACROSTUDY), a representation of the "real-world" setting, reported that pegvisomant normalized IGF-I levels in only 67.5 % of patients with acromegaly using a mean dose of 17.2 mg daily over 5 years [40]. These observations were consistent with the findings of country-specific data from the same pharmacoepidemiological surveillance database [24–26, 53, 54]. It was postulated that this discrepancy of the data with the higher efficacy in clinical trials might be related to insufficient dose titration as a consequence of "therapeutic inertia" by the treating physician, lack of availability of vials containing sufficiently high pegvisomant doses in the past, decreased patient adherence outside a clinical trial setting, AEs, and costs.

Recent outcome data from ACROSTUDY of the full cohort of 2221 acromegaly patients treated with pegvisomant reported that 75.4% of patients achieved IGF-I normalization at 10 years with increasing number of patients requiring at least

30 mg daily with time and 71.1% of patients with no changes in tumor size on MRI [26]. Importantly there were no new safety signals after long-term use and only 3% demonstrated transient transaminitis. Notably, improvements in all-cause mortality rates and small improvements in QoL and glycemia were observed when IGF-I level was normalized with pegvisomant therapy [26], indicating the overall favorable benefit-to-risk profile and effectiveness of pegvisomant as monotherapy and combination therapy with first-generation SRLs in the real-world setting. Long-term pegvisomant therapy has also been shown to accompany increases in visceral and subcutaneous adipose tissue mass that do not differ from stable skeletal muscle mass and no glycemic worsening [55]. When pegvisomant was combined with pasireotide LAR, this combination therapy only modestly improved glycemia in a small number of patients [56], presumably due to the greater hyperglycemic effects of pasireotide compared to first-generation SRLs in negating the beneficial effects of pegvisomant on glucose metabolism.

In patients with modest elevations of IGF-I levels ($\leq 2 \times$ ULN) but intolerant to SRLs, a trial of a dopamine agonist, usually cabergoline as the initial adjuvant medical therapy followed by combined therapy with low-dose pegvisomant has been suggested, as this combination has the potential to be more cost-effective with no deleterious effect on glucose metabolism. In a prospective clinical trial of 24 acromegaly patients treated for 18 weeks of dose titration to a maximum dose of 0.5 mg once daily, cabergoline monotherapy did not significantly reduce IGF-I levels, but the addition of 10 mg pegvisomant daily for 12 weeks significantly reduced IGF-I levels, with 68% of patients achieving IGF-I normalization [46]. These data suggest that combination treatment with cabergoline and low-dose pegvisomant may be more effective at reducing IGF-I levels than either cabergoline or pegvisomant alone.

When to Consider Pegvisomant Therapy in Patients with Acromegaly

Current guidelines recommend using SRLs first after surgery has failed and consider pegvisomant (approved at doses of 10–30 mg daily) if first-generation SRLs has not controlled the disease, if patients develop AEs while on SRLs, or if there is clinically relevant glucose intolerance [9]. The use of pegvisomant as first-line therapy has recently been proposed due to its high efficacy rates [47], and this notion has been substantiated by Qiao et al. [57] in a meta-analysis that demonstrated that pegvisomant was more effective than first-generation SRLS in unselected patients in normalizing serum IGF-I levels, with a mean absolute serum IGF-I control of 40% to 60%.

Table 18.2 Factors that require higher doses of pegvisomant in the treatment of patients with acromegaly

Female gender
High basal IGF-I and GH
Younger age Increased body mass index
No previous radiotherapy

GH growth hormone, *IGF-I* insulin-like growth factor-I

Previous studies have shown that a higher baseline IGF-I or GH level, younger age, female gender, greater body mass index, and the presence of glucose intolerance are associated with higher pegvisomant doses required to achieve IGF-I normalization [58–60] (Table 18.2). When used as second-line monotherapy, body weight is the best predictor, with obese patients requiring higher doses and more rapid up-titration [61]. When used in combination with first-generation SRLs, body weight, younger age, and higher baseline IGF-I levels are also associated with higher pegvisomant dose requirements [62, 63]. Conversely, patients that have received radiation therapy appear to require lower pegvisomant doses, likely reflecting the effects of previous radiotherapy on somatotroph adenoma function [59]. Some patients may have a GH receptor polymorphism with a short isoform due to a deletion of exon 3 (d3GHR) [64] that increases the GH receptor (GHR) activation by GH, and it has been proposed that GHR isoforms may increase the response to pegvisomant. Initial studies of patients with the d3GHR isoform demonstrated that they had better response to pegvisomant treatment (lower doses and shorter treatment to normalize IGF-I levels) [65, 66], but these data have not been replicated in other studies of pegvisomant treatment between patients with the d3GHR and those with the full-length isoform [67, 68] and a study using combination therapy with pegvisomant and first-generation SRLs in patients with the different isoforms of GHR [69]. Therefore, current data do not support the use of d3GHR as a biomarker of response to pegvisomant. Other patients that may benefit from pegvisomant therapy include those with acromegaly whose tumors harbor mutations in the aryl hydrocarbon receptor-interacting protein gene [70, 71] and patients with McCune Albright syndrome, as they tend to be resistant to SRLs [72, 73], and children and adolescents with gigantism, including patients with the X-linked acrogigantism [74, 75]. Table 18.3 displays several special circumstances where pegvisomant may be considered in patients with acromegaly.

Table 18.3 Special circumstances where pegvisomant may be considered in patients with acromegaly

Special circumstances	Rationale or case scenarios
To relieve symptoms while awaiting surgery	In selected patients, optimization of management of current comorbidities (e.g., glucose intolerance, hypertension, and obstructive sleep apnea) while awaiting surgery
High surgical risk	High risk of postoperative cardiovascular or cerebrovascular events (e.g., myocardial infarction or stroke)
Multiple comorbid conditions	Uncontrolled diabetes mellitus and hypertension, and severe obstructive sleep apnea
Patient unwilling to undergo surgery during COVID-19 pandemic	Patient can be counselled to reconsider surgery when the COVID-19 pandemic improves
Patient declining surgery	To improve clinical signs and symptoms, reverse/control associated metabolic abnormalities (e.g., hypertension and diabetes mellitus), and potentially improve mortality
Persistence of disease	Adenoma mostly resected by pituitary surgeon with minimal or no adenoma visible on MRI
Recurrence of disease after surgical remission	Adenoma not visible on MRI due to persistence of microscopic disease
Persistent disease after completion of radiotherapy	Awaiting radiotherapy to take effect
Patient contemplating but not fully decided to undergo pituitary surgery	Awaiting first or repeat pituitary surgery

COVID-19 coronavirus disease 2019, *MRI* magnetic resonance imaging

Initiation, Titration, and Maintenance of Pegvisomant Therapy

Considering pegvisomant and initiating and maintaining effective therapeutic doses needs to be personalized based on individual patient characteristics and adjusted to normalize IGF-I levels. In the pivotal phase III clinical trial [36], when starting therapy, a loading pegvisomant dose was subcutaneously administered, but this practice is often not undertaken in clinical practice nowadays. Pegvisomant can then be initiated subcutaneously once daily, in accordance with how it was administered in the pivotal phase III clinical trial [36]. Additionally, due to its excellent efficacy profile and long half-life of 6 days [76], I may also consider less frequent (alternate day, once weekly, or twice weekly) pegvisomant administration [77, 78] in patients on many other injection therapies (e.g., insulin and testosterone injections) in order to simplify their treatment regimen. Patients with concurrent glucose intolerance and no tumor concerns on MRI, in my opinion, are particularly appropriate candidates for pegvisomant therapy.

Once treatment is initiated, IGF-I levels should be monitored regularly (4–6 weeks upon treatment initiation or after each dose titration, as well as periodically thereafter ranging from 3- to 6-month intervals), aiming at IGF-I normalization and, ideally, inducing symptomatic relief. By antagonizing GH action, GH levels are elevated rendering the measurement the levels clinically unhelpful. Furthermore, pegvisomant causes interference in several commercial immunoassays, which may underreport endogenous GH levels, as a consequence of antibody binding to pegvisomant, thereby limiting the antibody mass available for interaction with GH molecules being assayed [79].

In recent years, combination medical therapy has also gained traction to capitalize on the additive and synergistic effects [28] and lower side-effect profile due to lower doses used of each therapy that may also be more cost-effective [43]. The combination therapy involving pegvisomant that I tend to use is pegvisomant plus SRLs and pegvisomant plus cabergoline. I tend to combine pegvisomant with a low-dose first-generation SRL if SRL monotherapy has failed to normalize IGF-I levels, especially in a patient with concurrent glucose intolerance. We recently reported in a prospective study of 51 patients that low-dose monthly octreotide LAR (10 mg) or lanreotide (60 mg) combined with weekly pegvisomant (40–160 mg/week) achieved a biochemical control rate of 96% in controlled and uncontrolled patients at considerably lower cost compared with combination regimens of higher-dose SRL and weekly pegvisomant or low-dose SRL and daily pegvisomant [43]. If the patient on first-generation SRL is showing worsening glycemia, switching the patient to pegvisomant monotherapy can be considered if liver function tests permits and no tumor concerns on MRI, rather than switching the patient to pasireotide or combining pegvisomant with pasireotide. In the PAPE study [80, 81], 61 well-controlled patients on first-generation SRLs plus pegvisomant were switched to pasireotide with or without pegvisomant, following a 12-week run-in phase in which pegvisomant dose was reduced by 50%, and 15 (25%) biochemically controlled patients were switched to 60 mg pasireotide monotherapy, while 46 (75%) uncontrolled patients were switched to the same dose of pasireotide but continued the 50% reduced pegvisomant dose (mean dose: 61 mg/week). After 12 weeks of switching therapy, IGF-I normalized in 73.8% of patients, including 93% of patients in the monotherapy arm and 67% of patients in the combination arm, despite decreasing mean pegvisomant doses to 48 mg/week and pegvisomant discontinuation in 68% of patients. However, the rate of hyperglycemia was high, with significant increases in mean fasting plasma glucose (110–164 mg/dL), mean hemoglobin A1c (6.1–7.3%), and new-onset diabetes mellitus in 36.1% of patients.

On the other hand, if the patient has mild elevations of IGF-I, concurrent glucose intolerance, and AEs to SRLs, combining low-dose pegvisomant with cabergoline is a reasonable option, as this combination has three advantages. Firstly, cabergoline is well-tolerated, orally administered, and less costly than SRLs. Secondly, both pegvisomant and cabergoline have the potential to be administered less frequently on a twice or once weekly basis. Thirdly, this combination may reduce the need for pegvisomant dose escalation, thus reducing the cost of effectively treating acromegaly.

Personalized medical treatment in acromegaly demands knowledge about the size and extension of the pituitary tumor on MRI. In any patient with a pituitary tumor impinging the optic chiasm, SRLs have a stronger case than pegvisomant. Only when the tumor is not of a clinical concern on MRI that pegvisomant should be considered as first-line treatment because of its superior efficacy and better glycemic control. Table 18.4 summarizes some practical recommendations at different treatment phases when utilizing pegvisomant to treat acromegaly.

Table 18.4 Practical recommendations at different treatment phases when utilizing pegvisomant to treat acromegaly

Treatment phases	Practical recommendations
Before starting therapy	• Review concomitant medications to rule out possible drug-drug interactions – Patients on opioids often need higher pegvisomant doses to achieve appropriate IGF-I suppression compared with patients not receiving opioids • Counsel patients on symptoms associated with adverse events (e.g., liver transaminitis, injection-site reactions, and lipohypertrophy) – *Normal baseline LFTs:* check LFTs at monthly intervals during the first 6 months of treatment, quarterly for the next 6 months, and then biannually for the next year – *Abnormal LFTs < 3 × ULN:* monitor LFTs monthly for at least 1 year after initiation of therapy and then biannually for the next year – *Abnormal LFTs > 3 × ULN:* do not treat with pegvisomant until a comprehensive workup establishes the cause of the patient's liver dysfunction. Determine if cholelithiasis or choledocholithiasis is present, particularly in patients with a history of prior therapy with SRLs, and if pegvisomant is initiated, LFTs and clinical symptoms should be monitored very closely • If a patient develops LFT elevations, or any other signs or symptoms of liver dysfunction while receiving pegvisomant, the following patient management is recommended – *Abnormal LFTs 3–5 × ULN without signs/symptoms of hepatitis or other liver injury*: may continue pegvisomant therapy but monitor LFTs weekly and perform a comprehensive hepatic workup to discern if an alternative cause of liver dysfunction is present – *Abnormal LFTs > 5 x ULN*: discontinue pegvisomant immediately and refer to hepatology and when LFTs normalize, consider cautious reinitiation of pegvisomant therapy with weekly LFT monitoring for 4 weeks and then monthly for 3 months until LFTs normalization has stabilized – *Signs or symptoms suggestive of hepatitis or other liver injury (e.g., jaundice, bilirubinuria, fatigue, nausea, vomiting, right upper quadrant pain, ascites, unexplained edema)*: pegvisomant should be discontinued and consider referral to hepatology
Initiation phase of therapy	• Start dose of 10 mg daily (less frequent dosing can be considered in mild disease) • Based on serum IGF-I levels, patient's clinical symptoms, and tolerability, titrate dose by increasing in 5 mg increments if IGF-I still elevated and 5 mg decrements if IGF-I below reference range every 4–6 weeks to no more than 30 mg/day maintenance
Monitoring phase of therapy	• Monitor serum IGF-I levels, clinical symptoms, and patient tolerability every 4–6 weeks during dose titration or as indicated during the initiation phase of therapy • Once the maintenance dose is achieved, monitor serum IGF-I levels, clinical symptoms, and patient tolerability monthly or as indicated • Monitor for adverse effects • If treatment is interrupted, reinitiate at a lower dose when serum IGF-I levels are normalized and symptoms have resolved • Perform surveillance MRI of the pituitary periodically to monitor for changes in tumor size

IGF-I insulin-like growth factor-I, *LFT* liver function test, *MRI* magnetic resonance imaging, *ULN* upper limit of normal

Precautions When Using Pegvisomant

The side effects of pegvisomant are usually mild, transient, or self-limiting, with liver enzyme disturbances being the most common side effect [26, 82]. Liver transaminitis can occur both during pegvisomant therapy in combination with SRLs or during monotherapy. During combination therapy, liver transaminitis can range from 11 to 15% when alanine transaminase cut-off levels between 2 and 3 x ULN are used [83, 84], whereas in 5.2% of patients, transaminitis with ≥ 3 ULN were observed with monotherapy [85]. In the ACROSTUDY outcome data, only 3.2% of patients had abnormal alanine transaminase or aspartate transaminase levels, with over one third of patients receiving combination therapy [26]. It is possible that this incidence is underreported as patients in ACROSTUDY are not seen as frequently as being in a clinical trial resulting in LFTs not being measured frequently. The pathophysiology of transaminitis during pegvisomant therapy remains unclear. Lipohypertrophy is another side effect of pegvisomant, with a lower prevalence than liver transaminitis [82, 83, 86, 87], and frequent rotation of injection sites seems to reverse local lipohypertrophy or prevent it [83, 88]. Nevertheless, in some cases, resolution can take up to 8 months, necessitating treatment discontinuation [83].

Because of its mechanism of action, safety concerns have been raised about the potential risk of tumor size increase with pegvisomant. Despite the fact that there are a few reports of increase in tumor size during pegvisomant use, there is no clear evidence that it directly promotes tumor growth [25, 84]. In the ACROSTUDY outcome data of 2221 patients treated with pegvisomant for a median of 9.3 years and followed up for a median of 7.4 years, only 7.1% of patients has pituitary tumor size increase, while the majority (71.1%) of patients had no changes [26]. It is hypothesized that in some patients, this increase in tumor size may have caused by the withdrawal of SRL therapy or may have simply reflected the natural history of more aggressive pituitary adenomas. Currently, it is reasonable to conclude that pegvisomant has a neutral effect on the natural course of tumor growth; nevertheless, periodic pituitary MRI should still be performed in patients receiving long-term pegvisomant therapy.

Cost Considerations When Using Pegvisomant

The cost for 10, 15, 20, 25, and 30 mg pegvisomant subcutaneous injections are around $259, $383, $508, $632, and $757, respectively, for a supply of 1 powder for injection, making it the most costly of available medical therapies [89]. With an increasing array of medical therapy options, it is important to personalize management of patients with acromegaly based not only on unique disease characteristics and patient preference [30–33] but also on cost considerations. One strategy is to use lower doses of pegvisomant and combine it with SRLs to offset the high pegvisomant cost while still maintaining high biochemical control rates. In a randomized, open-label, parallel three-arm study of high-dose SRL (lanreotide 120 mg/octreotide LAR 30 mg) plus weekly pegvisomant (40–160 mg/week), low-dose SRL (lanreotide 60 mg/octreotide LAR 10 mg) plus weekly pegvisomant, and low-dose SRL plus daily pegvisomant (15–60 mg/day), Bonert et al. [43] demonstrated that low-dose SRL plus weekly pegvisomant provided a new therapeutic regimen that minimizes drug cost while maximizes treatment efficacy for patients with acromegaly requiring combination therapy. Using a regimen of weekly pegvisomant plus low-dose SRL may be just as efficacious as weekly pegvisomant plus high-dose SRL in uncontrolled acromegaly patients, suggesting that patients started on pegvisomant while maintaining maximal SRL dose may be unnecessarily costly and possibly overtreated.

Conclusion

Pegvisomant is an effective and safe medical option for many acromegaly patients, but its use still needs to be optimized. Starting and maintaining pegvisomant therapy needs to be personalized based on individual patient characteristics. The patient that would most benefit from pegvisomant would be the one with minimal to no tumor concerns on MRI with low Ki-67 and concurrent glucose intolerance (Fig. 18.1),

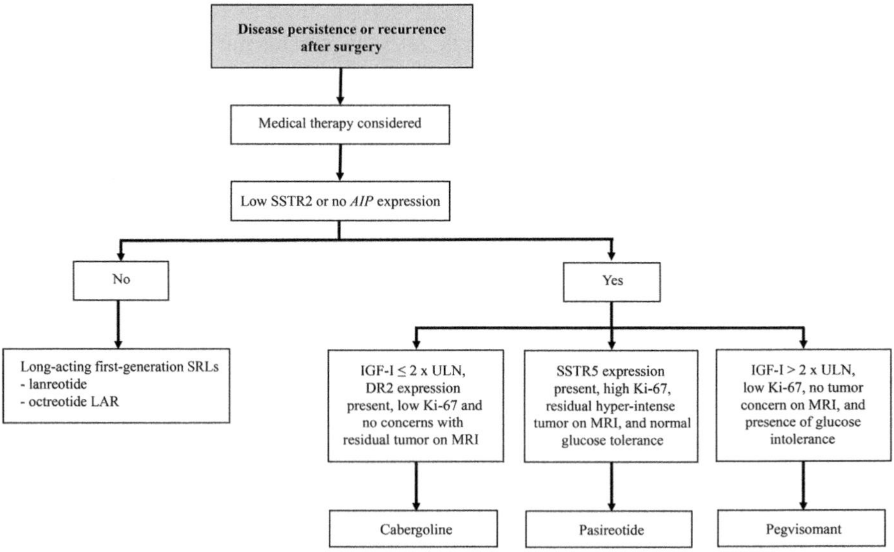

Fig. 18.1 How to position pegvisomant and other medical therapies for acromegaly guided by biochemical, molecular, histopathological, and radiological parameters. *AIP* aryl hydrocarbon receptor-interacting protein, *D2R* dopamine 2 receptor, *IGF-I* insulin-like growth factor-I, *Ki-67* marker of proliferation, *LAR* long-acting release, *MRI* magnetic resonance imaging, *SSTR2* somatostatin receptor 2, *SSTR5* somatostatin receptor 5, *ULN* upper limit of normal

where pegvisomant can be used either as first-line monotherapy or combined with cabergoline to minimize cost. In patients not adequately controlled by SRLs, pegvisomant can be added, but this combination therapy can be costly. However, when combined with SRLs, the dose of pegvisomant can be lowered while maintaining a similarly high degree of efficacy and minimizing drug cost. Another type of patient where pegvisomant can be added is patients controlled on SRLs but with poor QoL, as this combination can improve QoL, and young patients with genetic syndromes. Side effects related to pegvisomant are rare and mainly transient. Elevated transaminases are more common with combination therapy than monotherapy, but no reliable predictive factors are known. Long-term follow-up of patients on pegvisomant therapy have not demonstrated a risk of pituitary tumor growth, but periodic surveillance MRIs remains imperative.

Conflicts of Interest KCJY is an investigator on a research grant to St. Joseph's Hospital Medical Center from Amryt and has consulted for Amryt, Ipsen, Crinetics, and Pfizer on advisory board meetings.

References

1. Colao A, Grasso LFS, Giustina A, Melmed S, Chanson P, Pereira AM, Pivonello R. Acromegaly. Nat Rev Dis Primers. 2019;5(1):20.
2. Kreitschmann-Andermahr I, Buchfelder M, Kleist B, Kohlmann J, Menzel C, Buslei R, Kołtowska-Häggsträm M, Strasburger C, Siegel S. Predictors of quality of life in 165 patients with acromegaly: results from a single-center study. Endocr Pract. 2017;23(1):79–88.
3. Petrossians P, Daly AF, Natchev E, Maione L, Blijdorp K, Sahnoun-Fathallah M, Auriemma R, Diallo AM, Hulting AL, Ferone D, Hana V Jr, Filipponi S, Sievers C, Nogueira C, Fajardo-Montanana C, Carvalho D, Hana V, Stalla GK, Jaffrain-Rea ML, Delemer B, Colao A, Brue T, Neggers S, Zacharieva S, Chanson P, Beckers A. Acromegaly at diagnosis in 3173 patients from the Liege Acromegaly Survey (LAS) database. Endocr Relat Cancer. 2017;24(10):505–18.
4. Ritvonen E, Loyttyniemi E, Jaatinen P, Ebeling T, Moilanen L, Nuutila P, Kauppinen-Makelin R, Schalin-Jantti C. Mortality in acromegaly: a 20-year follow-up study. Endocr Relat Cancer. 2016;23(6):469–80.
5. Sievers C, Sämann PG, Pfister H, Dimopoulou C, Czisch M, Roemmler J, Schopohl J, Stalla GK, Zihl J. Cognitive function in acromegaly: description and brain volumetric correlates. Pituitary. 2012;15(3):350–7.
6. Bolfi F, Neves AF, Boguszewski CL, Nunes-Nogueira VS. Mortality in acromegaly decreased in the last decade: a systematic review and meta-analysis. Eur J Endocrinol. 2018;179(1):59–71.
7. Fleseriu M, Biller BMK, Freda PU, Gadelha MR, Giustina A, Katznelson L, Molitch ME, Samson SL, Strasburger CJ, van der Lely AJ, Melmed S. A Pituitary Society update to acromegaly management guidelines. Pituitary. 2021;24(1):1–13.
8. Katznelson L, Laws ER Jr, Melmed S, Molitch ME, Murad MH, Utz A, Wass JA. Acromegaly: an endocrine society clinical practice guideline. J Clin Endocrinol Metab. 2014;99(11):3933–51.
9. Melmed S, Bronstein MD, Chanson P, Klibanski A, Casanueva FF, Wass JAH, Strasburger CJ, Luger A, Clemmons DR, Giustina A. A Consensus Statement on acromegaly therapeutic outcomes. Nat Rev Endocrinol. 2018;14(9):552–61.
10. Marazuela M, Ramos-Levi A, Sampedro-Nunez M, Bernabeu I. Cabergoline treatment in acromegaly: pros. Endocrine. 2014;46(2):215–9.
11. Sandret L, Maison P, Chanson P. Place of cabergoline in acromegaly: a meta-analysis. J Clin Endocrinol Metab. 2011;96(5):1327–35.

12. Moyes VJ, Metcalfe KA, Drake WM. Clinical use of cabergoline as primary and adjunctive treatment for acromegaly. Eur J Endocrinol. 2008;159(5):541–5.
13. Abs R, Verhelst J, Maiter D, Van Acker K, Nobels F, Coolens JL, Mahler C, Beckers A. Cabergoline in the treatment of acromegaly: a study in 64 patients. J Clin Endocrinol Metab. 1998;83(2):374–8.
14. SANDOSTATIN® LAR DEPOT Prescribing information. Novartis. 1988. https://www.novartis.us/sites/www.novartis.us/files/sandostatin_lar.pdf. Accessed April 7, 2022.
15. Colao A, Auriemma RS, Pivonello R. The effects of somatostatin analogue therapy on pituitary tumor volume in patients with acromegaly. Pituitary. 2016;19(2):210–21.
16. Colao A, Auriemma RS, Pivonello R, Kasuki L, Gadelha MR. Interpreting biochemical control response rates with first-generation somatostatin analogues in acromegaly. Pituitary. 2016;19(3):235–47.
17. Taboada GF, Luque RM, Bastos W, Guimaraes RF, Marcondes JB, Chimelli LM, Fontes R, Mata PJ, Filho PN, Carvalho DP, Kineman RD, Gadelha MR. Quantitative analysis of somatostatin receptor subtype (SSTR1-5) gene expression levels in somatotropinomas and nonfunctioning pituitary adenomas. Eur J Endocrinol. 2007;156(1):65–74.
18. Somatuline Autogel 60 mg, solution for injection with a prefilled syringe. Summary of product characteristics. Ipsen Ltd. 2001. https://www.medicines.org.uk/emc/product/4808/smpc. Accessed April 7, 2022.
19. SIGNIFOR® LAR (pasireotide) for injectable suspension, for intramuscular use. Prescribing information. Recordati. 2012. https://www.signiforlar.com/pdf/signifor-lar-pi.pdf. Accessed April 7, 2022.
20. Shimon I, Adnan Z, Gorshtein A, Baraf L, Saba Khazen N, Gershinsky M, Pauker Y, Abid A, Niven MJ, Shechner C, Greenman Y. Efficacy and safety of long-acting pasireotide in patients with somatostatin-resistant acromegaly: a multicenter study. Endocrine. 2018;62(2):448–55.
21. Fleseriu M, Dreval A, Bondar I, Vagapova G, Macut D, Pokramovich YG, Molitch ME, Leonova N, Raverot G, Grineva E, Poteshkin YE, Gilgun-Sherki Y, Ludlam WH, Patou G, Haviv A, Gordon MB, Biermasz NR, Melmed S, Strasburger CJ. Maintenance of response to oral octreotide compared with injectable somatostatin receptor ligands in patients with acromegaly: a phase 3, multicentre, randomised controlled trial. Lancet Diabetes Endocrinol. 2022;10(2):102–11.
22. Melmed S, Popovic V, Bidlingmaier M, Mercado M, van der Lely AJ, Biermasz N, Bolanowski M, Coculescu M, Schopohl J, Racz K, Glaser B, Goth M, Greenman Y, Trainer P, Mezosi E, Shimon I, Giustina A, Korbonits M, Bronstein MD, Kleinberg D, Teichman S, Gliko-Kabir I, Mamluk R, Haviv A, Strasburger C. Safety and efficacy of oral octreotide in acromegaly: results of a multicenter phase III trial. J Clin Endocrinol Metab. 2015;100(4):1699–708.
23. Samson SL, Nachtigall LB, Fleseriu M, Gordon MB, Bolanowski M, Labadzhyan A, Ur E, Molitch M, Ludlam WH, Patou G, Haviv A, Biermasz N, Giustina A, Trainer PJ, Strasburger CJ, Kennedy L, Melmed S. Maintenance of acromegaly control in patients switching from injectable somatostatin receptor ligands to oral octreotide. J Clin Endocrinol Metab. 2020;105(10):e3785.
24. Kuhn E, Caron P, Delemer B, Raingeard I, Lefebvre H, Raverot G, Cortet-Rudelli C, Desailloud R, Geffroy C, Henocque R, Brault Y, Brue T, Chanson P. Pegvisomant in combination or pegvisomant alone after failure of somatostatin analogs in acromegaly patients: an observational French ACROSTUDY cohort study. Endocrine. 2021;71(1):158–67.
25. Barraud S, Caron P, Raingeard I, Lefebvre H, Raverot G, Cortet-Rudelli C, Desailloud R, Henocque R, Brault Y, Brue T, Chanson P, Delemer B. Pegvisomant treatment in acromegaly in clinical practice: final results of the French ACROSTUDY (312 patients). Ann Endocrinol. 2021;82(6):582–9.
26. Fleseriu M, Fuhrer-Sakel D, van der Lely AJ, De Marinis L, Brue T, van der Lans-Bussemaker J, Hey-Hadavi J, Camacho-Hubner C, Wajnrajch MP, Valluri SR, Palladino AA, Gomez R, Salvatori R. More than a decade of real-world experience of pegvisomant for acromegaly: ACROSTUDY. Eur J Endocrinol. 2021;185(4):525–38.
27. Kuhn E, Chanson P. Cabergoline in acromegaly. Pituitary. 2017;20(1):121–8.

28. Strasburger CJ, Mattsson A, Wilton P, Aydin F, Hey-Hadavi J, Biller BMK. Increasing frequency of combination medical therapy in the treatment of acromegaly with the GH receptor antagonist pegvisomant. Eur J Endocrinol. 2018;178(4):321–9.
29. Giustina A, Barkhoudarian G, Beckers A, Ben-Shlomo A, Biermasz N, Biller B, Boguszewski C, Bolanowski M, Bollerslev J, Bonert V, Bronstein MD, Buchfelder M, Casanueva F, Chanson P, Clemmons D, Fleseriu M, Formenti AM, Freda P, Gadelha M, Geer E, Gurnell M, Heaney AP, Ho KKY, Ioachimescu AG, Lamberts S, Laws E, Losa M, Maffei P, Mamelak A, Mercado M, Molitch M, Mortini P, Pereira AM, Petersenn S, Post K, Puig-Domingo M, Salvatori R, Samson SL, Shimon I, Strasburger C, Swearingen B, Trainer P, Vance ML, Wass J, Wierman ME, Yuen KCJ, Zatelli MC, Melmed S. Multidisciplinary management of acromegaly: a consensus. Rev Endocr Metab Disord. 2020;21(4):667–78.
30. Ezzat S, Caspar-Bell GM, Chik CL, Denis M-C, Domingue M-E, Imran SA, Johnson MD, Lochman HA, Nyomba G, Prebtani A, Ridout R, Ramirez JAR, Van Uum S. Predictive markers for post-surgical medical management of acromegaly: a systematic review and consensus treatment guideline. Endocr Pract. 2019. https://doi.org/10.4145/EP-2018-0500.
31. Kasuki L, Wildemberg LE, Gadelha MR. Management of endocrine disease: personalized medicine in the treatment of acromegaly. Eur J Endocrinol. 2018;178(3):R89–R100.
32. Puig Domingo M. Treatment of acromegaly in the era of personalized and predictive medicine. Clin Endocrinol. 2015;83(1):3–14.
33. Yuen KCJ. Medical therapy for acromegaly: towards the practice of a personalized medicine approach. Endocr Pract. 2019;25(4):396–8.
34. Fleseriu M, Molitch M, Dreval A, Biermasz NR, Gordon MB, Crosby RD, Ludlam WH, Haviv A, Gilgun-Sherki Y, Mathias SD. Disease and treatment-related burden in patients with acromegaly who are biochemically controlled on injectable somatostatin receptor ligands. Front Endocrinol. 2021;12:627711.
35. Neggers SJ, Muhammad A, van der Lely AJ. Pegvisomant treatment in acromegaly. Neuroendocrinology. 2016;103(1):59–65.
36. Trainer PJ, Drake WM, Katznelson L, Freda PU, Herman-Bonert V, van der Lely AJ, Dimaraki EV, Stewart PM, Friend KE, Vance ML, Besser GM, Scarlett JA, Thorner MO, Parkinson C, Klibanski A, Powell JS, Barkan AL, Sheppard MC, Malsonado M, Rose DR, Clemmons DR, Johannsson G, Bengtsson BA, Stavrou S, Kleinberg DL, Cook DM, Phillips LS, Bidlingmaier M, Strasburger CJ, Hackett S, Zib K, Bennett WF, Davis RJ. Treatment of acromegaly with the growth hormone-receptor antagonist pegvisomant. N Engl J Med. 2000;342(16):1171–7.
37. Trainer PJ, Ezzat S, D'Souza GA, Layton G, Strasburger CJ. A randomized, controlled, multicentre trial comparing pegvisomant alone with combination therapy of pegvisomant and long-acting octreotide in patients with acromegaly. Clin Endocrinol. 2009;71(4):549–57.
38. US Food and Drug Administration. FDA approves pegvisomant. 2003. https://www.accessdata.fda.gov/drugsatfda_docs/nda/2003/021106_somavertcfm#:~:text=Approval%20Date%3A%203%2F25%2F2003. Accessed April 7, 2022.
39. European Medicines Agency. Somavert. 2002. https://www.ema.europa.eu/en/medicines/human/EPAR/somavert. Accessed April 7, 2022.
40. Freda PU, Gordon MB, Kelepouris N, Jonsson P, Koltowska-Haggstrom M, van der Lely AJ. Long-term treatment with pegvisomant as monotherapy in patients with acromegaly: experience from ACROSTUDY. Endocr Pract. 2015;21(3):264–74.
41. Shimatsu A, Nagashima M, Hashigaki S, Ohki N, Chihara K. Efficacy and safety of monotherapy by pegvisomant, a growth hormone receptor antagonist, in Japanese patients with acromegaly. Endocr J. 2016;63(4):337–47.
42. Tritos NA, Chanson P, Jimenez C, King D, Jonsson PJ, Klibanski A, Biller BM. Effectiveness of first-line pegvisomant monotherapy in acromegaly: an ACROSTUDY analysis. Eur J Endocrinol. 2017;176(2):213–20.
43. Bonert V, Mirocha J, Carmichael J, Yuen KCJ, Araki T, Melmed S. Cost-effectiveness and efficacy of a novel combination regimen in acromegaly: a prospective, randomized trial. J Clin Endocrinol Metab. 2020;105(9):444.

44. Ma L, Luo D, Yang T, Wu S, Li M, Chen C, Zhou S, Ma L, Wu Y, Zhou Y, Cui Y. Combined therapy of somatostatin analogues with pegvisomant for the treatment of acromegaly: a meta-analysis of prospective studies. BMC Endocr Disord. 2020;20(1):126.
45. Bernabeu I, Alvarez-Escola C, Paniagua AE, Lucas T, Pavon I, Cabezas-Agricola JM, Casanueva FF, Marazuela M. Pegvisomant and cabergoline combination therapy in acromegaly. Pituitary. 2013;16(1):101–8.
46. Higham CE, Atkinson AB, Aylwin S, Bidlingmaier M, Drake WM, Lewis A, Martin NM, Moyes V, Newell-Price J, Trainer PJ. Effective combination treatment with cabergoline and low-dose pegvisomant in active acromegaly: a prospective clinical trial. J Clin Endocrinol Metab. 2012;97(4):1187–93.
47. van der Lely AJ, Kuhn E, Muhammad A, Coopmans EC, Neggers SJ, Chanson P. Pegvisomant and not somatostatin receptor ligands (SRLs) is first-line medical therapy for acromegaly. Eur J Endocrinol. 2020;182(6):D17–29.
48. Kopchick JJ, Parkinson C, Stevens EC, Trainer PJ. Growth hormone receptor antagonists: discovery, development, and use in patients with acromegaly. Endocr Rev. 2002;23(5):623–46.
49. Ross RJ, Leung KC, Maamra M, Bennett W, Doyle N, Waters MJ, Ho KK. Binding and functional studies with the growth hormone receptor antagonist, B2036-PEG (pegvisomant), reveal effects of pegylation and evidence that it binds to a receptor dimer. J Clin Endocrinol Metab. 2001;86(4):1716–23.
50. Thorner MO, Strasburger CJ, Wu Z, Straume M, Bidlingmaier M, Pezzoli SS, Zib K, Scarlett JC, Bennett WF. Growth hormone (GH) receptor blockade with a PEG-modified GH (B2036-PEG) lowers serum insulin-like growth factor-I but does not acutely stimulate serum GH. J Clin Endocrinol Metab. 1999;84(6):2098–103.
51. van der Lely AJ, Hutson RK, Trainer PJ, Besser GM, Barkan AL, Katznelson L, Klibanski A, Herman-Bonert V, Melmed S, Vance ML, Freda PU, Stewart PM, Friend KE, Clemmons DR, Johannsson G, Stavrou S, Cook DM, Phillips LS, Strasburger CJ, Hackett S, Zib KA, Davis RJ, Scarlett JA, Thorner MO. Long-term treatment of acromegaly with pegvisomant, a growth hormone receptor antagonist. Lancet. 2001;358(9295):1754–9.
52. Neggers SJ, van Aken MO, de Herder WW, Feelders RA, Janssen JA, Badia X, Webb SM, van der Lely AJ. Quality of life in acromegalic patients during long-term somatostatin analog treatment with and without pegvisomant. J Clin Endocrinol Metab. 2008;93(10):3853–9.
53. Cannavo S, Bogazzi F, Colao A, De Marinis L, Maffei P, Gomez R, Graziano E, Monterubbianesi M, Grottoli S, Italian Acrostudy G. Does pegvisomant treatment expertise improve control of resistant acromegaly? The Italian ACROSTUDY experience. J Endocrinol Investig. 2015;38(10):1099–109.
54. Chanson P, Brue T, Delemer B, Caron P, Borson-Chazot F, Zouater H, Medecins de l'Etude A. Pegvisomant treatment in patients with acromegaly in clinical practice: The French ACROSTUDY. Ann Endocrinol. 2015;76(6):664–70.
55. Kuker AP, Shen W, Jin Z, Singh S, Chen J, Bruce JN, Freda PU. Body composition changes with long-term pegvisomant therapy of acromegaly. J Endocr Soc. 2021;5(3):4.
56. Chiloiro S, Giampietro A, Visconti F, Rossi L, Donfrancesco F, Fleseriu CM, Mirra F, Pontecorvi A, Giustina A, Fleseriu M, De Marinis L, Bianchi A. Glucose metabolism outcomes in acromegaly patients on treatment with pasireotide-LAR or pasireotide-LAR plus Pegvisomant. Endocrine. 2021;73(3):658–66.
57. Qiao N, He M, Shen M, Zhang Q, Zhang Z, Shou X, Wang Y, Zhao Y, Tritos NA. Comparative efficacy of medical treatment for acromegaly: a systematic review and network meta-analysis of integrated randomized trials and observational studies. Endocr Pract. 2020;26(4):454–62.
58. Droste M, Domberg J, Buchfelder M, Mann K, Schwanke A, Stalla G, Strasburger CJ. Therapy of acromegalic patients exacerbated by concomitant type 2 diabetes requires higher pegvisomant doses to normalise IGF1 levels. Eur J Endocrinol. 2014;171(1):59–68.
59. Parkinson C, Burman P, Messig M, Trainer PJ. Gender, body weight, disease activity, and previous radiotherapy influence the response to pegvisomant. J Clin Endocrinol Metab. 2007;92(1):190–5.

60. van der Lely AJ, Jonsson P, Wilton P, Akerblad AC, Cara J, Ghigo E. Treatment with high doses of pegvisomant in 56 patients with acromegaly: experience from ACROSTUDY. Eur J Endocrinol. 2016;175(4):239–45.
61. Ragonese M, Grottoli S, Maffei P, Alibrandi A, Ambrosio MR, Arnaldi G, Bianchi A, Puglisi S, Zatelli MC, De Marinis L, Ghigo E, Giustina A, Maffezzoni F, Martini C, Trementino L, Cannavo S. How to improve effectiveness of pegvisomant treatment in acromegalic patients. J Endocrinol Investig. 2018;41(5):575–81.
62. Franck SE, Korevaar TIM, Petrossians P, Daly AF, Chanson P, Jaffrain-Rea ML, Brue T, Stalla GK, Carvalho D, Colao A, Hana V, Delemer B, Fajardo C, van der Lely AJ, Beckers A, Neggers S. A multivariable prediction model for pegvisomant dosing: monotherapy and in combination with long-acting somatostatin analogues. Eur J Endocrinol. 2017;176(4):421–31.
63. Sievers C, Baur DM, Schwanke A, Buchfelder M, Droste M, Mann K, Stalla GK. Prediction of therapy response in acromegalic patients under pegvisomant therapy within the German ACROSTUDY cohort. Pituitary. 2015;18(6):916–23.
64. Pantel J, Machinis K, Sobrier ML, Duquesnoy P, Goossens M, Amselem S. Species-specific alternative splice mimicry at the growth hormone receptor locus revealed by the lineage of retroelements during primate evolution. J Biol Chem. 2000;275(25):18664–9.
65. Bernabeu I, Alvarez-Escola C, Quinteiro C, Lucas T, Puig-Domingo M, Luque-Ramirez M, de Miguel-Novoa P, Fernandez-Rodriguez E, Halperin I, Loidi L, Casanueva FF, Marazuela M. The exon 3-deleted growth hormone receptor is associated with better response to pegvisomant therapy in acromegaly. J Clin Endocrinol Metab. 2010;95(1):222–9.
66. Bianchi A, Mazziotti G, Tilaro L, Cimino V, Veltri F, Gaetani E, Pecorini G, Pontecorvi A, Giustina A, De Marinis L. Growth hormone receptor polymorphism and the effects of pegvisomant in acromegaly. Pituitary. 2009;12(3):196–9.
67. Filopanti M, Olgiati L, Mantovani G, Corbetta S, Arosio M, Gasco V, De Marinis L, Martini C, Bogazzi F, Cannavo S, Colao A, Ferone D, Arnaldi G, Pigliaru F, Peri A, Angeletti G, Jaffrain-Rea ML, Lania AG, Spada A. Growth hormone receptor variants and response to pegvisomant in monotherapy or in combination with somatostatin analogs in acromegalic patients: a multicenter study. J Clin Endocrinol Metab. 2012;97(2):E165–72.
68. Kasuki L, Machado EO, Ogino LL, Coelho MC, Silva CM, Wildemberg LE, Lima CH, Gadelha MR. Experience with pegvisomant treatment in acromegaly in a single Brazilian tertiary reference center: efficacy, safety and predictors of response. Arch Endocrinol Metab. 2016;60(5):479–85.
69. Franck SE, van der Lely AJ, Delhanty PJ, Jorgensen JO, Neggers SJ. Pegvisomant in combination with long-acting somatostatin analogues in acromegaly: the role of the GH receptor deletion of exon 3. Eur J Endocrinol. 2015;173(5):553–61.
70. Joshi K, Daly AF, Beckers A, Zacharin M. Resistant paediatric somatotropinomas due to AIP mutations: role of pegvisomant. Horm Res Paediatr. 2018;90(3):196–202.
71. Oriola J, Lucas T, Halperin I, Mora M, Perales MJ, Alvarez-Escola C, Paz de MN, Diaz Soto G, Salinas I, Julian MT, Olaizola I, Bernabeu I, Marazuela M, Puig-Domingo M. Germline mutations of AIP gene in somatotropinomas resistant to somatostatin analogues. Eur J Endocrinol. 2013;168(1):9–13.
72. Galland F, Kamenicky P, Affres H, Reznik Y, Pontvert D, Le Bouc Y, Young J, Chanson P. McCune-Albright syndrome and acromegaly: effects of hypothalamopituitary radiotherapy and/or pegvisomant in somatostatin analog-resistant patients. J Clin Endocrinol Metab. 2006;91(12):4957–61.
73. Salenave S, Boyce AM, Collins MT, Chanson P. Acromegaly and McCune-Albright syndrome. J Clin Endocrinol Metab. 2014;99(6):1955–69.
74. Beckers A, Lodish MB, Trivellin G, Rostomyan L, Lee M, Faucz FR, Yuan B, Choong CS, Caberg JH, Verrua E, Naves LA, Cheetham TD, Young J, Lysy PA, Petrossians P, Cotterill A, Shah NS, Metzger D, Castermans E, Ambrosio MR, Villa C, Strebkova N, Mazerkina N, Gaillard S, Barra GB, Casulari LA, Neggers SJ, Salvatori R, Jaffrain-Rea ML, Zacharin M, Santamaria BL, Zacharieva S, Lim EM, Mantovani G, Zatelli MC, Collins MT, Bonneville

JF, Quezado M, Chittiboina P, Oldfield EH, Bours V, Liu P, WdH W, Pellegata N, Lupski JR, Daly AF, Stratakis CA. X-linked acrogigantism syndrome: clinical profile and therapeutic responses. Endocr Relat Cancer. 2015;22(3):353–67.

75. Rix M, Laurberg P, Hoejberg AS, Brock-Jacobsen B. Pegvisomant therapy in pituitary gigantism: successful treatment in a 12-year-old girl. Eur J Endocrinol. 2005;153(2):195–201.
76. Somavert Prescribing Information. Pfizer. 2012. https://www.accessdata.fda.gov/drugsatfda_docs/label/2012/021106s031lbl.pdf. Accessed April 7, 2022.
77. Higham CE, Thomas JD, Bidlingmaier M, Drake WM, Trainer PJ. Successful use of weekly pegvisomant administration in patients with acromegaly. Eur J Endocrinol. 2009;161(1):21–5.
78. Jehle S, Reyes CM, Sundeen RE, Freda PU. Alternate-day administration of pegvisomant maintains normal serum insulin-like growth factor-I levels in patients with acromegaly. J Clin Endocrinol Metab. 2005;90(3):1588–93.
79. Paisley AN, Hayden K, Ellis A, Anderson J, Wieringa G, Trainer PJ. Pegvisomant interference in GH assays results in underestimation of GH levels. Eur J Endocrinol. 2007;156(3):315–9.
80. Muhammad A, Coopmans EC, Delhanty PJD, Dallenga AHG, Haitsma IK, Janssen J, van der Lely AJ, Neggers S. Efficacy and safety of switching to pasireotide in acromegaly patients controlled with pegvisomant and somatostatin analogues: PAPE extension study. Eur J Endocrinol. 2018;179(5):269–77.
81. Muhammad A, van der Lely AJ, Delhanty PJD, Dallenga AHG, Haitsma IK, Janssen J, Neggers S. Efficacy and safety of switching to pasireotide in patients with acromegaly controlled with pegvisomant and first-generation somatostatin analogues (PAPE study). J Clin Endocrinol Metab. 2018;103(2):586–95.
82. van der Lely AJ, Biller BM, Brue T, Buchfelder M, Ghigo E, Gomez R, Hey-Hadavi J, Lundgren F, Rajicic N, Strasburger CJ, Webb SM, Koltowska-Haggstrom M. Long-term safety of pegvisomant in patients with acromegaly: comprehensive review of 1288 subjects in ACROSTUDY. J Clin Endocrinol Metab. 2012;97(5):1589–97.
83. Neggers SJ, Franck SE, de Rooij FW, Dallenga AH, Poublon RM, Feelders RA, Janssen JA, Buchfelder M, Hofland LJ, Jorgensen JO, van der Lely AJ. Long-term efficacy and safety of pegvisomant in combination with long-acting somatostatin analogs in acromegaly. J Clin Endocrinol Metab. 2014;99(10):3644–52.
84. van der Lely AJ, Bernabeu I, Cap J, Caron P, Colao A, Marek J, Neggers S, Birman P. Coadministration of lanreotide Autogel and pegvisomant normalizes IGF1 levels and is well tolerated in patients with acromegaly partially controlled by somatostatin analogs alone. Eur J Endocrinol. 2011;164(3):325–33.
85. Schreiber I, Buchfelder M, Droste M, Forssmann K, Mann K, Saller B, Strasburger CJ, German Pegvisomant I. Treatment of acromegaly with the GH receptor antagonist pegvisomant in clinical practice: safety and efficacy evaluation from the German Pegvisomant Observational Study. Eur J Endocrinol. 2007;156(1):75–82.
86. Bonert VS, Kennedy L, Petersenn S, Barkan A, Carmichael J, Melmed S. Lipodystrophy in patients with acromegaly receiving pegvisomant. J Clin Endocrinol Metab. 2008;93(9):3515–8.
87. Maffei P, Martini C, Pagano C, Sicolo N, Corbetti F. Lipohypertrophy in acromegaly induced by the new growth hormone receptor antagonist pegvisomant. Ann Intern Med. 2006;145(4):310–2.
88. Neggers SJ, de Herder WW, Janssen JA, Feelders RA, van der Lely AJ. Combined treatment for acromegaly with long-acting somatostatin analogs and pegvisomant: long-term safety for up to 4.5 years (median 2.2 years) of follow-up in 86 patients. Eur J Endocrinol. 2009;160(4):529–33.
89. Marko NF, LaSota E, Hamrahian AH, Weil RJ. Comparative effectiveness review of treatment options for pituitary microadenomas in acromegaly. J Neurosurg. 2012;117(3):522–38.

Chapter 19
Perspectives on Combination Medical Therapy in the Treatment of Acromegaly

Dawn Shao Ting Lim and Maria Fleseriu

Introduction

The goals of acromegaly treatment include insulin-like growth factor-1 (IGF-1) normalization, reduction in growth hormone (GH) levels (to <1.0 μg/L), decrease in tumor volume, and improvement in clinical symptoms [1–4]. Surgical pituitary tumor removal is the first-line treatment of choice. However, GH excess remains uncontrolled in 15–20% of patients who have microadenomas and is as high as 60% in patients with a macroadenomas [5, 6]. Medical therapy is indicated for persistent disease after surgery. Radiotherapy is usually reserved as a third-line treatment option in patients who have persistent disease or tumor growth despite surgery or medical therapy [1].

Somatostatin receptor ligands (SRLs) are the cornerstone of medical therapy [1]. However, as monotherapy, SRLs achieve IGF-1 normalization in only approximately 17–35% of unselected cases [7–9], with no differences in efficacy between the two first-generation, long-acting release (LAR) preparations, octreotide (OCT), and lanreotide (LAN) autogel (ATG) [10]. These SRLs have highest affinity to somatostatin receptor subtype 2 (SSTR2). When used as adjunct therapy after surgery, tumor volume reduction is observed in 30–40% of cases [11]. Several tumor characteristics, including sparsely granulated somatotroph adenomas [12, 13], a lack of somatostatin receptor (SSTR) expression [12], and high Ki67, have been shown to predict SRL resistance, affecting approximately 10% of acromegaly patients [14].

D. S. T. Lim
Departments of Endocrinology, Singapore General Hospital, Singapore, Singapore

M. Fleseriu (✉)
Departments of Medicine (Endocrinology, Diabetes and Clinical Nutrition), and Neurological Surgery, and Pituitary Center, Oregon Health & Science University, Portland, OR, USA
e-mail: fleseriu@ohsu.edu

L. S. Blevins Jr., M. K. Aghi (eds.), *Acromegaly*, Contemporary Endocrinology,
https://doi.org/10.1007/978-3-031-16258-9_19

Pasireotide LAR (PAS) is a multireceptor-targeting SRL with higher affinity to SSTR5 compared to SSTR2, SSTR3, and SSTR1. Approximately 20% of patients who are resistant to maximum doses of OCT LAR or LAN ATG achieve biochemical control with PAS [15, 16]. As such PAS is an option for patients who do not respond to first-generation SRLs [17]. The GH receptor antagonist, pegvisomant (PEG), and the dopamine agonist (DA), cabergoline, may also be used as monotherapy. Pegvisomant clinical trial data suggests disease control is achieved in more than 90% of patients with daily subcutaneous (s.c.) PEG injections. However, in longer-term "real-life" studies, IGF-1 normalization is observed in 75% of patients at 2 years and in two thirds at 5 years [18–20]. Results of a recent meta-analysis are consistent with disease control in 72% (64–78.4% [95% confidence interval; CI]) of patients [21]. Conversely, due to a modest effect, cabergoline is considered mainly in patients with mildly elevated IGF-1 (levels up to two times above the upper limit of normal; ULN) [1, 17, 22].

Combination medical therapy is therefore an approach that should be considered when managing those patients who are inadequately controlled after surgery and who are poor SRL monotherapy responders [23, 24]. Additive and possibly synergistic mechanisms are the aim of a combined medical treatment strategy. Results include improved efficacy, while minimizing individual medication side effects, potential dose decreases and/or less frequent s.c. injections, and thereby reduced cost. Combination therapy has also been suggested to be efficacious in selected elderly acromegaly patients [25].

Somatostatin Receptor Ligand and Dopamine Agonist Combination Treatment

Dopamine-2 receptor (D2R) is expressed on both somatomammotroph and pure GH-secreting adenomas and DAs suppress GH secretion in acromegaly. Of the two commercially available DAs, only cabergoline is considered an acromegaly medical treatment as bromocriptine normalizes IGF-1 in only 10% of cases [26]. In contrast, based on a 2011 meta-analysis of five studies, cabergoline monotherapy normalizes IGF-1 in 34% of patients [22]. Greater efficacy was observed in patients with mild IGF-1 elevations, <1.5 times above the ULN.

Several small studies undertaken between the years of 2000 and 2010 demonstrated a beneficial effect of adding cabergoline to SRL treatment in patients with persistent GH excess while on SRL monotherapy [27–31]. Normalization of IGF-1 was observed in 42–56% of patients. Similarly, in the aforementioned meta-analysis, based on individual data derived from 77 patients, IGF-1 normalization was observed in more than half of patients, with a 30% reduction in IGF-1 after 6 months. The addition of cabergoline resulted in a further 22% reduction in IGF-1 beyond that attributable to SRL monotherapy [22]. Similar to monotherapy, a lower baseline IGF-1 was the best predictor of efficacy. Cabergoline doses required in the treatment of acromegaly are, however, two to five times higher (mean 2.5 mg/week) than the usual recommended dose for hyperprolactinemia (0.5–1.0 mg/week).

Some retrospective observational studies have demonstrated more conservative IGF-1 normalization rates of 25–48% with SRL-cabergoline combination therapy [32–34]. Data from prospective studies also suggest lower efficacy rates of between 30 and 40%. In a study by Mattar et al. [35], IGF-1 normalized in 7 of 19 patients (37%) when cabergoline was added, at a maximum dose of 3.5 mg/week, to OCT LAR treatment, with effects persisting at 18 months (range 12–27 months). In another prospective study, Vilar et al. [36] demonstrated IGF-1 normalization in 21 of 52 patients (40.4%) at 6 months, which was sustained at 12 months. Mean cabergoline dose required was 2.2 mg/week, with some patients requiring up to 3 mg/week. Similar to previous studies, a lower baseline IGF-1 of up to 2.2-fold above the ULN was associated with better outcomes.

There is limited data related to tumor volume reduction in patients who are on a combined SRL-cabergoline treatment, and mechanisms resulting in GH suppression are unclear. Baseline prolactin levels, positive immunohistochemical staining for prolactin, and D2R expression have not been shown to predict treatment efficacy [34–36]. Importantly, the efficacy of cabergoline appears to wane with time [37]. This phenomenon was recently highlighted in a large retrospective single-center study of patients treated with cabergoline either as monotherapy or in combination with SRLs. At a median of 34 months (range 3–88 months), disease control was demonstrated in 20/62 patients (32%) on combination therapy with cabergoline (median 2.5 mg/week, range 1.5–2.5 mg/week) and SRLs. However, treatment escape was seen in in six patients (30%) after 38 months (range 10–55 months). Overall, long-term disease control was only observed in 23% at 60 months (range 20–88 months) [38]. Interestingly, in this study, pre-treatment GH, but not IGF-1 levels, predicted response to combination treatment.

Results of a combination study that evaluates oral octreotide capsule (OOC) and cabergoline are published (https://clinicaltrials.gov/ct2/show/NCT02685709) [39, 40]. This is a phase 3, randomized open-label study of patients well controlled on injectable SRLs, who switch to OOC. The study will assess in a sub-analysis, the effectiveness OOC-cabergoline combination in those with inadequate biochemical control on OOC alone in the run-in phase. If successful, this will represent the first available oral combination therapy that may be suitable for some patients.

The synergistic effect of SRLs and DAs has also led to the development of chimeric compounds that bind to both D2R and SSTRs, particularly SSTR2 and SSTR5. A chimeric compound BIM-23A760 was found to suppress GH more effectively than OCT, cabergoline, or the SRL-cabergoline combination, when used in vitro. Further studies, however, demonstrated that it produced interfering metabolites that compete with intrinsic drug activity, resulting in decreased efficacy with repeated injections [41, 42]. Another chimeric compound, BIM-065, has greater potency and efficacy and lacks interfering metabolites. In in vitro studies, BIM-065 has been found to decrease GH secretion and decrease cell viability in GH-secreting adenomas, via increased apoptosis [43]. Further studies in acromegaly patients are needed, but this novel compound may prove to be a promising new option for acromegaly treatment.

Adverse Effects

Adverse effects that are most commonly reported for SRL-cabergoline combination therapy include nausea, headache, postural hypotension, and dizziness. Despite high doses of cabergoline used to treat acromegaly and an inherently increased risk of valvular disease with GH excess, no association has been found between the use of cabergoline and the development of clinically relevant cardiac valve disease (CRVD). In a large cross-sectional and a 4-year longitudinal study, compared to acromegalic controls, patients who received cabergoline did not have a higher prevalence or incidence of valvular regurgitation [44]. Valvular abnormalities seem to be more likely related to acromegaly disease itself than to cabergoline use [2, 45].

Somatostatin Receptor Ligand and Growth Hormone Receptor Antagonist Combined Treatment

Greater efficacy has been reported with a SRL-PEG than a SRL-DA combined treatment therapy, likely owing to the direct effect of GH receptor antagonism in blocking peripheral IGF-1 production. The newest addition to the armamentarium of treatment options is the combination of PAS and PEG. First-generation SRL-PEG and PAS-PEG studies are highlighted in Table 19.1.

Long-Acting First-Generation Somatostatin Receptor Ligands and Pegvisomant (SRL-PEG)

Primary Efficacy Endpoints

In patients with acromegaly who are inadequately controlled with high-dose long-acting SRLs, the addition of PEG at a median once-weekly dose of 60 mg (range 40–80 mg) was first reported in 2005 to normalize IGF-1 at any point in 95% of patients [46]. Subsequently, in one of the largest studies to date, Neggers et al. [47] reported the outcome of 141 patients (mean IGF-1 1.9 × ULN) who had PEG added to SRL their treatment regime and were treated for a median of 4.9 years. Normalization of IGF-1 at any point was observed in 97% of patients with the addition of a median weekly PEG dose of 80 mg (range 60–120 mg). Treatment outcomes were similar in patients who had undergone surgery and in those patients receiving primary medical therapy.

Other multicenter studies, however, have reported lower efficacy rates of 60% at 6–12 months. Van de Lely et al. [48] reported IGF-1 normalization in 79% at any point in the study, but 58% at the 28-week study ended with PEG-LAN. Similarly, in a prospective randomized controlled trial, Trainer et al. [49] demonstrated that

Table 19.1 First-generation somatostatin receptor ligand (SRL)-pegvisomant (PEG) and pasireotide LAR (PAS)-PEG combination studies (adapted from Lim and Fleseriu [24])

Study (year) (patient *n*)	Study design	Prior SRL treatment at time of enrollment	Treatment groups	Study treatments		Insulin-like growth factor-1 normalization[a] (%)		Median weekly effective PEG dose (mg)	Tumor size	Glycemic control	QoL/ symptom improvement	>Threefold elevation in hepatic enzyme with SRL-PEG (%)
				SRL	Pegvisomant	At any time	At study end					
Somatostatin receptor ligand-Pegvisomant add on therapy studies												
Feenstra (2005) (26)	Prospective, OL Duration: 42 weeks Objective: dose-finding, efficacy	≥ 6 months inadequate control	SRL-PEG	LAN 120 mg/ month or OCT 30 mg/ month	Starting dose: 25 mg/week (adjusted q6 weeks until IGF-1 is normal) Maximum dose: 80 mg/week	95	NA	60 (40–80)	No tumor growth seen in all 19 patients with available MRIs	NA	NA	19.2
Neggers (2007) (32)	Prospective, OL Duration: median 138 weeks (range: 35–149) Objective: efficacy and safety	≥ 6 months inadequate control	SRL-PEG	LAN 120 mg/ month or OCT 30 mg/ month	Starting dose: 40 mg/week (adjusted q6weeks until IGF-1 is normal) *Dose reduced if IGF-1 level falls in the lowest quartile* Maximum dose: 160 mg/week	100	NA	60 (range: 40–160)	>25% decrease in 13%[b] No change in size in the remaining	9/10 patients with DM had significant HbA1c decrease that continued after IGF-1 stabilized	Yes	15.6

(continued)

Table 19.1 (continued)

Study (year) (patient n)	Study design	Prior SRL treatment at time of enrollment	Treatment groups	Study treatments		Insulin-like growth factor-1 normalization[a] (%)		Median weekly effective PEG dose (mg)	Tumor size	Glycemic control	QoL/ symptom improvement	>Threefold elevation in hepatic enzyme with SRL-PEG (%)
				SRL	Pegvisomant	At any time	At study end					
Neggers (2009) (86)	Prospective, OL Duration: up to 4.5 years Objective: safety	≥ 6 months inadequate control (n = 63)	SRL-PEG	LAN 120 mg/ month or OCT 30 mg/ month	Starting dose 25 mg/week (n = 19) 40 mg/week (n = 13) Variable starting dose guided by baseline IGF-1 (n = 26)	NA	NA	NA	≥20% decrease in 19%[c] No increase in any patients	NA	NA	15.1
		Controlled on SRL monotherapy (n = 23)			PEG added for QoL Starting dose: 20 mg/week Median dose: 60 mg/week							
van der Lely (2011) (57)	Prospective, OL Duration: up to 28 weeks Objective: efficacy and QoL improvement	≥ 6 months inadequate control[d] (confirmed on a 4-month run-in period)	SRL-PEG	LAN 120 mg/ month	Starting dose: 60 mg/week (adjusted q8weeks until IGF-1 is normal) Maximum dose: 120 mg/week	78.9	57.9	60[e]	>20% decrease in 13.2% >20% increase in 24.5%	Decrease in mean fasting insulin in nondiabetic patients after combination	Yes	11[f]

Neggers (2014) (141)	Prospective, OL Duration: Median 4.9 years (0.5–9.2 years) Objective: long-term efficacy and safety	≥ 6 months inadequate control (n = 112)	SRL-PEG	LAN 120 mg/month or OCT 30 mg/month	Starting dose 25 mg/week (n = 27) 40 mg/week (n = 18) Variable starting dose guided by baseline IGF-1 (n = 67) (adjusted q6–8 weeks until IGF-1 is normal)	97.3	NA	80 (range: 60–120)	≥20% decrease in 16.9%[g] Significant tumor growth In 1 patient who required TSS, followed by RT	NA	NA	15.6
		Controlled on SRL monotherapy (n = 29)			PEG added for QoL Starting dose: 20 mg/week Median dose: 60 mg/week							
Somatostatin receptor ligand-pegvisomant or pasireotide-pegvisomant vs monotherapy comparison studies												
Trainer (2009) (84)	Prospective, OL, randomized Duration: up to 40 weeks Objective: efficacy and safety	≥ 6 months inadequate control	PEG-SRL (n = 29)	OCT varying doses (median 30 mg/month)	Starting dose: 10 mg/day (adjusted in 5mg increments q8weeks until IGF-1 normal) Maximum dose: 30 mg/day Minimum dose: 5 mg/day	73	62	105	≥20% increase in 1 patient on PEG monotherapy	Mean fasting and post-OGTT glucose an HbA1c significantly Lower only in monotherapy group No change in combo group	Yes, in both groups	13.8[h]
		≥ 6 months inadequate control	PEG monotherapy (n = 27)	–		60 (ns)[i]	58 (ns)	140				
		Controlled on SRL monotherapy	SRL monotherapy (n = 28)	OCT varying doses (median 20 mg/month)	–	–		NA				

(continued)

Table 19.1 (continued)

Study (year) (patient *n*)	Study design	Prior SRL treatment at time of enrollment	Treatment groups	Study treatments: SRL	Study treatments: Pegvisomant	Insulin-like growth factor-1 normalization[a] (%): At any time	Insulin-like growth factor-1 normalization[a] (%): At study end	Median weekly effective PEG dose (mg)	Tumor size	Glycemic control	QoL/ symptom improvement	>Threefold elevation in hepatic enzyme with SRL-PEG (%)
Madsen (2011) (18)	Prospective, OL Duration: 24 weeks Objective: Efficacy with reduced SRL dose	Well controlled on SRL monotherapy	SRL monotherapy	LAN 80 mg/ month or OCT 10–30 mg/month	–	NA (comparable IGF-1 at baseline and end of study in both groups)		NA	NA	Similar in both groups	Similar in both groups	17
			SRL-PEG with SRL dose halved	Baseline SRL dose halved	15–30 mg 2×/week			52.5 (range: 30–60)				
Bianchi (2013) (62)	Retrospective, observational, real-life study Duration: 6 years Objective: efficacy and safety	≥ 12 months inadequate control	PEG-SRL (n = 27)	LAN 120 mg/ month or OCT 30 mg/ month	Starting dose: 10 mg/day (adjusted according to IGF-1 by individual managing physicians)	66.7	55.5	140	Decrease: 3.7% vs 0 (ns)	NA	NA	11.1[j]
			PEG monotherapy (*n* = 35)	–		82.8 (ns)	80 (p <0.05)	105 (ns)				
Muhammad (2018) (61)	Prospective, OL Duration: 24 weeks Objective: efficacy of PAS monotherapy or PAS-PEG in patients previously well controlled on SRL-PEG	Well controlled with SRL-PEG (mean 134 mg/ week)	PAS monotherapy	PAS 60 mg/ month	–	93.3		PEG sparing effect of 66%	NA	Rise in FBG (6.1–9.1 mmol/L) Rise in HbA1c (6.1–7.3%) Incidence of DM: 33–69%	NA	Nil
			PAS-PEG	PAS 60 mg/ month	61 mg/week (50% reduction from baseline)	67.4						

Somatostatin receptor ligand-pegvisomant cost-effectiveness studies											
Bonert (2020) (52)	Prospective, randomized Duration: 24–32 weeks Objective: cost-effectiveness of SRL-PEG combination	≥ 3 months controlled on SRL monotherapy (63%) inadequate control (37%)	High-dose SRL + Weekly PEG	LAN 120 mg/month or OCT 30 mg/month	40–160 mg/week	End of study: 93.3	NA	NA	Similar in all groups	NA	5.8
			Low-dose SRL + Weekly PEG	LAN 60 mg/month or OCT 10 mg/month	40–160 mg/week	95.7					
			Low-dose SRL + Daily PEG	LAN 60 mg/month or OCT 10 mg/month	15–60 mg/day	100					
			PAS-PEG	PAS 60 mg/month	61 mg/week (50% reduction from baseline)	67.4					

PAS pasireotide LAR, *PEG* pegvisomant, *SRL* long-acting somatostatin receptor ligand, *QoL* quality of life, *OL* open-label, *LAN* lanreotide, *OCT* octreotide LAR, *OGTT* 75 g oral glucose tolerance test, *NA* not applicable, *ns* not significant

[a]Different study criteria for IGF-1 normalization: defined by either end-of-study IGF-1, or lowest IGF-1 achieved

[b]Previous pituitary surgery: 1/4; primary medical therapy: 3/4; none had radiotherapy

[c]Previous pituitary surgery: 2/14; primary medical therapy: 11/14; one patient had radiotherapy

[d]Inclusion criteria: responders to daily PEG monotherapy (presumed previously uncontrolled on SRL therapy) or partial responders to the highest marketed doses of either PEG at 3 months or SRL at 6 months

[e]Post hoc analysis: eight patients whose mean IGF-1 levels were similar while on pegvisomant monotherapy and during the co-administration period were able to reduce their weekly pegvisomant dose by 50%

[f]Defined as >2 × ULN in this study

[g]None had radiotherapy

[h]2/3 patients with elevations >10 × ULN received OCT 60 mg/28 days; vs 3.7 and 3.5 for PEG and OCT monotherapy, respectively

[i]12/21 patients who did not achieve normal IGF-1 received PEG <20 mg/day

[j]Vs. 14.3 in PEG monotherapy group (ns)

62% of patients on PEG-OCT LAR had a normal IGF-1 at 40 weeks. Interestingly, in this study, there was no difference in efficacy between this group and those randomized to PEG monotherapy. In a recent analysis of the ACROSTUDY (a long-term international observational study of patients taking PEG combined with SRLs), IGF-1 was normal in 62% of patients at 4 years [50]. Of note, however, is that in this real-world clinical study, patients could switch treatment categories, and at 7 years after the start of PEG, only 44% of patients remained in the original PEG-SRL treatment category.

Differences in treatment and efficacy definitions may account for differences in the reported study outcomes. In particular, studies differed with respect to criteria for normal IGF-1 (below 1.2 × ULN vs below 1.0 × ULN) and with regard to efficacy endpoints. Some studies used lowest IGF-1 achieved at any time point during treatment [46, 47], while others used fixed time point or end of study IGF-1 to define efficacy [48–50]. Furthermore, varying study protocols, patient inclusion criteria, dosing regimens, and lack of SRL dose escalation [51] and IGF-1 assays may also have contributed to the observed differences.

Secondary Efficacy Endpoints

One advantage of SRL-PEG combination therapy over switching from SRL to PEG monotherapy is the potential to reduce the PEG dose needed to normalize IGF-1 levels. In the aforementioned randomized controlled trial by Trainer et al., PEG doses were 5 mg/day less (15 mg/day vs 20 mg/day) when used as part of combination therapy, as compared to monotherapy [49]. Van der Lely et al. [48] also showed in post hoc analyses that weekly PEG doses could also be reduced by about half in patients whose IGF-1 levels were similar during PEG monotherapy and combination therapy. In a similar fashion, SRL dosing may also be reduced when PEG is introduced. In one study, the addition of PEG (median dose 52.5 mg/week) allowed a 50% reduction in SRL dose in patients previously well controlled on SRL monotherapy [52]. There is, however, significant inter-individual variation in the PEG dose required to normalize IGF-1 in patients with acromegaly with limited clinical data to specifically guide dosing and titration when PEG is added to a SRL treatment regime. Recently, based on a multivariable prediction model, IGF-1 x ULN (but not GH) and body weight beyond a threshold of 100 kg were found to be positively associated with the normalization dose in patients on combination therapy [53].

The cost effectiveness of SRL-PEG combination therapy has been evaluated in a prospective, randomized, open-label, parallel arm study [54]. Sixty patients stratified by SRL dose required for IGF-1 normalization were randomized to three arms: (Arm A) high-dose SRL (LAN 120 mg or OCT LAR 30 mg, monthly) plus weekly PEG 40–160 mg/week, (Arm B) low-dose SRL (LAN 60 mg or OCT LAR 10 mg, monthly) plus weekly PEG 40–160 mg/week, and (Arm C) low-dose SRL (LAN 60 mg or OCT LAR 10 mg, monthly) plus daily PEG (15–60 mg/day). Low-dose SRL plus weekly PEG was the most cost-effective, achieving IGF-1 normalization in 95.7%, a rate that was independent of previous SRL-responsiveness and similar to the two other treatment arms (93.3% and 100% in Arms A and C, respectively).

Another advantage of a SRL-PEG combination treatment is tumor shrinkage or tumor control [47]. Significant tumor volume reduction (TVR) of >20% has been reported in 13–19% of patients [47, 55–57]. This is in contrast to PEG monotherapy whereby tumor growth has been reported, albeit in the minority of patients [21].

In addition, first-generation SRLs have been found to be effective in reducing headache, and in patients who remain biochemically uncontrolled, the addition of PEG may achieve the goal of IGF-1 normalization, while maintaining the benefits of symptom relief with SRLs [58]. Furthermore, one study showed that the addition of PEG at a weekly dose of 40 mg resulted in improvement in quality of life (QoL) scores in patients already biochemically controlled on first-generation SRLs [59]. In this double-blind, placebo-controlled cross-over study, the addition of PEG improved acromegaly-specific QoL despite an absence of significant IGF-1 changes.

The effects of medical therapies on acromegaly complications are less well established. Most studies demonstrate a modest negative impact of first-generation SRLs on glucose homeostasis [60, 61]. Meta-analyses of prospective interventional studies showed that though the effect on fasting plasma glucose (FPG) was neutral, SRL treatment reduced insulin levels and increased after-load glucose, leading to increased hemoglobin A1c, an effect that was proportionate to IGF-1 and GH lowering [62]. Conversely, PEG improves FPG, glucose tolerance, and hemoglobin A1c in patients when used as monotherapy and in those switched from SRLs to PEG [63–65]. Of note, in a meta-analysis of 13 prospective interventional studies of PEG monotherapy treatment, Feola et al. demonstrated that these positive effects on glucose metabolism were independent of disease control [66].

Compared to SRL monotherapy, several small studies have demonstrated improvements in glucose tolerance with the addition of PEG, but no significant differences in FPG, hemoglobin A1c, insulin resistance, or beta-cell function [52, 67, 68]. In one prospective study of 50 patients, FPG levels were lower during SRL-PEG combination therapy than PEG monotherapy among patients biochemically controlled, declining further with withdrawal of SRL therapy and maintenance of PEG monotherapy. A similar effect on glucose tolerance was observed in patients with active disease [69]. However, in the aforementioned meta-analysis by Feola et al. [66], based on five SRL-PEG studies, besides a decrease in fasting plasma insulin, there was no significant effect on other parameters, signifying that overall, adding PEG may mitigate the negative effect of SRLs on glucose metabolism toward a neutral balance. Somatostatin receptor ligand-PEG combination may therefore be especially beneficial in patients with diabetes who have persistently elevated IGF-1 with either drug when used as monotherapy.

Auriemma et al. [70] reported significant improvement in left ventricular mass index (LVMi) and diastolic function with the addition of PEG to SRL treatment, both at 12 months, and in the long term (5 years). Cardiac structure and performance correlated with PEG dose, but not IGF-1 levels, suggesting a potentially intrinsic role of PEG in blocking cardiac GH receptors, over and above the effects of IGF-1 normalization and improvement in metabolic parameters, with regard to acromegalic cardiomyopathy. The significance of this finding needs further investigation.

Adverse Effects

Transient two- to threefold elevation in liver enzymes has been reported in 11–15% of patients on SRL-PEG combination treatment [47, 48], significantly >1.5–5.2% risk reported with PEG monotherapy in clinical practice studies [18, 19]. Incidence is highest particularly in the first year following treatment and especially in patients on high-dose SRLs [49]. No correlation has, however, been observed between PEG dose and the degree of transaminitis [46, 47]. It is hypothesized that the increase in intrahepatic fat content with combination therapy may account for elevated liver enzymes [52]. Patients with elevations >3 × ULN need close monitoring, and cholelithiasis should be ruled out. Discontinuation of therapy and a liver biopsy is recommended if liver enzymes are more than tenfold elevated [47].

Pasireotide Long-Acting Release and Pegvisomant (PAS-PEG)

Twenty percent of patients resistant to maximum doses of first-generation SRLs may benefit from a switch to PAS monotherapy, achieving biochemical control and an improvement in acromegaly symptom scores [15, 16]. Consistent GH and IGF-1 lowering is seen for up to 6 years [71], and tumor volume reduction is equal or slightly superior compared to the first-generation SRLs [16, 72].

Primary Efficacy Endpoints

A combination of PAS-PEG may, therefore, confer an additional advantage over SRL-PEG. Recently, a PEG-sparing effect has been demonstrated in patients on PAS-PEG combination therapy, as compared to first-generation SRL-PEG combination. In a prospective open-label Pegvisomant and First-Generation Somatostatin Analogues (PAPE Study), patients who were well controlled with SRL-PEG (IGF-1 <1.2 × ULN) were switched to either PAS as monotherapy or a combination with PEG [73]. Mean PEG dose was 134 mg/week at baseline. After a 50% reduction in PEG weekly dose to 60 mg/week, 46/61 (75.4%) patients had elevated IGF-1 (1.59 × ULN), following, which first-generation SRLs were switched to monthly PAS 60 mg. Normalization of IGF-1 was achieved in 31/46 patients (67.4%) at 24 weeks despite the reduced PEG dose. This increased to 71.7% at 48 weeks in an extension study, albeit with 40% achieving <50% PEG dose reduction at that time point [74].

Overall, at 24 weeks, a cumulative 66% PEG-sparing effect was observed with the switch from first-generation SRLs to PAS, which reduced to 52% at 48 weeks.

Secondary Efficacy Endpoints

There is limited data on tumor response with PAS-PEG combination therapy. However, PAS monotherapy studies show that TVR occurs more frequently in patients using PAS than in patients whose disease is inadequately controlled on first-generation SRLs (54% vs 42%), with a 25% TVR observed in the former and 18% reduction observed in the latter [16]. Theoretically, there may, therefore, be a beneficial effect on tumor response compared to patients on SRL-PEG combination [75].

In the PAPE study, authors observed a significant improvement in global AcroQoL with greatest improvements observed in the physical dimension; improvement in QoL was associated mainly with improvement in symptoms of fatigue and headache [75].

A published small case series also highlights the role of PAS-PEG in treatment-resistant acromegaly. Six patients with giant, invasive pituitary adenomas and persistent disease resistant to first-generation SRLs received second-line medical therapy, including SRL-PEG and PAS monotherapy. After failure of all other treatments, biochemical control was finally achieved only through combination therapy with PAS and PEG [76]. Of note, in this case series, a greater SSTR5 and lower SSTR2 expression in the pituitary adenoma was found in those responsive to this combination, as compared to a control of patients resistant to SRLs but controlled with other treatments such as PAS monotherapy, PEG monotherapy, or SRL-PEG. Though in vitro studies suggest a lower SST2/SSTR5 expression in PAS-responders [77], an in vivo study demonstrated that the IGF-1 lowering effects of PAS treatment seemed to be mainly driven by SSTR2 expression as opposed to SSTR5 [78]. Further studies are needed to ascertain which patients will benefit the most from PAS-PEG combination.

Triple combination therapy is rare; however, a combination of PAS, PEG, and cabergoline has been reported to be effective in IGF-1 normalization in a patient resistant to all other treatments [79].

Adverse Effects

While the PAS safety profile is otherwise comparable to first-generation SRLs, PAS is associated with a greater frequency and degree of hyperglycemia-related adverse events [16, 72, 80] that can be explained by its affinity binding. Glucagon-producing pancreatic α-cells predominantly express SSTR2, whereas insulin-producing β-cells mainly express SSTR2 and SSTR5. By binding with high affinity to SSTR5, PAS suppresses insulin secretion, but only modestly inhibits glucagon secretion [81], leading to hyperglycemia. As in PAS monotherapy, hyperglycemia is also commonly encountered with PAS-PEG treatment. In the PAPE study, FPG increased significantly after the start of PAS treatment, rising from 6.1 mmol/L (95% CI 5.9–6.3) to 9.1 mmol/L (95% CI 8.1–10.1), and hemoglobin A1c rising from 6.1% (95% CI 5.9–6.3) to 7.3% (95% CI 6.9–7.7). The incidence of diabetes mellitus doubled from 33% at baseline to 69% after 24 weeks, with baseline hemoglobin A1c being the most important predictor for development of diabetes. Incidence of diabetes increased further to 77% at 48 weeks of treatment. Most patients required treatment with a combination of metformin and a dipeptidyl peptidase 4 (DPP-4) inhibitor. Nine of 59 patients discontinued PAS-LAR due to severe hyperglycemia, which improved after switching back to first-generation SRL-PEG treatment [73, 74]. Of note, no significant elevation in liver enzymes was observed in patients in the PAPE study.

Therefore, the PEG-sparing effect of PAS may be most beneficial to patients without diabetes using low PEG doses (≤80 mg/week) during combination therapy with first-generation SRLs. Close monitoring for hyperglycemia is recommended in all patients treated with PAS. Patients whose disease is biochemically controlled with first-generation SRL-PEG but who develop symptoms toward the fourth week after SRL administration may also have symptomatic relief after switching to PAS-PEG combination [75].

Cabergoline and Pegvisomant Combination Treatment

Limited data is available on cabergoline-PEG (CAB-PEG) combination therapy. In the only prospective trial to date, this combination therapy was found to be more effective than either drug used alone [82]. Twenty-four patients with active disease (mean IGF-1 1.8 × ULN) on no treatment or after withdrawal of DAs or SRLs were treated with cabergoline monotherapy titrated to a maximum dose of 3.5 mg/week. Only two achieved normal IGF-1 levels after 18 weeks. The addition of PEG 10 mg/day for 12 weeks normalized IGF-1 in 13 (68%). When cabergoline was withdrawn, only five patients (26%) continued to have normal IGF-1 levels and demonstrated greater efficacy with the combination than either treatment as monotherapy.

In another retrospective observational study, 14 patients partially resistant to first-generation SRLs and with elevated IGF-1 (median 1.6 × ULN) were placed on PEG monotherapy (mean 20 mg/day) [83]. The addition of cabergoline (final dose 1.5 mg/week) normalized IGF-1 in 4 patients (28%) after 18 months. It should be noted that all four had received prior radiotherapy. The relatively lower dose of cabergoline used, as compared to that commonly required in acromegaly, may account for the lower efficacy observed in this study. The nadir IGF-1 achieved, but not the rate of IGF-1 normalization was significantly associated with baseline prolactin levels. No significant TVR was observed in this study. Based on the ACROSTUDY [50], at 4 years, IGF-1 normalization in patients on CAB-PEG was similar to patients on SRL-PEG combination treatments (63% and 62%, respectively), though as previously noted, patients could switch between treatment categories.

Overall, as compared to PEG monotherapy, an increased use of combination therapy with SRLs or DA has increased, from 20% in 2003 to 54% in 2012. No significant impact on hepatic function has been reported with this CAB-PEG combination treatment and, overall, appears to be well-tolerated [82, 83]. While no data is available, based on PEG monotherapy studies, a CAB-PEG combination treatment is likely to have a neutral, if not positive, effect on glycemic control.

Conclusion

The management of patients with acromegaly who are inadequately controlled after surgery and first-line medical therapy with first-generation SRLs remains challenging. While further SRL dose optimization, tumor debulking, or switching to PAS or PEG monotherapy may be options, combination therapy should also be considered. In particular, first-generation SRL-PEG combination treatment leads to good biochemical control in the majority and is recommended in patients with no significant response to first-generation SRLs. In those who respond well, reduction in individual drug dosage and frequency of subcutaneous PEG injections may be possible thereafter, which may be both cost-effective and improve QoL. Availability of OOC might increase combination therapy use as patients will only require one injectable therapy. Furthermore, in patients with mild deterioration in glycemic control with first-generation SRLs, the addition of PEG may negate this effect. As compared to PEG monotherapy, this combination may also provide additional symptom relief and TVR and may be considered in patients with large remnant tumor volumes.

In patients with uncontrolled disease, tumor growth, or persistent symptoms despite high doses of first-generation SRL-PEG, switching to PAS-PEG is a viable option. A PEG-sparing effect may also be observed in patients taking SRL-PEG on low PEG doses of 80 mg/week or less, if switched to PAS-PEG. This again allows for a reduction in PEG dose and injection frequency. These benefits, however, have to be balanced against the propensity of the PAS-PEG combination to worsen glycemic control and may not be suitable in patients with underlying diabetes mellitus.

The addition of the relatively inexpensive, well-tolerated, and orally administered cabergoline to SRL treatment is most likely to be effective in patients with mild IGF-1 elevations 1.5–2 × ULN, though patients will need to be monitored for treatment escape. While less data is available, the combination of PEG and cabergoline may be useful in a subset of patients with mild IGF-1 elevations, particularly in the setting of SRL-intolerance, if the cost of SRL-PEG is prohibitive, or in patients with poorly controlled diabetes.

Ultimately, individualization remains key to the management of patients with acromegaly and patient characteristics, including disease activity, tumor volume and location, symptoms and comorbidities, patient preferences, and QoL, and the cost effectiveness of combination therapy needs to be considered [84].

Conflict of Interest MF has received research support to OHSU as a principal investigator from Chiasma, Crinetics, Ionis, Novartis and has received occasional scientific consulting from Chiasma, Crinetics, Ionis, Ipsen, Novartis, Pfizer, Recordati.

DSTL has no conflict of interests.

Funding No funding was received for this work.

References

1. Katznelson L, Laws ER Jr, Melmed S, Molitch ME, Murad MH, Utz A, et al. Acromegaly: an endocrine society clinical practice guideline. J Clin Endocrinol Metab. 2014;99(11):3933–51.
2. Gadelha MR, Kasuki L, Lim DST, Fleseriu M. Systemic complications of acromegaly and the impact of the current treatment landscape: an update. Endocr Rev. 2019;40(1):268–332.
3. Melmed S. Acromegaly pathogenesis and treatment. J Clin Invest. 2009;119(11):3189–202.
4. Melmed S. Pituitary-tumor endocrinopathies. N Engl J Med. 2020;382(10):937–50.
5. Jane JA Jr, Starke RM, Elzoghby MA, Reames DL, Payne SC, Thorner MO, et al. Endoscopic transsphenoidal surgery for acromegaly: remission using modern criteria, complications, and predictors of outcome. J Clin Endocrinol Metab. 2011;96(9):2732–40.
6. Starke RM, Raper DM, Payne SC, Vance ML, Oldfield EH, Jane JA Jr. Endoscopic vs microsurgical transsphenoidal surgery for acromegaly: outcomes in a concurrent series of patients using modern criteria for remission. J Clin Endocrinol Metab. 2013;98(8):3190–8.
7. Caron PJ, Bevan JS, Petersenn S, Flanagan D, Tabarin A, Prevost G, et al. Tumor shrinkage with lanreotide Autogel 120 mg as primary therapy in acromegaly: results of a prospective multicenter clinical trial. J Clin Endocrinol Metab. 2014;99(4):1282–90.
8. Howlett TA, Willis D, Walker G, Wass JA, Trainer PJ, Group UKARS. Control of growth hormone and IGF1 in patients with acromegaly in the UK: responses to medical treatment with somatostatin analogues and dopamine agonists. Clin Endocrinol. 2013;79(5):689–99.
9. Mercado M, Borges F, Bouterfa H, Chang TC, Chervin A, Farrall AJ, et al. A prospective, multicentre study to investigate the efficacy, safety and tolerability of octreotide LAR (long-acting repeatable octreotide) in the primary therapy of patients with acromegaly. Clin Endocrinol. 2007;66(6):859–68.
10. Carmichael JD, Bonert VS, Nuno M, Ly D, Melmed S. Acromegaly clinical trial methodology impact on reported biochemical efficacy rates of somatostatin receptor ligand treatments: a meta-analysis. J Clin Endocrinol Metab. 2014;99(5):1825–33.
11. Mazziotti G, Giustina A. Effects of lanreotide SR and Autogel on tumor mass in patients with acromegaly: a systematic review. Pituitary. 2010;13(1):60–7.
12. Brzana J, Yedinak CG, Gultekin SH, Delashaw JB, Fleseriu M. Growth hormone granulation pattern and somatostatin receptor subtype 2A correlate with postoperative somatostatin receptor ligand response in acromegaly: a large single center experience. Pituitary. 2013;16(4):490–8.
13. Varlamov EV, Wood MD, Netto JP, Thiessen J, Kim J, Lim DST, et al. Cystic appearance on magnetic resonance imaging in bihormonal growth hormone and prolactin tumors in acromegaly. Pituitary. 2020;23(6):672–80.
14. Colao A, Auriemma RS, Lombardi G, Pivonello R. Resistance to somatostatin analogs in acromegaly. Endocr Rev. 2011;32(2):247–71.
15. Bronstein MD, Fleseriu M, Neggers S, Colao A, Sheppard M, Gu F, et al. Switching patients with acromegaly from octreotide to pasireotide improves biochemical control: crossover extension to a randomized, double-blind, Phase III study. BMC Endocr Disord. 2016;16:16.
16. Gadelha MR, Bronstein MD, Brue T, Coculescu M, Fleseriu M, Guitelman M, et al. Pasireotide versus continued treatment with octreotide or lanreotide in patients with inadequately controlled acromegaly (PAOLA): a randomised, phase 3 trial. Lancet Diabetes Endocrinol. 2014;2(11):875–84.

17. Melmed S, Bronstein MD, Chanson P, Klibanski A, Casanueva FF, Wass JAH, et al. A consensus statement on acromegaly therapeutic outcomes. Nat Rev Endocrinol. 2018;14(9):552–61.
18. Freda PU, Gordon MB, Kelepouris N, Jonsson P, Koltowska-Haggstrom M, van der Lely AJ. Long-term treatment with pegvisomant as monotherapy in patients with acromegaly: experience from acrostudy. Endocr Pract. 2015;21(3):264–74.
19. Schreiber I, Buchfelder M, Droste M, Forssmann K, Mann K, Saller B, et al. Treatment of acromegaly with the GH receptor antagonist pegvisomant in clinical practice: safety and efficacy evaluation from the German Pegvisomant Observational Study. Eur J Endocrinol. 2007;156(1):75–82.
20. van der Lely AJ, Hutson RK, Trainer PJ, Besser GM, Barkan AL, Katznelson L, et al. Long-term treatment of acromegaly with pegvisomant, a growth hormone receptor antagonist. Lancet. 2001;358(9295):1754–9.
21. Leonart LP, Tonin FS, Ferreira VL, Fernandez-Llimos F, Pontarolo R. Effectiveness and safety of pegvisomant: a systematic review and meta-analysis of observational longitudinal studies. Endocrine. 2019;63(1):18–26.
22. Sandret L, Maison P, Chanson P. Place of cabergoline in acromegaly: a meta-analysis. J Clin Endocrinol Metab. 2011;96(5):1327–35.
23. Fleseriu M. The role of combination medical therapy in acromegaly: hope for the nonresponsive patient. Curr Opin Endocrinol Diabetes Obes. 2013;20(4):321–9.
24. Lim DS, Fleseriu M. The role of combination medical therapy in the treatment of acromegaly. Pituitary. 2017;20(1):136–48.
25. Ambrosio MR, Gagliardi I, Chiloiro S, Ferreira AG, Bondanelli M, Giampietro A, et al. Acromegaly in the elderly patients. Endocrine. 2020;68(1):16–31.
26. Jaffe CA, Barkan AL. Treatment of acromegaly with dopamine agonists. Endocrinol Metab Clin N Am. 1992;21(3):713–35.
27. Cozzi R, Attanasio R, Lodrini S, Lasio G. Cabergoline addition to depot somatostatin analogues in resistant acromegalic patients: efficacy and lack of predictive value of prolactin status. Clin Endocrinol. 2004;61(2):209–15.
28. Gatta B, Hau DH, Catargi B, Roger P, Tabarin A. Re-evaluation of the efficacy of the association of cabergoline to somatostatin analogues in acromegalic patients. Clin Endocrinol. 2005;63(4):477–8.
29. Jallad RS, Bronstein MD. Optimizing medical therapy of acromegaly: beneficial effects of cabergoline in patients uncontrolled with long-acting release octreotide. Neuroendocrinology. 2009;90(1):82–92.
30. Marzullo P, Ferone D, Di Somma C, Pivonello R, Filippella M, Lombardi G, et al. Efficacy of combined treatment with lanreotide and cabergoline in selected therapy-resistant acromegalic patients. Pituitary. 1999;1(2):115–20.
31. Selvarajah D, Webster J, Ross R, Newell-Price J. Effectiveness of adding dopamine agonist therapy to long-acting somatostatin analogues in the management of acromegaly. Eur J Endocrinol. 2005;152(4):569–74.
32. Puig-Domingo M, Soto A, Venegas E, Vilchez R, Blanco C, Cordido F, et al. Use of lanreotide in combination with cabergoline or pegvisomant in patients with acromegaly in the clinical practice: the ACROCOMB study. Endocrinol Nutr. 2016;63(8):397–408.
33. Vandeva S, Elenkova A, Natchev E, Kirilov G, Tcharaktchiev D, Yaneva M, et al. Treatment outcome results from the Bulgarian Acromegaly Database: adjuvant dopamine agonist therapy is efficient in less than one fifth of non-irradiated patients. Exp Clin Endocrinol Diabetes. 2015;123(1):66–71.
34. Suda K, Inoshita N, Iguchi G, Fukuoka H, Takahashi M, Nishizawa H, et al. Efficacy of combined octreotide and cabergoline treatment in patients with acromegaly: a retrospective clinical study and review of the literature. Endocr J. 2013;60(4):507–15.
35. Mattar P, Alves Martins MR, Abucham J. Short- and long-term efficacy of combined cabergoline and octreotide treatment in controlling igf-I levels in acromegaly. Neuroendocrinology. 2010;92(2):120–7.

36. Vilar L, Azevedo MF, Naves LA, Casulari LA, Albuquerque JL, Montenegro RM, et al. Role of the addition of cabergoline to the management of acromegalic patients resistant to longterm treatment with octreotide LAR. Pituitary. 2011;14(2):148–56.
37. Freda PU, Reyes CM, Nuruzzaman AT, Sundeen RE, Khandji AG, Post KD. Cabergoline therapy of growth hormone & growth hormone/prolactin secreting pituitary tumors. Pituitary. 2004;7(1):21–30.
38. Kasuki L, Dalmolin MD, Wildemberg LE, Gadelha MR. Treatment escape reduces the effectiveness of cabergoline during long-term treatment of acromegaly in monotherapy or in association with first-generation somatostatin receptor ligands. Clin Endocrinol. 2018;88(6):889–95.
39. Fleseriu M, Katznelson L, Clemmons DR, Trainer P, Biermasz NR, Strasburger CJ, et al. Mpowered: study design of a phase 3 head-to-head trial evaluating oral octreotide capsules versus injectable somatostatin analogs in patients with acromegaly. Endocr Pract. 2016;22(2):193–226.
40. https://pubmed.ncbi.nlm.nih.gov/34953531/.
41. Ferone D, Saveanu A, Culler MD, Arvigo M, Rebora A, Gatto F, et al. Novel chimeric somatostatin analogs: facts and perspectives. Eur J Endocrinol. 2007;156(1):S23–8.
42. Jaquet P, Gunz G, Saveanu A, Barlier A, Dufour H, Taylor J, et al. BIM-23A760, a chimeric molecule directed towards somatostatin and dopamine receptors, vs universal somatostatin receptors ligands in GH-secreting pituitary adenomas partial responders to octreotide. J Endocrinol Investig. 2005;28(11):21–7.
43. Vázquez-Borrego MC, Gálvez-Moreno MA, Fuentes-Fayos AC, Venegas-Moreno E, Herrera-Martínez AD, et al. A new generation somatostatin-dopamine analogue exerts potent antitumoral actions on pituitary neuroendocrine tumor cells. Neuroendocrinology. 2020;110(1-2):70–82.
44. Maione L, Garcia C, Bouchachi A, Kallel N, Maison P, Salenave S, et al. No evidence of a detrimental effect of cabergoline therapy on cardiac valves in patients with acromegaly. J Clin Endocrinol Metab. 2012;97(9):1714–9.
45. Kuhn E, Chanson P. Cabergoline in acromegaly. Pituitary. 2017;20(1):121–8.
46. Feenstra J, de Herder WW, ten Have SM, van den Beld AW, Feelders RA, Janssen JA, et al. Combined therapy with somatostatin analogues and weekly pegvisomant in active acromegaly. Lancet. 2005;365(9471):1644–6.
47. Neggers SJ, Franck SE, de Rooij FW, Dallenga AH, Poublon RM, Feelders RA, et al. Long-term efficacy and safety of pegvisomant in combination with long-acting somatostatin analogs in acromegaly. J Clin Endocrinol Metab. 2014;99(10):3644–52.
48. van der Lely AJ, Bernabeu I, Cap J, Caron P, Colao A, Marek J, et al. Coadministration of lanreotide Autogel and pegvisomant normalizes IGF1 levels and is well tolerated in patients with acromegaly partially controlled by somatostatin analogs alone. Eur J Endocrinol. 2011;164(3):325–33.
49. Trainer PJ, Ezzat S, D'Souza GA, Layton G, Strasburger CJ. A randomized, controlled, multicentre trial comparing pegvisomant alone with combination therapy of pegvisomant and long-acting octreotide in patients with acromegaly. Clin Endocrinol. 2009;71(4):549–57.
50. Strasburger CJ, Mattsson A, Wilton P, Aydin F, Hey-Hadavi J, Biller BMK. Increasing frequency of combination medical therapy in the treatment of acromegaly with the GH receptor antagonist pegvisomant. Eur J Endocrinol. 2018;178(4):321–9.
51. Fleseriu M. Clinical efficacy and safety results for dose escalation of somatostatin receptor ligands in patients with acromegaly: a literature review. Pituitary. 2011;14(2):184–93.
52. Madsen M, Poulsen PL, Orskov H, Moller N, Jorgensen JO. Cotreatment with pegvisomant and a somatostatin analog (SA) in SA-responsive acromegalic patients. J Clin Endocrinol Metab. 2011;96(8):2405–13.
53. Franck SE, Korevaar TIM, Petrossians P, Daly AF, Chanson P, Jaffrain-Rea ML, et al. A multivariable prediction model for pegvisomant dosing: monotherapy and in combination with long-acting somatostatin analogues. Eur J Endocrinol. 2017;176(4):421–31.
54. Bonert V, Mirocha J, Carmichael J, Yuen KCJ, Araki T, Melmed S. Cost-effectiveness and efficacy of a novel combination regimen in acromegaly: a prospective, randomized trial. J Clin Endocrinol Metab. 2020;105(9):444.

55. Bianchi A, Valentini F, Iuorio R, Poggi M, Baldelli R, Passeri M, et al. Long-term treatment of somatostatin analog-refractory growth hormone-secreting pituitary tumors with pegvisomant alone or combined with long-acting somatostatin analogs: a retrospective analysis of clinical practice and outcomes. J Exp Clin Cancer Res. 2013;32:40.
56. Neggers SJ, de Herder WW, Janssen JA, Feelders RA, van der Lely AJ. Combined treatment for acromegaly with long-acting somatostatin analogs and pegvisomant: long-term safety for up to 4.5 years (median 2.2 years) of follow-up in 86 patients. Eur J Endocrinol. 2009;160(4):529–33.
57. Neggers SJ, van Aken MO, Janssen JA, Feelders RA, de Herder WW, van der Lely AJ. Long-term efficacy and safety of combined treatment of somatostatin analogs and pegvisomant in acromegaly. J Clin Endocrinol Metab. 2007;92(12):4598–601.
58. Kreitschmann-Andermahr I, Siegel S, Weber Carneiro R, Maubach JM, Harbeck B, Brabant G. Headache and pituitary disease: a systematic review. Clin Endocrinol. 2013;79(6):760–9.
59. Neggers SJ, van Aken MO, de Herder WW, Feelders RA, Janssen JA, Badia X, et al. Quality of life in acromegalic patients during long-term somatostatin analog treatment with and without pegvisomant. J Clin Endocrinol Metab. 2008;93(10):3853–9.
60. Grasso LF, Auriemma RS, Pivonello R, Colao A. Adverse events associated with somatostatin analogs in acromegaly. Expert Opin Drug Saf. 2015;14(8):1213–26.
61. Mazziotti G, Floriani I, Bonadonna S, Torri V, Chanson P, Giustina A. Effects of somatostatin analogs on glucose homeostasis: a metaanalysis of acromegaly studies. J Clin Endocrinol Metab. 2009;94(5):1500–8.
62. Cozzolino A, Feola T, Simonelli I, Puliani G, Pozza C, Giannetta E, et al. Somatostatin analogs and glucose metabolism in acromegaly: a meta-analysis of prospective interventional studies. J Clin Endocrinol Metab. 2018. https://doi.org/10.1210/jc.2017-02566
63. Barkan AL, Burman P, Clemmons DR, Drake WM, Gagel RF, Harris PE, et al. Glucose homeostasis and safety in patients with acromegaly converted from long-acting octreotide to pegvisomant. J Clin Endocrinol Metab. 2005;90(10):5684–91.
64. Drake WM, Rowles SV, Roberts ME, Fode FK, Besser GM, Monson JP, et al. Insulin sensitivity and glucose tolerance improve in patients with acromegaly converted from depot octreotide to pegvisomant. Eur J Endocrinol. 2003;149(6):521–7.
65. Higham CE, Rowles S, Russell-Jones D, Umpleby AM, Trainer PJ. Pegvisomant improves insulin sensitivity and reduces overnight free fatty acid concentrations in patients with acromegaly. J Clin Endocrinol Metab. 2009;94(7):2459–63.
66. Feola T, Cozzolino A, Simonelli I, Sbardella E, Pozza C, Giannetta E, et al. Pegvisomant improves glucose metabolism in acromegaly: a meta-analysis of prospective interventional studies. J Clin Endocrinol Metab. 2019;104(7):2892–902.
67. De Marinis L, Bianchi A, Fusco A, Cimino V, Mormando M, Tilaro L, et al. Long-term effects of the combination of pegvisomant with somatostatin analogs (SSA) on glucose homeostasis in non-diabetic patients with active acromegaly partially resistant to SSA. Pituitary. 2007;10(3):227–32.
68. Jorgensen JO, Feldt-Rasmussen U, Frystyk J, Chen JW, Kristensen LO, Hagen C, et al. Cotreatment of acromegaly with a somatostatin analog and a growth hormone receptor antagonist. J Clin Endocrinol Metab. 2005;90(10):5627–31.
69. Urbani C, Sardella C, Calevro A, Rossi G, Scattina I, Lombardi M, et al. Effects of medical therapies for acromegaly on glucose metabolism. Eur J Endocrinol. 2013;169(1):99–108.
70. Auriemma RS, Grasso LF, Galdiero M, Galderisi M, Pivonello C, Simeoli C, et al. Effects of long-term combined treatment with somatostatin analogues and pegvisomant on cardiac structure and performance in acromegaly. Endocrine. 2017;55(3):872–84.
71. Colao A, Bronstein MD, Brue T, De Marinis L, Fleseriu M, Guitelman M, et al. Pasireotide for acromegaly: long-term outcomes from an extension to the Phase III PAOLA study. Eur J Endocrinol. 2020;182(6):583.
72. Colao A, Bronstein MD, Freda P, Gu F, Shen CC, Gadelha M, et al. Pasireotide versus octreotide in acromegaly: a head-to-head superiority study. J Clin Endocrinol Metab. 2014;99(3):791–9.

73. Muhammad A, van der Lely AJ, Delhanty PJD, Dallenga AHG, Haitsma IK, Janssen J, et al. Efficacy and safety of switching to pasireotide in patients with acromegaly controlled with pegvisomant and first-generation somatostatin analogues (PAPE Study). J Clin Endocrinol Metab. 2018;103(2):586–95.
74. Muhammad A, Coopmans EC, Delhanty PJD, Dallenga AHG, Haitsma IK, Janssen J, et al. Efficacy and safety of switching to pasireotide in acromegaly patients controlled with pegvisomant and somatostatin analogues: PAPE extension study. Eur J Endocrinol. 2018;179(5):269–77.
75. Coopmans EC, Muhammad A, van der Lely AJ, Janssen J, Neggers S. How to position pasireotide LAR treatment in acromegaly. J Clin Endocrinol Metab. 2019;104(6):1978–88.
76. Chiloiro S, Bima C, Tartaglione T, Giampietro A, Gessi M, Lauretti L, et al. Pasireotide and pegvisomant combination treatment in acromegaly resistant to second-line therapies: a longitudinal study. J Clin Endocrinol Metab. 2019;104(11):5478–82.
77. Gatto F, Feelders RA, Franck SE, van Koetsveld PM, Dogan F, Kros JM, et al. In vitro head-to-head comparison between octreotide and pasireotide in GH-secreting pituitary adenomas. J Clin Endocrinol Metab. 2017;102(6):2009–18.
78. Muhammad A, Coopmans EC, Gatto F, Franck SE, Janssen J, van der Lely AJ, et al. Pasireotide responsiveness in acromegaly is mainly driven by somatostatin receptor subtype 2 expression. J Clin Endocrinol Metab. 2019;104(3):915–24.
79. Ciresi A, Radellini S, Guarnotta V, Giordano C. Efficacy of combined treatment with pasireotide, pegvisomant and cabergoline in an acromegalic patient resistant to other treatments: a case report. BMC Endocr Disord. 2018;18(1):2.
80. Fleseriu M, Rusch E, Geer EB, Investigators AS. Safety and tolerability of pasireotide long-acting release in acromegaly-results from the acromegaly, open-label, multicenter, safety monitoring program for treating patients who have a need to receive medical therapy (ACCESS) study. Endocrine. 2017;55(1):247–55.
81. Henry RR, Ciaraldi TP, Armstrong D, Burke P, Ligueros-Saylan M, Mudaliar S. Hyperglycemia associated with pasireotide: results from a mechanistic study in healthy volunteers. J Clin Endocrinol Metab. 2013;98(8):3446–53.
82. Higham CE, Atkinson AB, Aylwin S, Bidlingmaier M, Drake WM, Lewis A, et al. Effective combination treatment with cabergoline and low-dose pegvisomant in active acromegaly: a prospective clinical trial. J Clin Endocrinol Metab. 2012;97(4):1187–93.
83. Bernabeu I, Alvarez-Escola C, Paniagua AE, Lucas T, Pavon I, Cabezas-Agricola JM, et al. Pegvisomant and cabergoline combination therapy in acromegaly. Pituitary. 2013;16(1):101–8.
84. https://pubmed.ncbi.nlm.nih.gov/33079318/.

Chapter 20
Long-Term Follow-up of Patients with Acromegaly

Lewis S. Blevins Jr.

A lot has changed in the more than three decades since I first started caring for patients with acromegaly. In the early 1990s, most patients underwent surgery and received radiotherapy as adjuvant treatment. Bromocriptine was then the only drug available to treat patients with residual and recurrent disease, and it normalized IGF-1 levels in only about 15% of patients [1]. Long-term follow-up and management focused on control of tumor and, mostly, management of the comorbidities of disease in those with active acromegaly. Today, because of a combination of advances in surgical therapy leading to improved remission rates, radiotherapy to control residual tumor, and with several classes of drugs available to treat patients with residual and recurrent disease, we are now able to achieve and maintain control of tumor growth and GH and IGF-1 levels in a majority of patients. These abilities are despite current recommendations that call for tighter control than was required three decades ago. The natural history of treated acromegaly has changed. While we still see occasional patients with significant morbidity due to the disorder, one encounters these dastardly complications with less frequency due to the development of effective treatments. In fact, most of my recent patients with cardiac disorders or severe arthropathy requiring joint replacement had complications because of a considerable delay in diagnosis rather than due to persistent disease after treatment. I will say, however, that all patients with acromegaly, whether they enter remission after initial surgery or have residual or recurrent disease requiring multimodal therapy, require long-term follow-up (lifetime) for several important reasons.

There are several reasons it is difficult to gain true estimates regarding the remission and recurrence rates after surgery in patients with acromegaly. Much of the variance in the literature is related to the experience levels of the surgeon's reporting their outcomes. Some of the differences are related to the variable criteria used to define a successful surgical procedure. Laboratory assays employed over time also

L. S. Blevins Jr. (✉)
Department of Neurological Surgery, University of California, San Francisco, CA, USA
e-mail: lewis.blevins@ucsf.edu

L. S. Blevins Jr., M. K. Aghi (eds.), *Acromegaly*, Contemporary Endocrinology,
https://doi.org/10.1007/978-3-031-16258-9_20

affect the results. Further, longitudinal follow-up studies are of different lengths of time, and many are not of sufficient duration to make any real inferences as to actual recurrence rates. Silverstein wrote "a substantial number of patients (48.0–72.4%) will have persistent acromegaly despite treatment with surgery, medical therapy, and/or radiotherapy and ~2–8% of patients who achieve remission with surgery will experience disease recurrence within 5 years" [2]. So, what do we tell our patients? How do we proceed? It's actually very simple and straightforward. I tell all patients they may have residual or recurrent disease after surgery, and they require lifetime follow-up. I am, however, able to make some generalizations based on my experiences with a small number of excellent surgeons. I have included these estimates in Table 20.1 as an example of the information that I provide to my patients so that I may manage their expectations. While most patients with acromegaly experience recurrences within 5 years, I've seen patients recur more than a decade after initial successful surgery illustrating the need for long-term follow-up.

Responses to radiotherapy in patients with acromegaly are highly variable and seem to depend on tumor size, biology, and other unknown factors. It is conceivable that success and even the time to normalization of IGF-1 is also dependent on whether the entire tumor was irradiated as there are patients who have recurrent disease in an area of the original tumor bed where stereotactic radiosurgery to residual disease might have not been administered. It's tempting to compare stereotactic radiosurgery to conventional radiotherapy, but there is inherent bias in patient selection for one modality or the other based on tumor size and proximity to vital structures, so the comparisons are invalid. In general, three-fourths of patients who receive conventional radiotherapy will normalize IGF-1 levels within a 10- to 20-year period after treatment [3]. Following Gamma Knife radiosurgery, as many as three-fourths of patients will normalize IGF-1 levels within 15 years and half will do so by about 7 years after treatment. I have seen patients with minimal disease treated with Gamma Knife radiosurgery who have required medical therapy for 12 years and others with large tumors who received conventional radiotherapy who required therapy for less than 5 years. Long-term tumor control is achieved in most patients provided that all viable residual or recurrent tumor is irradiated. These approximations are useful in educating patients and in planning for ongoing assessments of disease activity in medically treated patients. My approach in these patients has been to follow the IGF-1 level at 6-month intervals once stability on medical therapy has been achieved. When the IGF-1 starts to decline from a treatment

Table 20.1 Likelihood of remission in acromegaly after surgery based on tumor characteristics

Tumor characteristics	Likelihood of remission (%)
Intrasellar microadenoma	92–97
Intrasellar macroadenoma	87–95
Suprasellar macroadenoma	70–90
Macroadenoma invading medial cavernous sinus	40–50
Macroadenoma invading lateral to carotid artery	0
Macroadenoma >4 cm	0

average level, I presume the patient is responding to radiotherapy. Then, I taper medical therapy as able, and, when the IGF-1 level remains controlled on the lowest dose of medication, I discontinue therapy and follow the IGF-1 at monthly intervals for a year then twice a year thereafter. If the level rises to above the third quartile of the normal range and the patient develops symptoms of active acromegaly, I reinitiate medical treatment at the lowest dose that was providing control. Obviously, treatment is resumed in those patients in whom the IGF-1 exceeds the upper limit of normal during a period of follow-up. I usually discontinue medical therapy and reassess over time in those patients whose IGF-1 levels fall below the lower limit of the normal range. Once a patient has demonstrated a response but still requires medical therapy, I often withdraw therapy annually and assess the need for continued medical therapy. Invariably, a patient will simply no longer require medical therapy and then can be followed every 6 months for a couple of years and then annually provided they maintain normal IGF-1 levels.

Magnetic resonance imaging of the sella should be performed only when clinically indicated [4]. In patients with residual or recurrent disease, I tend to perform imaging studies only when it is necessary to assess for tumor growth or else regression in response to treatment. Frankly, the choice to do imaging should be made according to need; there are no specific guidelines for performance of serial imaging in these patients since every single patient is different from the others affected with acromegaly. In patients who have been rendered disease free or are in remission, I favor deciding on follow-up imaging based on the results of GH and IGF-1 levels. A rise or elevation in one of these parameters of disease activity and, especially, if there is failure of GH to suppress in response to oral glucose should prompt imaging to assess for recurrent tumor. I am more inclined to do regular imaging in those in remission after treatment of residual or recurrent disease.

I tend to follow GH and IGF-1 levels every 6 months for a few years then annually for life in patients who achieve remission after therapy. I've learned that biochemical presence of disease oft precedes any abnormalities that may be seen on imaging studies. Rises in GH alone are evaluated further with the assessment of GH after an oral glucose load. IGF-1 levels that continue to rise through the normal range, and, especially, if associated with symptoms consistent with acromegaly, should be considered as a sign of recurrent disease. Patients with discordant IGF-1 and GH levels should be evaluated carefully and followed long-term to determine the best time to intervene [5]. These biochemical parameters are assessed more regularly but on an as-needed basis in patients on medical therapy.

The long-term follow-up of patients with acromegaly should also include periodic assessments for complications of treatment. Hypopituitarism and diabetes insipidus are just two of the common complications that may result from surgery and necessitate treatment [6]. Patients who have received radiotherapy and especially in the setting of having had large tumors and multiple surgical procedures should undergo annual screening to evaluate pituitary functions since there is a risk of radiation-induced hypopituitarism in a significant number of patients. Replacement therapy may be required, and treatment should be assessed in a manner, combining clinical and laboratory assessments, to ensure that specific hormone replacement therapy is optimized. Some patients develop clinically important GH deficiency, and replacement therapy should be considered in the absence of contraindications to treatment. Though rare, second neoplasm and vascular malformations may complicate radiotherapy and should be considered in symptomatic patients who received conventional radiotherapy. Medications used to treat acromegaly are not without side effects. Treating physicians should familiarize themselves with the relevant side effects and assess treated patients regularly for symptoms and signs of a variety of complications specific to the drugs employed in the management of these patients.

Importantly, follow-up must include surveillance for complications of long-standing or poorly controlled acromegaly [7]. Many patients in remission for will require treatment for one or more comorbidities of their disease as the consequences of GH and IGF = 1 excess are not fully reversed after successful treatment. In fact, many of these, such as the arthropathies, inexorably progress despite remission. Some patients require ongoing evaluation and management of conditions such as diabetes mellitus, hypertension, osteopenia, osteoporosis, nephrolithiasis, cardiac failure, colon polyposis, sleep apnea, and psychosocial consequences of their disorder. I've seen patients with acromegaly who have suffered from various malignancies including those of the skin, gastrointestinal tract, genitourinary tract, lung, and breast. While I don't recommend any particular screening schedules for malignancy, treating physicians should individualize their recommendations to individual patients based on factors such as age, other risk factors and disease processes, family history, duration of disease, etc.

References

1. Jaffe CA, Barkan AL. Treatment of acromegaly with dopamine agonists. Endocrinol Metab Clin N Am. 1992;21:713–35.
2. Silverstein JM. Need for improved monitoring in patients with acromegaly. Endocr Connect. 2015;4:59–67.
3. Knappe UJ, Petroff D, Quinkler M, Schmid SM, Schofl C, Schopohl J, Stieg MR, Tonjes A. Fractionated radiotherapy and radiosurgery in acromegaly: analysis of 352 patients from the German Acromegaly Registry. Eur J Endocrinol. 2020;182:275–84.
4. Puig-Domingo M, Resmini E, Gomez-Anson B, Nicolau J, Mora M, Palomera E, Marti C, Halperin I, Webb SW. Magnetic resonance imaging as a predictor of response to somatostatin analogs in acromegaly after surgical failure. J Clin Endocrinol Metab. 2010;95:4973–8.
5. Brzana JA, Yedinak CG, Delashaw JB, Gultelkin HS, Cook D, Fleseriu M. Discordant growth hormone and IGF-1 levels post pituitary surgery in patients with acromegaly naïve to medical therapy and radiation: what to follow, GH or IGF-1 values? Pituitary. 2012;15:562–70.
6. Goldfine ID, Lawrence AM. Hypopituitarism in acromegaly. Arch Intern Med. 1972;130:720–3.
7. Rolla M, Jawiarczyk-przybtowska A, Halupczok-Zyla J, Kaluzny M, Knopka BM, Bloniecka I, Zielinski G, Bolanowski M. Complications and comorbidities of acromegaly-retrospective study in polish center. Front Endocrinol. 2021;12:642131. https://doi.org/10.3389/fendo.2021.642131.

Chapter 21
Acromegaly from the Perspective of a Patient

Jorge D. Faccinetti

A Perspective

Perhaps, one of the more fascinating things about living with acromegaly, as well as the journey you embark on when you have this disease, is that the farther away you move on from the day of diagnosis, at least for me, the least you feel like a patient. You either get used to it, or you forget what it is like not to have it. Not sure which one. Regardless, early on, I knew I would have to adapt my life to a new normal. Gone were the days of long hikes, tennis, biking in the mountains, skiing, and other sports. Understanding early in the disease process that life would not be the same worked well for me. I adapted. It is not that I don't often experience the disease's effect: the tiredness, the joint pain, the slow metabolism that makes weight management a struggle, the daily injection, the surgeries, and the physical therapy. I suppose you can say that pretending it's not there is not smart. I think it is more like I know you are there, but I'm ignoring you, and to the extent that is possible, it makes it easier to get on with your life with as few challenges as possible. And by what I can gather from my personal experience and listening to virtually thousands of people with acromegaly, a much healthier way to deal with everything that comes with it. It is better than spending your life lamenting you have it. But listen, it's always best to look at the positives in everything. Right? I always looked for the positive side in any situation and this disease wasn't going to change it. Whining, complaining, and feeling sorry for myself was not going to happen. Not in this lifetime.

Which brings me to the word lamenting; it reminds me of the Pope. I'm not particularly religious, but I have a great deal of respect and admiration for Francis, the Pope. He is simple and direct. No nonsense. Not sure where this admiration comes from since I've never been particularly fond of Popes.

J. D. Faccinetti (✉)
Pituitary World News (is a Publication Dedicated to Pituitary Diseases),
San Francisco, CA, USA
e-mail: jdfaccinetti@pituitaryworldnews.com

L. S. Blevins Jr., M. K. Aghi (eds.), *Acromegaly*, Contemporary Endocrinology,
https://doi.org/10.1007/978-3-031-16258-9_21

I grew up with Italian Catholic paternal and Scottish Protestant maternal grandparents, so organized religion has never been an essential part of my life. It was more like an annoyance peppered with people telling me how to think, convinced that their views are better than the others. So, I opted very early in my life not to give religion too much importance. Curiously, the Pope and I have a few things in common: our first name is Jorge. We were both born in Argentina, the Pope in 1936, I in 1954 (I emigrated to the USA in 1973). Both our paternal families were Italian, and coincidentally, we both have the same sign in our homes: the Pope's is a placard, in Italian, that says "Vietato Lamentarsi," which translates as "forbidden to complain" [1]. Mine is a little rock carved with two words: "No Whining," which means the same thing. I don't know how long the Pope has had this emblem, but mine has been there for 30 years. It was handy during my two sons' teenage years. The Pope's sign, roughly translated from Italian, goes on to say, "violators are subject to a syndrome of always feeling like a victim and the consequent reduction of sense of humor and capacity to solve problems." The "vietato lamentarsi," no whining, mantra has been in my home for quite a long time.

Acromegaly is a disease that requires problem-solving, so you're going to need an ethos that allows you to be positively engaged. And it is not the same for everyone. I remember early on in a conversation with Dr. Blevins, where he said, "You know, you can have 150 people with acromegaly in a room and you will find 150 different disease states." And that means that acromegaly affects everyone differently. That stuck with me and it's been very helpful in my ability to understand it and, through that process of understanding, relate to other people who have it.

When I was diagnosed with acromegaly in 2010, the first order of business was to learn the facts about the disease. I clearly understood that even though it comes with a whole host of complications, it is treatable and manageable. The second order of business was to get over the shock of it all and wrap my mind around the fact that my condition was missed by everyone and could have potentially been "cured" if someone would have recognized it earlier. Many doctors and other healthcare professionals, say a dentist or physical therapist, didn't recognize the signs and symptoms and my diagnosis was delayed for 28 years. I've heard literally thousands of people with acromegaly describe their stories and journeys and they are all very similar to mine: things start growing, blood pressure goes up, blood sugar goes up, teeth start moving, energy goes down, and bones and joints start hurting; doctors and other healthcare providers in positions to recognize the symptoms don't recognize them, so it takes an average of *10 years* to diagnose acromegaly and that is preposterous. It is senseless because an early diagnosis would preclude many of the *related* conditions—or to use a medical term, "comorbidities"—from happening. Quality of life would be considerably better, even if the condition remains chronic and you have to manage it with medication. I should add that typically you would only require medication if you have a residual tumor, and obviously a residual tumor happens if the surgeon can't resect it all. The longer you have the disease unrecognized, the bigger the tumor, the tougher it is to resect. You get the picture.

The third order of business was to *stop whining* and do something. So, after many San Francisco Café discussions with Lewis Blevins M.D., we created Pituitary

World News, a doctor-patient collaboration with two basic goals in mind: one, to work to, through basic awareness strategies, try to reduce the time it takes for someone to get diagnosed properly and, two, to connect through leaders with patients, and, in doing so, provide a platform for collaboration that would result in creative, innovative ways of solving problems and make life better for people that have to deal with this disease. I'll tell you more about this effort later in the chapter.

The Diagnosis Story

For me, it all started early spring 2010, when I couldn't stand for more than 10 min or walk a few blocks without feeling intense, sharp pain. The pain moved from the lower back to the groin to the legs. It was worse on the right side. A few calls to my primary care doc yielded a "humm those hips look pretty bad" and a referral to the local Lake Tahoe orthopedist group where I live. A great group of physicians if you have a ski injury but frankly not very good at anything else. I immediately called friends, did some research, and ended up at Dr. John Dearborn's office at the Institute for Join Restoration in Menlo Park, California, just South of San Francisco in the famous Silicon Valley.

John Dearborn, M.D., has a stellar reputation and has performed thousands of these operations. He immediately recommended a hip replacement. After showing me the X-ray and pointing out where the bone hit the bone, he explained exactly where they pain was coming from and how it typically moves through your body. It's called referred pain. Where it hurts is not actually where the injury is. My hips didn't really hurt. It was everything around it that felt like it was going to explode. He proceeded to explain how he noticed unusual bone plates and how the femoral head had grown too big for the socket, called the acetabulum, and "by the way," "I think you have a condition called Acromegaly," he said. That was the first time I had heard the word. Well, actually, I had heard it before in a documentary about the Irish Giants. But that's beside the point. The simple truth was that it was the furthest thing I could have imagined. Not on the radar, at all. I think he had a few more questions. He mentioned something about growth hormone and whether I was aware of other issues. Through the shock of it all, I really don't remember what he said after that. I never, ever thought I could have something like acromegaly. "I was no giant," I reasoned, although I had gained weight, my shoe size increased a few sizes, and could no longer play my guitar. My fingers had gotten so big I could no longer do basic chords. He told me what it was and what causes it. I must have looked at him in horror because immediately after he felt compelled to tell me I was not going to die and, I think to make me feel better, then proceeded to explain how a colleague of his had Acromegaly and had had a golf ball-size tumor removed from his pituitary gland. "This is serious but treatable," I remember him saying. "You really should see an endocrinologist if you haven't done so already," he added. "You need to see someone now" he said. It was like a bucket of cold water in your face. Strangely, somewhere during that whole surreal event with Dr. Dearborn, I remembered that a few months before one of my dearest friends, a neurologist, had asked me if I had ever had my hormones checked. Ah, of course, I now realized that's what my friend Evye was telling me. I remember that moment to this day, but at the time I dismissed it, not sure why. Likely because somewhere in my unconscious, and I really don't want to get too Freudian here, I didn't want to deal with it. Honestly that is the best I can do to offer an explanation as to why I didn't pay much attention to what she told me. To this day, I wonder why I reacted the way I did, and really did nothing. Now, in retrospect, I know now exactly what she meant. I remember thinking there were several signs. It was so farfetched that something like a hormonal condition could be affecting me that I just didn't react.

And there were more early signs. A high school friend, whom I had not seen in decades, during a reunion dinner in 1996 in Argentina, made a comment about growth hormone. You see, he knew me when I was 18 years old and weighed 119 pounds, which incidentally was the last time had I had seen him before I immigrated to the USA in 1973. He is a physician, so he knew what he was looking at during that reunion. Many years later, he told me he had suspected a problem, but he never said, "Hey, there is something wrong with you! You need to get checked." I told him in a recent conversation about this book and asked him if he remembered our conversation. He told me he clearly remembered briefly telling me, albeit timidly, about his suspicion. At the time, I didn't process it. After all, this was dinner with my dearest high school friends, a night where we celebrated seeing each other after 25 years of being away, full of anecdotes, remembrances, and camaraderie where it often felt we were still 16. Whatever he said, I sadly didn't hear it, or simply dismissed it.

I started gaining muscle in my late 20s. I could run for miles and bike all day long.

I could hit the hell out of a tennis ball and play all day. I didn't spend too much time at the gym working out. It was like the workout ferry had touched me "you must be doing something right," I kept thinking. I didn't have an ounce of fat in my body. But then, in my early 40s the pain started. First the lower back, then ankles, then the knees, and then I think everything that could hurt did. I remember many days getting up in the morning and thinking, "Humm, I didn't know you could hurt there." It was a clear as a bell. I know now what Dr. Charlie Craig, my pediatrician friend in Argentina, and my dear friend Dr. Evye Szanto asking about my hormone had meant. It made total sense. But I, in a sea of naivete, reasoned I was aging, and when you age, you change, and to me, that was normal.

I remember getting home after my appointment with Dr. Dearborn and Googling "Acromegaly," as we all do when we have no clue about something, and *there it was!* "How is this possible," I thought. People that looked like me filled the screen. I read through the symptoms and started checking each one of them – high blood pressure, check! High blood sugar, check! Skin tags, check! Tired, check! Joint pain, check! Fatigue, muscle weakness, check! "I have almost every symptom listed," I screamed loud enough for my wife to hear me three rooms away. "You mean to tell me other people are running around with this?" "I have most of the physical characteristics!" I added. "Wait a second, Andre the Giant has acromegaly? Don't any of these doctors I've seen for 30 years know about this?" "My grandmother could have diagnosed me. I could have diagnosed it," I thought angrily. It was so evident to me!

I felt ignorant, then angry, then depressed. But I also realized then and there that I should have been more aware as a patient. Perhaps, if I had been more aware of potential pituitary conditions, I could have asked better questions and helped the doctors focus on a diagnosis earlier. Then, the symptoms and the changes would have registered as not normal and usual. Particularly since my doctors treated the symptoms and never once questioned an underlined reason. I knew things would get better, but growing for 30 years had done irreversible damage to my bones and joints. That was the end of some of my favorite things: tennis, backpacking, hiking, and even standing and walking for long periods. I was going to have to adjust to all of that.

The Surgery and Treatment

I met Dr. Lewis Blevins and Dr. Sandeep Kunwar for the first time at UCSF Center for Pituitary Disorders on a dreary, grey, drippy November San Francisco morning in 2010. "How fitting," I thought; when you're going to get bad news, it is usually a day like today, wet, windy, and miserable. But, in sharp contrast to my expectation of bad news, they were amazingly reassuring, particularly to my wife Carol, who was very worried. After all, it is not every day someone tells you you have a tumor in your head. Yet, for some strange reason, I was as calm as I've ever been. Finally, knowing what had been bothering me for so many years was like a 5000-pound rock lifted off my back. "Well," Dr. Blevins said, "you've been growing for 30 years, and we're going stop that." "You are going to be feeling much better," he said. As I listened to their explanations, the surgery, medical treatment steps, and what the future would hold, I was as reassured as anyone could ever be and could not wait to get this thing out of my head. I felt fortunate to be where I was.

After transsphenoidal surgery removed 95% of the pituitary adenoma, I remember thinking I wanted to do something to help raise the awareness of acromegaly and pituitary disorders. "People should be diagnosed early and properly. I can use my skills to do this," I thought. I studied communication and marketing and later specialized in qualitative research, which meant that I could glean insight from people and collect information that could help us understand how best to communicate. I spent 35 years working with advertising firms and national and international clients, helping their marketing department understand the different ways to get their stories and products known.

My perception at the time was that many people were spending a lot of time trying to educate the world about pituitary disorders. But it was also evident that the word was not getting out fast and efficiently enough. Too many people are still without a proper diagnosis because the disease is not recognized or suspected early enough. There was a real need here. Early diagnosis would mean real tangible impacts in this patient population.

In one of my follow-up meetings with the UCSF team, I told Dr. Blevins I wanted to help and get involved, and he immediately connected me with many people and organizations. Dr. Blevins and I have developed a great friendship over the past years. I have great admiration for his skills as a doctor and as a friend. We've spent many moons chatting about how and what to do to help educate and inform.

Pituitary World News

The online e-magazine Pituitary World News was our first effort. The doctor-patient collaborative approach would be very helpful to communicate, not just the medical and scientific knowledge but also what it is like to live with a chronic condition, right from the horse's mouth. We also wanted to give patients and their perspectives a seat at the table. We started publishing articles of general interest, medical knowledge, updates, opinions, insight, resources, and helpful reading so people could manage their disease. Importantly, we wanted to provide ideas and knowledge for people to improve the way they work with their physicians and healthcare teams. The simple idea was to generate conversation and amplify pituitary disease scientifically based content. But when we started in 2014, we really weren't sure what and how we were going to do it. I knew, because of my background that awareness was key. But awareness is not just talking about something. How you talk about it matters. Messages have to break through; people have to want to read them. That takes effort, knowledge, and an understanding of the audience. Yes, we did have a strategy, but I can honestly tell you, we didn't have a clue how it was going to develop or if it was going to take off at all. Let's just get started, we thought, and stop talking about it. Let's give anyone that wants to work with us an opportunity to frame their issues and experiences in their own words, we said to ourselves.

I always thought that it was better to "Just do it" [2], to steal the great Nike advertising tag line, and learn, fine-tune, make it better, ask for opinions, try new things, rather than planning until you're green and leaving ideas in a file somewhere, never to see the light of day. Many great initiatives die in the concept stage because they are never tried; they are never tested in the real world because some focus group somewhere has a few negative comments or opinions. I can't tell you how many times I've seen so called marketing research kill great ideas. In the communications business, unlike the scientific, medical world, if you're going to test ideas, you do it as you go. This is exactly what Nike did, and they became one of the most powerful brands in the world. Like I was saying, we had a strategy, and the logic went something like this: if we could, through our communications and content development efforts, provide relevant information and amplify the conversation, so these diseases become better known, how they affect someone, we may be able to affect diagnosis times. We think that if patients know more about the disease their questions may focus the physician to think about the possibility of a pituitary disease, and conversely, with more awareness of the disease, the Doctor will have it on the radar and inevitably put it on the list of possibilities sooner, or at the very least suspect it. If anything close to that dynamic would have happened with me, I could have possibly been diagnosed ten or fifteen years earlier. The signs were all there. All it would have taken is someone to recognize it and send me to get an IGF-1 test. It's that simple!

Pituitary World News grew as a communication and publishing platform. It evolved and is still evolving into a platform where industry experts, pharmaceutical company executives, medical personnel, physicians, scientists, patients, patient advocate groups, families, and everyone who has been touched by a pituitary disorder can collaborate for the greater good of patients, their families, and the healthcare community in general. Since our founding in September 2014, we've been writing about pituitary disease and listening to people's experiences, through their comments and feedback, about their journey with diagnosis and treatment. We have been learning from the many voices of the people affected by this tough disease and its many related conditions. As patients, doctors, communicators, and publishers, we work to understand the importance of our collective experiences to find solutions that are effective, sustainable, and long-lasting. We have written hundreds of articles and produced audio podcasts and video educational series on these devastating conditions.

A big piece of the solution, we learned, is rather simple; listening to patients' voices will advance care and, most critically, aid in the development of new treatments. The good news is it seems these channels of communication and collaboration are taking shape. Many patient advocacy organizations, physicians, healthcare professionals, industry, and governmental organizations have joined us by sharing the content we produce and contributing to the effort with opinions, articles, and awareness initiatives.

The role of awareness and strategic communication is well understood in the business and marketing academic literature [3]. Further the role of strategic communications is well documented in successful efforts to affect behavior change and adherence to social causes. Strategic communications can make a difference, but it has to be done right.

Language and imagery are critical to the impact content can have. Stigmatized images, particularly the ones associated with pituitary disease, especially with acromegaly, affect how people perceive the disease. Take, for example, Andre the Giant. A recent documentary about Andre the Giant caught my attention specifically how the producers treated his gigantism and acromegaly [4]. Andre Roussimoff, that was his real name, was a French professional wrestler who suffered from gigantism and later acromegaly. He was once called the 8th wonder of the world. This was an intense documentary about the crazy world of professional wrestling and the tragic life of a person with an "extreme," let me say that again, an "extreme" case of gigantism and acromegaly who did not get or, according to the producers, refused treatment.

Throughout the film, I could feel his sorrow. It made me angry and sad, so much so that several times I couldn't help but flip the channel and walk away. I eventually resorted to the "On Demand" feature to watch it in its entirety. "If I'm going to have an opinion about this, I need to sit through it," but I kept thinking, *Andre the Giant is the last thing I want people to think about when they think about or hear the word acromegaly*. Here I was watching someone with a debilitating disease that I know all too well and have, unfortunately, firsthand experience with, and all I could see was a sad human being far, very far from the reality of the thousands of people that deal with the disease. It was unfortunate acromegaly was even mentioned in the documentary, which concluded with a segment about the inevitability of his fate when he died of a heart attack at age 46.

For those of us who are in the business of increasing awareness, educating, and informing people about pituitary disease, this documentary underlined the stigma of the illness. Let me try to explain what I mean. When all people see are extreme cases, they think this could never happen to them, and, in my humble opinion, there is a good chance they will ignore it. I can't remember what I knew or felt about acromegaly before my diagnosis, but the thought that I could have what Andre had was so far from the possibility of ever happening to me, or so I thought, the disease didn't register even for a nanosecond.

Most people with acromegaly look very much like everyone else. Early in their disease process, most people don't have the unusual physical characteristics so often photographed in the medical and popular literature. Perhaps, if we paid less attention to the physical issues and more to other signs of the disease, we'd be catching it earlier before it starts wracking havoc with people's physiques and metabolism. Typically, once physical changes manifest themselves, the disease has taken a firm hold in a person. And, if all we are looking for are the physical manifestations, we will never achieve meaningful change to significantly reduce the time it takes to recognize it and diagnose it.

The Work and the Learning Continues

A pituitary disease diagnosis gives you perspective. Suddenly, you are immersed in knowledge that you didn't have a clue about before. The science is fascinating; hormones, the pituitary gland, genetics, therapies, research, and the everyday life new things you are force to think about are endless. I often ask my friends who have experience with acromegaly what they would do if faced with this scenario: imagine you're sitting at an airport, I tell them, suddenly someone sits next to you. You look. Then look again. The features. The hands. "Yes, I think this person has acromegaly," you say to yourself. "Or, maybe not. Hmm, not sure. But it sure looks like it. I should know; I have it! Once you know acromegaly, you can't miss it, right?" Hmm, what to do? Do you say something? Of course, you do! Or do you? But what? How do you approach it? How do you walk up to a complete stranger and tell them you think they have a disease—maybe you should say "condition," that sounds a bit better, you say to yourself—and by the way, who the hell are you to get involved? What makes you an expert? Are you a doctor? Are you nuts? This may very well be the response you get, but you can't just leave it alone! How do you start this conversation? All this goes through your head in a split second. But in the end, you just can't let this person disappear. What if they don't know? How much longer will it be until someone else notices? Will they suffer for 10 or, worse yet, 25 years, wondering what's wrong with them? This scenario is not that uncommon. It happens pretty frequently.

I have run into it twice since my diagnosis. The first encounter was so evident, but I didn't know what to do or how to approach it. My hesitation was not knowing how to verbalize it clearly. Maybe say, "I was recently diagnosed with a disease called acromegaly and you look like you have some of the physical characteristics of the condition. This is a tough disease but it's very manageable once you are treated, and sometimes you can be totally cured. Early detection is key. And so many people go undetected by their physicians. Here's a number you can call." I hesitated and hesitated and hesitated. Every time I decided to approach this person, my heart would start pounding and a rush of what felt like gallons of adrenaline rushing through my body. Shame on me, I thought, and in the end, I did nothing. Needless to say, I could not get this person out of my head for months. I still think about it and want to kick myself for not saying anything.

The second time was at an airport frequent flyer lounge. As I gathered enough mustard to go, the same feelings of insecurity and stress came over me and I hesitated. "I'll go get a cup of coffee, gather some courage then talk to him," I thought. When I returned, he had gone. Couldn't find him.

In sharp contrast, sometime later my son mentioned he had met someone whose features looked eerily similar to mine, and without skipping a beat, he told him to go see a Doctor. This person was diagnosed immediately, had very successful surgery, and today is in total remission. Not a peep of the tumor. So, my advice: don't walk away. Don't over think it. Say something!'

About Insights

In the awareness business, coming up with new, fresh, creative ideas is essential to get messages across. However, breaking through the clutter can be challenging, expensive, and, yes, very often, frustrating.

I try to tell people about acromegaly and, without boring them to tears, give them a quick explanation. For this, you need an "elevator pitch," which assumes that you only have the time it takes to ride an elevator, usually a minute or 2, to tell your story. Therefore, whatever you say has to be memorable, relatable, and, above all, brief.

Learning how other people talk about their disease gives perspective and insight, so, in preparation for this project, I asked our readers to tell us what it is like to have acromegaly. How does it affect their life, goals, hobbies, and perspectives?

Usually, the best answers are straightforward: "A rollercoaster," someone once said to me.

Here are a few more:

As I wake each morning, I am hopeful that *this will be the morning my energy returns*. That I will be able to jump out of bed at my "usual" 5:30 AM, get a 3-mile mountain run in or a 1500 m swim at the rec pool. I will then work an 8–10-h day, followed by 60 min of crossfit or a 20-mile bike ride. After running a few errands on the way home, I cook dinner, catch up on phone calls, take the dogs for a walk, complete a few chores, watch a show with my husband, and read a few chapters before bed. This was my past life, pre-diagnosis, but it is far from my present reality. My husband's alarm goes off at 6:30 AM. There is no way my eyes can open yet. My lids are so heavy it feels like they're weighted down with bean bags. My mind is aware that I need to get up and start my day, but my body is telling me "hell no!".

It is a battle with your body. You look at yourself and the person looking back isn't you. Your appearance has changed, your character has changed. Every aspect of your life is impacted on. You are in constant pain, whether it is the permanent headache that peaks at various points of the day, or the bone pain and nerve pain due to the years of being undiagnosed taking its toll. The mood swings. Depression, anxiety, zero patience.

I was blindsided with the diagnosis of Acromegaly in 2012 after I went to an endocrinologist referral for diabetes. I didn't know what this disease was but when I left her office, I got home and quickly did my research. After almost 8 years, I have to say that I feel I am probably in the minority of patients with Acromegaly that finds it has not had horrible impact on my life. After 4 MRIs over the past 8 years, a tumor still cannot be seen, but all the clinical tests indicate I have acromegaly. Looking back, I was lucky to be diagnosed early and now I can see the symptoms that I mistook for aging annoyances as being the symptoms of Acromegaly.

Acromegaly is coming to terms with the unknown. There are days where I feel like my "old" self again, and I can partake in physically demanding activities, such as rearrange an entire room or garden, without having my joints lock up. There are days where I can stay awake for the entire day and feel like I can contribute to my household. Then there are days where I can't do anything. I have headaches that last all day long, I forget what I'm saying in the middle of my sentence, or I can hardly walk due to the joint inflammation throughout my body. These days are the hardest because I know what I used to be like previous to the diagnosis, and I mourn for that on occasion. Having acromegaly is almost like a rebirth of yourself because so many things change in a short period of time.

Acromegaly has a duality to it because you can look so healthy but feel so unhealthy; you can have so much wrong with you yet no one can see it. Or, conversely, you can appear so unusual to others, yet no one knows the changes you've gone through. It's silent but visceral. It's never- ending, from daily shots and monthly doctor visits to regular battles with insurance and pharmaceutical companies just to get and afford your medication. It's humbling, it's scary, and it's frustrating. It teaches you things, like self-awareness and how to be your own advocate. The side effects and symptoms can be depressing and alter how you interact with the world (or how you don't).

Frustrating....my body doesn't work like it used to but my brain has a hard time processing how broken it is because my brain says I can still do everything. I spend way too much time, money, and energy dealing with medications. I hate anytime I have to see a new doctor of any kind and explain what acromegaly is and how long I've been dealing with it.

Often, when people affected by Acromegaly talk about their experiences with the disease, it usually includes a discussion into what some people call the diagnosis journey: when were you diagnosed? How long did it take? It goes something like this: "boy, it took forever for someone to figure it out"; "I kept bouncing between doctors"; "I kept gaining weight"; "they told me to stop eating, exercise more"; "my primary care doc never put it together"; "they kept giving me pills;" "I had to see many different doctors for each of my symptoms." You get the jest. The conversation inevitably moves to the symptoms and signs that brought you in to see the doctor in the first place and often end in a comment like "finally someone recognized it!" Yes, those are the same symptoms and signs that eventually lead to a proper diagnosis.

On Family and Genetics

Carol Mackie Passera (Passera is her married name) is my second cousin. Our maternal grandmothers were sisters. Their families immigrated from Scotland and Wales to Argentina in different waves in the mid-1800s to the early 1900s when many European immigrants came to the Southlands to seek opportunities and a better life. Not unlike the many people that came to the USA during the same period in search of the same things: happiness and opportunity.

Early settlers from my grandmother's maternal family arrived in the now famous, cold, inhospitable, mysterious, but beautiful Patagonia region. If you want to learn about this spectacular place, visit Carol's eco-travel business at Causana Viajes and browse through the pages; I guarantee you'll want to go there tomorrow and experience some of these incredible places.

I honestly can't tell you when was the last time Carol and I saw each other. We were probably 10 years old. Perhaps we saw each other one or two more times after that, but I really can't remember. I came to the USA in 1973. I had just turned 18 years old. I haven't seen or heard of Carol and her family since. But with the advent of technology and social media, I reconnected with that side of my family, and after a series of conversations and coincidences, I learned Carol has acromegaly. Talk about a shock!

After sharing the news with my wife, my first call was to my Pituitary World News partner, doc, and friend, Dr. Lewis Blevins. He was amazed! My second call was to Dr. Marta Korbonits at St. Bart's and the London Medical School in the UK, whom I met through Dr. Blevins a few years back in San Francisco. For those who don't know, Dr. Korbonits is an expert in the genetics of acromegaly. She researched the acromegaly AIP gene mutation and the FIPA (Familial Isolated Pituitary Adenoma) gene. If you haven't read about Dr. Korbonits and her work, here it is. Please give it a read. It is well worth the time [5].

Carol and I are the same age. We both started noticing changes in our early 30s.

Carol and I met a few years ago in person after 50 plus years in what was an emotional almost surreal experience. Her story is very similar to mine, but then again, all of our stories are. We shared our lives and our experiences, and after all these years, we became closer through the magic of technology and, unimaginably, acromegaly.

The coincidences are concerning because acromegaly is a familial disease, and current knowledge tell us it occurs in clusters. My take on this: although science has made tremendous inroads in understanding genetics and the genome, we don't know enough about the specifics of the genetics of these diseases to be sure of anything. So, keep a close eye on your family and close relatives if you can, and at the first-ever slight sign, have them checked.

How Awareness Works: One Story

A few years after starting PWN, the impact of awareness became crystal clear. Involvement, engagement, and conversation on a significant scale work in what sometimes seems magic ways. Case in point. My primary care doc of many years, for this story, I'm going to call him Larry, and I had a fantastic experience. I started seeing Larry in 1990, and for 20 years, he treated everything from wellness visits to my aches and pains. He prescribed the one-a-day aspirin, hypertension, the prediabetes medication, we did all the stress tests, and as I aged, he continued to see me. But, together with the other doctors in the group, he never even once suggested or sadly suspected there was an underlying disease affecting me. I think Larry really enjoyed seeing me, and so did I. We had great chats during my office visits and occasional social events. But post-diagnosis, I kept trying to understand how you can go for 28 years without anyone noticing some connection. Is it a failure of the medical education system or how we practice primary care medicine today? You know, the 15-min visits, the constant typing on the keyboard. It isn't easy to understand the whys. I've heard many physicians say acromegaly is a disease you miss only once. That's why awareness is critical, and this story perfectly illustrates it.

I got over being mad and feeling sorry for myself and kept seeing Larry for minor aches and pains and checks, and to this day, I consider him one of the best doctors I ever had. We had the opportunity to talk things out. I had a chance to get it off my chest. He was candid and frank with me. "I never saw an acromegaly case before." "You were my first patient ever." "I just did not put it together," he said. His honesty was heartfelt, and that was enough for me. We moved on.

One morning, a few years after my diagnosis, I got a call from Larry. He tells me he had just seen a patient he immediately suspected had acromegaly. He confirmed his suspicion, and I would mind talking to him about my experiences with the disease; "Chat with him," he suggested. I jumped at the opportunity. This gentleman had brought his elderly father for an appointment and came into the treatment room. Larry noticed his features immediately, "there was no doubt in my mind," he told me. "And it's all because of you. I don't think I would have recognized his acromegaly if I hadn't had that experience with you," he added. So, I met with Larry's second-in-less-than-a-year-acromegaly patient after 28 years of no acromegaly patients. I advised his newly minted acromegaly patient where to go and what to expect. Dr. Blevins and the team at UCSF treated him. His adenoma was successfully resected, and today he is in total remission. That, my acromegaly and pituitary friends and colleagues, was an indescribable feeling!

Shortly after, the New York Times Magazine published an article about this story. The article "The Patient Had Pain When He Walked, but There Was a More

Telling Change" illustrates a narrative that we, unfortunately, often hear [6]. People across the globe go undiagnosed for long periods; research tells us, on average, 8–10 years from the onset of symptoms. In most pituitary diseases, the underlying condition can be successfully treated. Still, the effect of long delays in diagnosis means that many related illnesses continue to progress. It is a poignant article about the realities of life with pituitary disease, and it clearly illustrates why our mission to increase awareness is so critical. In that New York Times article, renowned author Lisa Sanders M.D., who pens the popular Diagnosis column for the New York Times Magazine, said acromegaly is a disease you miss once! This is an excerpt of the article:

> As a primary-care doctor, I had my own [Larry] moment. One of my patients, a 50-something woman, suffered from what in my own mind I call "the usual"—obesity, diabetes, and hypertension. I'd cared for her for several years. And then, when I was away on vacation, a colleague saw her, and at the end of their encounter, she asked my patient if she had an old photo of herself or driver's license. The patient did and that was enough to allow my colleague to diagnose acromegaly. The patient was kind when I saw her. But I wasn't surprised when she moved her care to continue with the doctor who figured it out.
>
> How could I have missed this? Like [Larry], I asked myself that a thousand times. I'd assumed that was the way the patient looked. But acromegaly is a disorder you miss only once. Recently, I saw a patient with one of my trainees. He had the familiar set of problems—obesity, diabetes, hypertension. But I recognized the broad, square forehead and wide, flat nose that I saw in my old patient. I suggested to the resident that we check for a pituitary tumor. I still haven't heard. But I'm pretty sure of the diagnosis.

Life, like acromegaly, has taught me a few lessons.

You live every day in the present; the past is gone; the future has never happened. You make the best out of every day. You have fun doing it. Despite the disruption a disease like this one brings, it also brings gifts, the opportunity to serve, give, and use one's skills to do some good.

Lewis Blevins and I undertook this challenge to move the needle, however insignificantly. One person with acromegaly undiagnosed is one too many.

I want to thank Lewis for the opportunity to ramble in this book. Lots of work to do, please get in touch, get involved. I hope you find the insight enlightening and helpful.

References

1. Reuters PP. Pope tacks sign on his apartment door: 'No Whining'. Vatican City. 2017.
2. Nayak T. Nike "just do it" ad campaing: the case of Nike Inc. Globsyn Manage J. 2017;11(1/2):59–66.
3. Making strategic communications work to prevent elder abuse JD Faccinetti - Journal of Elder Abuse & Neglect, 2002 - Taylor & Francis Strategic communications - K Bonk - The Jossey-Bass handbook of nonprofit leadership and… 2010. books.google.com.
4. Andre the Giant: Directed by Jason Hehir. With Cary Elwes, Arnold Schwarzenegger, Robin Wright, Billy Crystal. A look at the life and career of professional wrestler André Roussimoff, who gained notoriety in the 1980s as Andre the Giant. https://www.imdb.com/title/tt6543420/.

5. Korbonits M. https://www.qmul.ac.uk/fipa-patients/ A tall story: unravelling the genetics behind Charles Byrne. https://www.youtube.com/watch?v=IWaPgnk1-Kc&t=4s
6. Sanders L. Diagnosis. New York Times Magazine. The patient had pain when he walked, but there was a more telling change. 2018. https://www.nytimes.com/2018/06/27/magazine/the-patient-had-pain-when-he-walked-but-there-was-a-more-telling-change.html.

Index

L. S. Blevins Jr., M. K. Aghi (eds.), *Acromegaly*, Contemporary Endocrinology,
https://doi.org/10.1007/978-3-031-16258-9

T

GPSR Compliance

The European Union's (EU) General Product Safety Regulation (GPSR) is a set of rules that requires consumer products to be safe and our obligations to ensure this.

If you have any concerns about our products, you can contact us on ProductSafety@springernature.com

In case Publisher is established outside the EU, the EU authorized representative is:

Springer Nature Customer Service Center GmbH
Europaplatz 3
69115 Heidelberg, Germany

Batch number: 10726135

Printed by Printforce, the Netherlands